CDT 2023

Coding Companion

MORE THAN 300 CODING EXAMPLES

Training Guide for the Dental Team

Book ISBN: 978-1-68447-175-1

E-book ISBN: 978-1-68447-176-8

ADA Product No.: J453BT

Acknowledgements

The ADA would like to acknowledge contributions made by the following individuals to this publication, in addition to the chapter authors:

Council on Dental Benefit Programs' Coding and Transactions Subcommittee
Dr. Roderick Adams; Dr. J. Luke Andrews; Dr. Adrian Carrington; Dr. Kevin Dens (ex-officio); Dr. Stacey Gardner; Dr. Rodney Hill; Dr. Mark Moats; Dr. M. Eddie Ramirez; Dr. King Scott; and Dr. Jessica Stilley-Mallah (ex-officio)

ADA Practice Institute – Center for Dental Benefits, Coding and Quality
Dr. Krishna Aravamudhan, Senior Director; Afton Dunsmoor, Manager; Dennis McHugh, Manager; Frank Pokorny, MBA, FACD (hon.), Senior Manager; and Stacy Starnes, Coordinator

ADA Department of Product Development and Sales
Caitlin Wilson, Manager/Editor, Product Development and Sales, and Pamela Woolf, Senior Manager, Product Development

We also want to acknowledge the permissions to reprint:

- Artwork provided by Glidewell Laboratories used in the discussion of Implant procedures, which are captioned: "Image courtesy of Glidewell Laboratories."

- Artwork provided by Zest Dental Solutions used in the discussion of Implant procedures, which are captioned: "Image courtesy of Zest Dental Solutions."

CDT 2023 Coding Companion
Table of Contents

Foreword

Proper dental procedure coding is an essential skill for dentists and their dental practice staff. Done correctly, it helps ensure accurate record keeping and proper communication with payors. If done incorrectly, it can create confusion, delay or decrease reimbursement, and, at worst, create serious legal issues.

Over the last decade and a half, we have worked hard to help guide dentists in the correct use of Current Dental Terminology (CDT) with our series of reference books and the Insurance Solutions Newsletter. There are changes to the CDT every year, and dentists and their teams must stay abreast of these changes. When we update our materials each year, we always reach for the ADA's annual *CDT Coding Companion: Training Guide for the Dental Team*. The *Coding Companion* is vetted each year by ADA staff and the Council on Dental Benefit programs. When we reference this publication, we are citing the guidance from the "definitive source" of CDT coding.

The *Coding Companion* provides key definitions and concepts, pertinent changes and updates to the CDT for each year. It includes questions and answers, and a large number of clinical coding scenarios that help clarify correct code reporting. There are also tips and advice for any office submitting to insurance, and many useful tables for reference. Whenever we are working to understand and interpret a dental code, new or old, we often find our answer within its pages.

Whether you are a dentist, a dental team member, or an insurance company employee, the *CDT Coding Companion* will be one of the top resources you'll reach for to help sort through confusing reporting situations.

Charles Blair, DDS
Founder, Practice Booster®

Greg Grobmyer, DDS
Editor, *Coding with Confidence*

Section 1
The CDT Code: What It Is and How to Use It

A Brief History

The CDT Code was first published in 1969 as the "Uniform Code on Dental Procedures and Nomenclature" in the *Journal of the American Dental Association.* It originally consisted of numbers and a brief name, or nomenclature. Since 1990, the CDT Code has been published in the American Dental Association's dental reference manual titled *Current Dental Terminology* (CDT). The CDT Code version published in CDT-1 (1990) was marked by the addition of descriptors (a written narrative that provides further definition and the intended use of a dental procedure code) for most of the procedure codes.

The American Dental Association is the copyright owner and publisher of the CDT Code. New versions are published every year and become effective January 1st.

Federal regulations and legislation arising from the Health Insurance Portability and Accountability Act of 1996 (HIPAA) require all payers to accept HIPAA standard electronic dental claim. One data element on the electronic dental claim is the dental procedure code, which must be from the CDT Code – specifically the version that is in effect on the date of service.

Purpose

The CDT Code supports uniform, consistent, and accurate documentation of services delivered. This information is used in several ways:

- To provide for the efficient processing of dental claims
- To populate an electronic health record (EHR)
- To record services to be delivered in a treatment plan

Note: Treatment plans must be developed according to professional standards, not according to provisions of the dental benefit contract. Always keep in mind that the existence of a procedure code does not guarantee that the procedure is a covered service.

Categories of Service

The CDT Code is organized into twelve categories of service, each with its own series of five-digit alphanumeric codes. These categories:

- Exist solely as a means to organize the CDT Code.

- Reflect dental services that are considered similar in purpose.

- Contain CDT codes that are available to document services delivered by anyone acting within the scope of their state law (for example, a dentist in general practice uses D7140 that is found in the oral and maxillofacial surgery category to document an extraction).

#	Name	Code Range	Description in Commonly Used Terms*
I.	Diagnostic	D0100–D0999	Examinations, X-rays, pathology lab procedures
II.	Preventive	D1000–D1999	Cleanings (prophy), fluoride, sealants
III.	Restorative	D2000–D2999	Fillings, crowns and other related procedures
IV.	Endodontics	D3000–D3999	Root canals
V.	Periodontics	D4000–D4999	Surgical and non-surgical treatments of the gums and tooth supporting bone
VI.	Prosthodontics – removable	D5000–D5899	Dentures – partials and "flippers"
VII.	Maxillofacial Prosthetics	D5900–D5999	Facial, ocular and various other prostheses.
VIII.	Implant Services	D6000–D6199	Implants and implant restorations
IX.	Prosthodontics – fixed	D6200–D6999	Cemented bridges
X.	Oral & Maxillofacial Surgery	D7000–D7999	Extractions, surgical procedures, biopsies, treatment of fractures and injuries
XI.	Orthodontics	D8000–D8999	Braces
XII.	Adjunctive General Services	D9000–D9999	Miscellaneous services including anesthesia, professional visits, therapeutic drugs, bleaching, occlusal adjustment

* The language used in the "description" column has been simplified using common non-clinical terms. It is not technical terminology.

Note: Documentation of services provided may necessitate selection of CDT codes from different categories of service. Two illustrative scenarios follow. Section 4 "Alphabetic Index to the CDT Code" in *CDT 2023: Current Dental Terminology* will also help you locate an applicable procedure code.

Scenario Description	Procedure Delivered	Category of Service
1. Implant Case – Four-unit Fixed Partial Denture	Radiographs	Diagnostic D0100–D0999
	Implant body placement	Implant Services D6000–D6199
	Implant supported retainers	
	Pontics	Prosthodontics, fixed D6200–D6999
2. Orthodontic Case – Treatment Planning	Pre-treatment examination	Orthodontics D8000–D8999
	Radiographs	Diagnostic D0100–D0999
	Diagnostic casts	
	Case presentation	Adjunctive General Services D9000–D9999

Subcategories

All CDT Code categories of service are subdivided into one or more subcategories to aid navigation through the code set. For example, subcategories in the Diagnostic category of service include:

- Clinical Oral Evaluations
- Diagnostic Imaging
- Tests and Examinations

Note: CDT Code entries are not always in numerical order within a category of service or subcategory. As the CDT Code grows and evolves, there are times when there is no sequential number available for a new entry that is related to an existing code.

Components of a CDT Code Entry

Every dental procedure code within a category of service has at least the first two and sometimes all three of the following components:

Procedure Code – A five-character alphanumeric code beginning with the letter "D" that identifies a specific dental procedure. Each procedure code is printed in **boldface** type in the CDT manual and cannot be changed or abbreviated.

Dental Procedure Code – five character alphanumeric beginning with "D"

D1351   **sealant – per tooth**
Mechanically and/or chemically prepared enamel
surface sealed to prevent decay.

Nomenclature – The written, literal definition of a procedure code. Each code has a nomenclature that is printed in **boldface** type in the CDT manual. Nomenclature may be abbreviated only when printed on claim forms or other documents that are subject to space limitation. Any such abbreviation does not constitute a change to the nomenclature.

Nomenclature (name) – written title of the procedure

D1351   sealant – per tooth
Mechanically and/or chemically prepared enamel
surface sealed to prevent decay.

Descriptor – A written narrative providing further definition and describing clinical aspects of the procedure. A descriptor is not provided for every procedure code. Descriptors that apply to a series of procedure codes may precede that series of codes; otherwise a descriptor will follow the applicable procedure code and its nomenclature. When present, descriptors are printed in regular typeface in the CDT manual. Descriptors as published cannot be added, abbreviated, or otherwise changed.

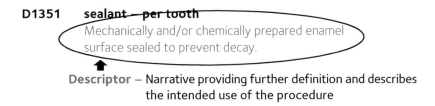

D1351   ~~sealant – per tooth~~
Mechanically and/or chemically prepared enamel surface sealed to prevent decay.

Descriptor – Narrative providing further definition and describes the intended use of the procedure

Descriptors are a very important component. Understanding the descriptor can help determine whether the procedure code accurately describes the service provided to a patient. This information can also help resolve questions about the accuracy of claim submissions.

Note: Your practice management software may not include entire CDT Code entries as some, due to space limitations, truncate nomenclatures and omit descriptors. With the current CDT Manual at hand you will have the complete entries for all CDT codes, which will help you select the appropriate code to document and report the service delivered.

What If There Is No Code Describing a Procedure?

The complete CDT Code entry, described above, published in *CDT 2023: Current Dental Terminology,* is used to determine the procedure code for documenting and reporting a service provided to a patient. But, what if there is no CDT code that, in the dentist's opinion, is applicable to the service? The available and appropriate option is to use an "unspecified procedure, by report" code, also known as a "999" code. These codes (e.g., **D2999 unspecified restorative procedure, by report**) are in every category of service, and when used must include a supporting narrative that explains the service provided.

A third-party payer may request additional documentation of certain procedures regardless of the presence of the narrative. Note, too, that dental benefit plan coverage limitations and exclusions, and where applicable the provisions of a participating provider agreement, affect third-party payer claim adjudication and reimbursement.

Narratives for "By Report" Codes

There are two types of CDT codes that require an explanatory narrative. The first and most readily known type are the "unspecified...procedure, by report" codes found in every category of service. Second are those codes in several categories that include "by report" in their nomenclatures, as seen in the following three examples:

D5862 **precision attachment, by report**
Each pair of components is one precision attachment.
Describe the type of attachment used.

D0321 **other temporomandibular joint radiographic images, by report**

D6190 **radiographic/surgical implant index, by report**
An appliance, designed to relate osteotomy or fixture position to existing anatomic structures, to be utilized during radiographic exposure for treatment planning and/or during osteotomy creation for fixture installation.

When preparing a narrative report, first try to put yourself in the claim examiner's position. Your goal is to describe what you did and why, in a writing style and tone of an explanation to a friendly colleague. A good report is a clear and concise narrative that includes, as needed:

- Clinical condition of the oral cavity
- Description of the procedure performed
- Specific reasons why the procedure was needed, or extra time or material was needed
- How new technology enabled delivery
- Specific information required by a participating provider contract

Both the ADA Dental Claim Form and the HIPAA standard electronic dental claim transaction support transmittal of your narrative. If the "Remarks" field on the paper form does not provide enough space for you to say what you need to say, additional sheets may be included. Check with your practice management system vendor to learn how a narrative is included on your electronic claim submission.

Clarity is crucial. Do not assume that the reader will be familiar with acronyms or abbreviations you use on your patient records. Be sure to proofread the text before inclusion with the claim submission.

What do you think of this "by report" narrative?

> ½ carp anestetic 4% w/10.5 epinephrine administered. Explained procedure with patient's mother. Laser gingivectomy #8 and #9 and frenulectomy for max ant. Patient tolerated procedure well. Coagulation observed. Removed 2 mm of hyperplastic gingival #8 and 1.5 mm on #9 in facial and contured interseptal region. Raised max labial attendant 5 mm. Coagulation observed. POIG. Patient given rinse and cold sore meds for topical anesthisia.

It is a real-life example — shown exactly as submitted — that looks more like quickly written notes from the patient's record, with acronyms, misspellings, and abbreviations that may confuse the reader. The entire claim was returned unprocessed.

Acronyms, abbreviations, and misspelled words hinder understanding. Narrative templates should be avoided, but, if used, the dentist remains obligated to review and approve the completed work before submission.

Now let's look at how the returned report narrative might have looked if written clearly.

> Patient age 5 presented with hyperplastic gingival tissue, and short and taut lingual frenum. Parent stated that child suffered from Aichmophobia, which could be diminished by anesthesia and use of laser in lieu of scalpel.
>
> Administered ½ carpule 4% Citanest Forte DENTAL with epinephrine. Used laser to: 1) remove 2 mm of hyperplastic gingival tissue from #8 and 1.5 mm on #9; 2) excise lingual frenum; and 3) cauterize wound. Coagulation was observed.
>
> Patient received post-operative instructions, oral antibiotic (amoxicillin) and oral analgesic (benzocaine) before release. Procedures delivered were: D4211 (gingivectomy or gingivoplasty); D7962 (lingual frenectomy [frenulectomy]); D9215 (local anesthesia); D9630 (drugs dispensed for home use).

This is a clear and concise report that answers the "what and why" questions the claims reviewer will be asking. It establishes clinical need and the procedure's positive outcome as expected.

CDT Code Maintenance: Additions, Revisions, and Deletions

The ADA's Council on Dental Benefit Programs (CDBP) is responsible for CDT Code maintenance. In 2012, it established its Code Maintenance Committee (CMC), which convenes annually to vote on CDT Code action requests. Accepted requests are incorporated into the next version, which is effective on January 1st yearly.

Features of the maintenance process now in place are:

1. The CMC is a decision-making body comprised of 19 organizations representing diverse sectors of the dental community (such as third-party payers and dental specialties, including public health dentistry) that votes to accept, amend, or decline a CDT Code action request.

2. A summary of action requests to be addressed at each CMC meeting is posted for download on ADA.org/cdt, including information on how to obtain a copy of the complete request form.

3. During a CMC meeting, the chair encourages submitters of action requests and any other interested party to voice their comments on any requests to the committee's members.

4. During a CMC meeting the committee members discuss action requests and cast their votes.

5. The CMC Secretariat sends notices of action taken to each person or entity that submitted a CDT Code action request, and posts the results on *ADA.org/cdt*.

Please visit the ADA's web page *ADA.org/cdt* for more information.

The CDT Code changes for many reasons, including technology or materials that have led to new procedures not currently in the taxonomy, or the need to improve clarity and accuracy of nomenclature and descriptors. Anyone may submit an action request.

For further assistance please contact the ADA Member Service Center at 312.440.2500.

Dental Procedure Codes (CDT) and Diagnosis Codes (ICD)

Dentists, through education and experience, diagnose a patient's oral health prior to treatment plan preparation and delivery of necessary dental services. However, for diagnoses, codified clinical documentation or reporting on a dental claim is not a routine activity. Change is afoot and your colleagues on the ADA Council on Dental Benefit Programs offer a look ahead to help you prepare for documenting and reporting diagnosis codes if and when required.

Dentists and their staff are urged to familiarize themselves with the particulars of patients' dental benefits plans claim preparation and submission requirements. In addition, pay close attention to communications from dental plans regarding additional benefits for services connected to systemic health or about dental plans' intentions to require diagnostic codes on dental claim submissions.

Note: There is no immediate and universal mandate to include an ICD-10-CM code on all dental claims. We also emphasize that dental benefit plans are unlikely to establish identical diagnostic code reporting requirements in the foreseeable future. You should check with each plan for its requirements.

Both the ADA Dental Claim Form and the HIPAA standard electronic dental claim transaction are able to report up to four diagnosis codes. This capability was added to the claim forms with the expectation that International Classification of Diseases (ICD) would, at some point, become a required data element for dental claim adjudication. ICD-10-CM is the International Classification of Diseases, Tenth Revision, Clinical Modification, which is the USA's code set for medical diagnoses. ICD-10-CM became the HIPAA standard on October 1, 2015. It is a code set maintained by federal government agencies and available online at *www.cms.gov/Medicare/Coding/ICD10*. Most – but not all – diagnoses will be reported using an entry from the "Diseases of Oral Cavity and Salivary Glands" in ICD-10-CM (K00–K14 series).

Why should dentists be concerned with ICD codes when the ADA has developed SNODENT?

SNODENT is a clinical terminology designed for use with electronic health records, and it differs from ICD in three ways:

1. It is an input code set.
2. It has broader scope and specificity.
3. It may be mapped to ICD as needed on a dental claim.

Federal regulations published under the auspices of HIPAA's Administrative Simplification provisions specify only ICD-10-CM codes as valid on claim submissions.

Section 3 of this book contains the appendix titled "CDT Code to ICD (Diagnosis) Code Crosswalk," an aid to recordkeeping and claim preparation. Tables in this appendix link frequently reported CDT codes with one or more possible ICD-10-CM diagnostic codes. Please note that these tables are not all inclusive but do serve as a guide for commonly occurring conditions.

Dentists, by virtue of their clinical education, experience, and professional ethics, are the individuals responsible for diagnosis. As such, a dentist is also obligated to select the appropriate diagnosis code for patient records and claim submission. It is quite possible that other diagnoses and their associated codes may be appropriate for a given clinical scenario.

As you study these tables, please note:

1. Some address a single CDT code (e.g., preventive resin restoration), and others include a suite of related procedure codes (e.g., resin-based composite).

2. Likewise, the number of suggested ICD-10-CM diagnosis codes in a table can range from one (e.g., gingival recession for eight graft codes) to more than 10.

3. Several contain suggested diagnosis codes that are not from the "Diseases of the Oral Cavity and Salivary Glands" section ICD-10-CM; there are circumstances (e.g., vehicle accidents, workers compensation) where other sections of the ICD code set have pertinent entries.

4. Most of the frequently cited ICD codes applicable to dental procedures are found in the Kxx series (Diseases of Oral Cavity and Salivary Glands), and to a lesser degree from three other series – Rxx (Symptoms, Signs and Abnormal Clinical and Laboratory Findings, Not Elsewhere Classified); Sxx (Injury, Poisoning and Certain Other Consequences of External Causes); and Zxx (Factors Influencing Health Status and Contact with Health Services).

5. Some ICD code terms contain words that are not commonly used in the US. These words, identified by an asterisk (*), are defined in the ADA online glossary: ADA.org/CDTGlossary.

Additional CDT-to-ICD tables are posted on the ADA's CDT Code website at https://www.ADA.org/publications/cdt/icd-and-cdt-codes.

These online tables may be updated more frequently than those in print as changes to ICD-10-CM occur on an annual schedule that differs from the CDT Code's timetable.

Dental Procedure Codes vs. Medical Procedure Codes

The CDT Code is the source for procedure codes used when submitting claims to dental benefit plans on either the ADA Dental Claim Form or the HIPAA standard electronic dental claim transaction. There may be times when a dentist's services are submitted to a patient's medical benefit plan. When this happens, not only is there a different claim form, but there are also different procedure codes that must be used. None of these are developed or maintained by the ADA.

Filing claims with a patient's medical benefit plan can be done using the "1500" paper form or HIPAA electronic equivalent. Information on the 1500 Claim Form, including completion instructions, can be found at the American Medical Association's (AMA) National Uniform Claim Committee website *www.nucc.org.*

Medical procedure codes come from two sources, the AMA's Current Procedure Terminology (CPT) code set and the federal government's Healthcare Common Procedure Code Set (HCPCS). All medical diagnosis codes come from the federal government's International Classification of Diseases, 10th Revision, Clinical Modification (ICD-10-CM) code set.

Note: When selecting a medical procedure code, the rule of thumb is to first look at the CPT code set to determine if there is an appropriate code to use. If there is none, a HCPCS code may be used.

Sources for medical procedure codes include, but are not limited to:

- American Medical Association
  https://commerce.ama-assn.org/store
  800.621.8335

- Centers for Medicare and Medicaid Services (HCPCS)
  www.cms.hhs.gov/HCPCSReleaseCodeSets

Sources for ICD-10-CM diagnosis codes include, but are not limited to:

- National Center for Health Statistics, *https://www.cdc.gov/nchs/icd/index.htm*

- PMIC Coding and Compliance, *http://icd10coding.com*

- American Medical Association, *https://commerce.ama-assn.org/store*

Sources of dental to medical procedure cross coding include, but are not limited to:

- *Medical Dental Cross Coding with Confidence* by Charles Blair, D.D.S. available on *ADAstore.org* 800.947.4746

- *2023 Coding and Payment Guide for Dental Services* by Optum available on *ADAstore.org* 800.947.4746

Claim Rejection: Payer Misuse of the CDT Code or Something Else?

Some claims will be rejected by a third-party payer and the reason for denial helps determine what should be done next. "The existence of a dental procedure code does not mean that the procedure is a covered or reimbursed benefit," is a quote from the preface of the first (1990) and every later edition of the CDT manual. This is an important concept as available coverage is determined by dental benefit plan design. Plan limitations and exclusions vary, which means a procedure that is covered by one patient's benefit plan may not be covered by another patient's plan.

In August 2000, HIPAA (Health Insurance Portability and Accountability Act of 1996) Subtitle F (Administrative Simplification) regulations named the Code on Dental Procedures and Nomenclature (CDT Code) as the federal standard for reporting dental procedures on electronic dental claims. Some have interpreted this to mean that since the CDT Code is a national standard, payers must provide reimbursement for any valid procedure code reported on a claim. This is an erroneous interpretation as the HIPAA regulations are limited to four statements:

1. A standard electronic dental claim may only contain procedures found in the CDT Code.

2. A dentist must submit the procedure code that is valid on the date of service.

3. A payer may not refuse to accept for processing a claim with a valid procedure code.

4. A payer's benefit plan design and adjudication policies apply when processing a claim.

In other words, HIPAA establishes a standard for communicating information about services provided to a patient. HIPAA does not influence a payer's claim adjudication process (e.g., application of policies and benefit limitations and exclusions).

An explanation of benefits (EOB) that shows reimbursement for fewer services or for different procedure codes than reported on the claim raises eyebrows and prompts dentists to call the ADA and ask, "How can this happen? Isn't the third-party payer doing something wrong or illegal? It looks like the CDT Code is being misused." The first step in answering these questions and concerns is to look at what guidance is in place concerning CDT Code use:

- A third-party payer is supposed to use the code number (e.g., D0120), its nomenclature, and its descriptor as written.

- The ADA defines procedure code bundling as "the systematic combining of distinct dental procedures by third-party payers that results in a reduced benefit for the patient/beneficiary." Procedure code bundling is frowned upon by the ADA.

- However, dentists who have signed participating provider agreements with third-party payers may be bound to plan provisions that limit or exclude coverage for concurrent procedures.

- HIPAA requires the procedure code reported on a claim be from the CDT Code version that is effective on the date of service. Yet neither HIPAA, ADA policy, nor the CDT Code itself requires that a third-party payer cover every listed dental procedure.

- Covered dental procedures are identified in the contract between the plan purchaser and the third-party payer.

Many patients do not understand how dental benefit programs work and that coverage limitations and exclusions may limit reimbursement for necessary care. Such a misunderstanding is compounded when EOB language suggests that the dentist is at fault. Ensuring patients understand the limitations of their dental plan prior to treatment may help avoid problems and maintain a strong dentist-patient relationship.

Some dental claim adjudication practices are appropriate when based on plan design and should be clearly explained on the EOB to prevent misunderstandings. Other situations, where the EOB message suggests the dentist is in error, may pose problems. Each of these conditions is illustrated in the following examples:

- **Acceptable EOB explanation**: A claim for a full mouth debridement and a two-surface restoration is adjudicated, and only the D4355 is reimbursed. The EOB message states that the benefit plan has limitations and exclusions, one of which is that the plan does not cover any restorative procedure delivered on the same day as a D4355. In this example, the payer has not paid for the procedure due to benefit plan design limitations – there is no suggestion that the dentist has done anything improper.

- **Unacceptable EOB explanation**: The dentist reports a D1110 on the claim because the patient is 13 years old with predominantly adult dentition, but the EOB lists D1120 with a message that this is the correct code for a patient under the age of 15. In this example, the payer is wrong, as the message implies that the dentist reported the incorrect prophylaxis procedure code. Here, the payer ignored the CDT code's descriptor where dentition, not age, is the criterion for reporting an adult versus child prophylaxis. What the payer should do when the benefit plan specifies an age-based benefit limitation is accept the claim as submitted and note on the EOB that the claim has been adjudicated based on benefit plan design.

The second example illustrates why it is important that the dental office help the patient understand the clinical basis for treatment. In this case, the type of prophylaxis is determined by the state of the patient's dentition, not age, even though the patient's benefit may be determined by age.

Dental benefit plan limitations and exclusions affect how a claim is adjudicated and, as noted above, a payer may reject or not reimburse a claim in accordance with the benefit plan's provisions. Just as benefit plan designs vary, there is variation in participating provider contract provisions, and if you have one (or more), each must be reviewed to see how claim submission and processing may be affected. The ADA Contract Analysis Service, an ADA member benefit, can identify areas of provider contract provisions that may be of concern and be addressed before signing the contract. More information on the Contract Analysis Service is available here: *https://www.ADA.org/resources/practice/dental-insurance/dental-insurance-resources/dental-insurance-contract-issues*.

Participating provider contracts are between the dentist and payer. These contracts may include provisions that require you to accept least expensive alternative treatment (LEAT) reimbursement, or agree to reimbursement based on payer guidelines instead of specific procedure codes reported on a claim. A dentist who signs a participating provider contract is generally bound to its legally sound provisions. Likewise, the payer is also bound to the contract provisions and cannot obligate you to do something that is beyond the signed agreement.

It is appropriate to appeal the benefit decision if you think the claim has not been properly adjudicated. When appealing a claim, it is important to follow the specific instructions provided by the particular carrier including the submittal of the appeal in writing within the time allowed by the carrier. It is important to send it to the specified department of the carrier, and it must be in the required format. The word "appeal" should prominently appear in the title and text of the document, as well as in any cover letter that accompanies the appeal document.

Remember, the dentist consultant representing the carrier may only be looking at a dental claim form, and you will want to provide the consultant as much information as possible so that he or she will agree with your treatment plan and approve the appropriate benefits for your patient.

A proper appeal involves sending the carrier a written request to reconsider the claim. Additional documentation should be included to give the carrier a clearer picture of why you recommended the treatment. For example, the following claim attachments may assist in getting consideration for core buildup claims – radiographic evidence of the need for a buildup, pre- and post-photographs and a narrative description providing as much explanatory information as possible (even if this appears obvious to you). If you have further questions, it is best to give that carrier a call.

Remember, you are trying to have the dentist consultant understand the rationale for your recommended treatment plan so that your patient can receive the appropriate benefit from his or her plan.

It may help to ask the dentist consultant to call you if the claim is going to be denied. This way you can discuss the case with the dentist consultant on a professional level. You may want to leave a time and date when you will be available so that the consultant does not call while you are seeing patients.

Payers using the CDT Code must be licensed to do so – and abide by the copyright license. Any payer actions that do not adhere to contractual obligations may represent misuse, and be reason to seek redress. The copyright license does not dictate how a procedure code is to be reimbursed and cannot be used as a tool to force payers to use the CDT Code in a particular manner.

It is appropriate to appeal the benefit decision if you think the claim has not been properly adjudicated. Information on how to file an appeal (and more) is available online at *www.ADA.org/dentalinsurance*.

Note: The ADA Member Service Center (MSC) is your first point of contact when you have questions about the CDT Code and its use. Contact the MSC at 312.440.2500. Email inquiries concerning the CDT Code should be sent to *dentalcode@ADA.org*.

The "Golden Rules" of Procedure Coding

Correct coding, part and parcel of the following rules, demonstrates a dentist's adherence to the ADA's Principles of Ethics and Code of Professional Conduct, particularly "5.A. Representation of Care" that states "Dentists shall not represent the care being rendered to their patients in a false or misleading manner."

- "Code for what you do" is the fundamental rule to apply in all coding situations.
- After reading the full nomenclature and descriptor, select the code that matches the procedure delivered to the patient.
- If there is no applicable code, document the service using an unspecified, by report ("999") code, and include a clear and appropriate narrative.
- The existence of a procedure code does not mean that the procedure is a covered or reimbursed benefit in a dental benefit plan.
- Treatment planning is based on clinical need, not covered services.

If you have difficulty finding an appropriate CDT code, consider whether there may be another way to describe the procedure. The CDT manual's alphabetic index and the glossary of dental terms posted on *ADA.org* are likely to be helpful in these situations.

Code Changes in CDT 2023

The number and nature of annual CDT Code changes vary, as does their relevance to an individual dentist – primarily based on her or his type of practice. CDT 2023 incorporates a variety of CDT Code entry actions – 22 additions, 14 revisions, and two deletions – summarized in the following table.

Code	Change
Diagnostic	
D0210	Revision
D0351	Deletion
D0372	Addition
D0373	Addition
D0374	Addition
D0393	**Revision**
D0387	Addition
D0388	Addition
D0389	Addition
D0704	Deletion
D0709	**Revision**
D0801	Addition
D0802	Addition
D0803	Addition
D0804	Addition
Preventive	
D1781	Addition
D1782	Addition
D1783	Addition
Restorative	
None	
Endodontics	
D3333	**Revision**
Periodontics	
D4240	**Revision**
D4241	**Revision**
D4266	**Revision**
D4267	**Revision**
D4286	Addition
D4355	**Revision**
D4921	**Revision**

Code	Change
Prosthodontics (removable)	
None	
Maxillofacial Prosthetics	
None	
Implant Services	
D6105	Addition
D6106	Addition
D6107	Addition
D6197	Addition
Prosthodontics, fixed	
None	
Oral & Maxillofacial Surgery	
D7251	**Revision**
D7509	Addition
D7956	Addition
D7957	Addition
Orthodontics	
Category (descriptor) D8000–D8999	**Revision**
Adjunctive General Services	
D9110	**Revision**
D9450	**Revision**
D9953	Addition

Some of the CDT 2023 changes listed in this table are stand-alone and others – additions with associated revisions or deletions – are interrelated. These changes will be addressed in detail within the following chapters.

Special Note: During the CDT Code maintenance cycle in calendar year 2022, the Code Maintenance Committee approved the following seven procedure code additions for inclusion in CDT 2022. Therefore, they are considered continuing code entries in CDT 2023, which is why they are not in the above listing of CDT 2023 changes. Information about these codes and their use was published in 2022, and this guidance document is posted on the CDT's Coding Education page (*ADA.org/ CDTEducation*) titled *COVID-19 Vaccination Procedures* and is available to any member of the dental community.

D1708   **Pfizer-BioNTech Covid-19 vaccine administration – third dose**
SARSCOV2 COVID-19 VAC mRNA 30mcg/0.3mL IM DOSE 3

D1709   **Pfizer-BioNTech Covid-19 vaccine administration – booster dose**
SARSCOV2 COVID-19 VAC mRNA 30mcg/0.3mL IM DOSE BOOSTER

D1710   **Moderna Covid-19 vaccine administration – third dose**
SARSCOV2 COVID-19 VAC mRNA 100mcg/0.5mL IM DOSE 3

D1711   **Moderna Covid-19 vaccine administration – booster dose**
SARSCOV2 COVID-19 VAC mRNA 50mcg/0.25mL IM DOSE BOOSTER

D1712   **Janssen Covid-19 vaccine administration - booster dose**
SARSCOV2 COVID-19 VAC Ad26 5x1010 VP/.5mL IM DOSE BOOSTER

D1713   **Pfizer-BioNTech Covid-19 vaccine administration tris-sucrose pediatric – first dose**
SARSCOV2 COVID-19 VAC mRNA 10mcg/0.2mL tris-sucrose IM DOSE 1

D1714   **Pfizer-BioNTech Covid-19 vaccine administration tris-sucrose pediatric – second dose**
SARSCOV2 COVID-19 VAC mRNA 10mcg/0.2mL tris-sucrose IM DOSE 2

D0100–D0999 Diagnostic

Diagnostic Imaging

▲ **D0210** **intraoral – ~~complete~~ <u>comprehensive</u> series of radiographic images**
A radiographic survey of the whole mouth~~, usually consisting of 14–22 periapical and posterior bitewing images or~~ intended to display the crowns and roots of all teeth, periapical areas<u>,</u> <u>interproximal areas</u> and alveolar bone <u>including edentulous areas</u>.

Rationale for this change: The revisions clarifies the procedure's objective as a comprehensive survey and acknowledges that it is the dentist who determines the appropriate number and type of images necessary to safely achieve the objective for the individual patient. This revised wording is carried forward to the CDT Code's comparable procedure codes (e.g., D0709 for image capture only).

• **D0372** **intraoral tomosynthesis – comprehensive series of radiographic images**
A radiographic survey of the whole mouth intended to display the crowns and roots of all teeth, periapical areas, interproximal areas and alveolar bone including edentulous areas.

• **D0373** **intraoral tomosynthesis – bitewing radiographic image**

• **D0374** **intraoral tomosynthesis – periapical radiographic image**

Rationale for these changes: Tomosynthesis is a procedure whose image capture and reconstruction steps differ from single plane radiographic imaging reported with current CDT codes—comprehensive, bitewing, and periapical diagnostic imaging procedures.

• **D0801** **3D dental surface scan – direct**

• **D0802** **3D dental surface scan – indirect**
A surface scan of a diagnostic cast.

• **D0803** **3D facial surface scan – direct**

• **D0804** **3D facial surface scan – indirect**
A surface scan of constructed facial features.

Rationale for these changes: These new codes replace the current "D0351 3D photographic image" CDT Code entry (now deleted in CDT 2023) to enable greater specificity in procedure documentation and reporting and to recognize that inclusion of "photographic" in the nomenclature does not acknowledge other image capture technologies (e.g., digital scanning). In the nomenclatures, the term "direct" means that the patient is present when the image is captured, and "indirect" means the patient is not present when the image is captured.

D1000–D1999 Preventive

Vaccinations

- **D1781** vaccine administration – human papillomavirus – Dose 1
  Gardasil 9 0.5mL intramuscular vaccine injection.

- **D1782** vaccine administration – human papillomavirus – Dose 2
  Gardasil 9 0.5mL intramuscular vaccine injection.

- **D1783** vaccine administration – human papillomavirus – Dose 3
  Gardasil 9 0.5mL intramuscular vaccine injection.

Rationale for these changes: These new codes enable documentation and reporting delivery of this particular type of vaccine.

D4000–D4999 Periodontics

Surgical Services

- **D4286 removal of non-resorbable barrier**

Rationale for this change: This new code acknowledges that removal of a non-resorbable barrier is a distinct procedure that is delivered on a different date of service, and possibly by a different dentist or dental practice, than the initial placement. The addition also establishes that the guided tissue regeneration procedures (revised D4267 and new codes for "per implant" and "edentulous spaces"—effective in CDT 2023) that involve a non-resorbable barrier, include only membrane placement as part of these procedures.

- ▲ **D4355 full mouth debridement to enable a comprehensive** ~~oral~~
  __periodontal__ **evaluation and diagnosis on a subsequent visit**
  ~~Full mouth debridement involves the preliminary removal of plaque and calculus that interferes with the ability of the dentist to perform a comprehensive~~ oral evaluation. Not to be ~~completed on the same day as D0150, D0160, or D0180.~~

Rationale for this change: These revisions clarify that this full mouth debridement procedure is delivered when a periodontal evaluation and diagnosis occur on a different date of service. This time interval allows time for gingival tissue to heal so that the comprehensive periodontal evaluation procedure (reported separately), which includes periodontal probing and charting, will have accurate findings.

D6000–D6199 Implant Services

Surgical Services

- **D6106** **guided tissue regeneration – resorbable barrier, per implant**
  This procedure does not include flap entry and closure, or, when indicated, wound debridement, osseous contouring, bone replacement grafts, and placement of biologic materials to aid in osseous regeneration. This procedure is used for peri-implant defects and during implant placement.

- **D6107** **guided tissue regeneration – non-resorbable barrier, per implant**
  This procedure does not include flap entry and closure, or, when indicated, wound debridement, osseous contouring, bone replacement grafts, and placement of biologic materials to aid in osseous regeneration. This procedure is used for peri-implant defects and during implant placement.

Rationale for these changes: These new codes recognize the GTR procedures may be required for an implant case, and mirror similar procedure codes in the Periodontics category of service where GTR is delivered to a natural tooth.

D7000–D7999 Oral and Maxillofacial Surgery

Other Repair Procedures

- **D7956** **guided tissue regeneration, edentulous area – resorbable barrier, per site**
  This procedure does not include flap entry and closure, or, when indicated, wound debridement, osseous contouring, bone replacement grafts, and placement of biologic materials to aid in osseous regeneration. This procedure may be used for ridge augmentation, sinus lift procedures, and after tooth extraction.

- **D7957** **guided tissue regeneration, edentulous area – non-resorbable barrier, per site**
  This procedure does not include flap entry and closure, or, when indicated, wound debridement, osseous contouring, bone replacement grafts, and placement of biologic materials to aid in osseous regeneration. This procedure may be used for ridge augmentation, sinus lift procedures, and after tooth extraction.

Rationale for these changes: These new codes recognize the GTR procedures may be required for a patient with an edentulous area of the oral cavity. They mirror similar procedure codes in the Periodontics category of service, where GTR is delivered to a natural tooth, and in the Implant Services category to resolve peri-implant defects or at the time of implant placement.

D8000–D8999 Orthodontics

All of the following orthodontic treatment codes may be used more than once for the treatment of a particular patient depending on the particular circumstance. A patient may require ~~more than one interceptive procedure or~~ more than one limited or comprehensive procedure depending on their particular problems.

Rationale for this change: This revision is prompted by CDT 2022's deletion of the Interceptive subcategory and codes. It reinforces that there are clinical reasons for repeated delivery of Limited or Comprehensive treatment procedures.

D9000–D9999 Adjunctive General Services

Unclassified Treatment

▲ **D9110** **palliative ~~(emergency)~~ treatment of dental pain ~~— minor procedure~~ – per visit**
Treatment that relieves pain but is not curative; services provided do not have distinct procedure codes. ~~This is typically reported on a "per-visit" basis for emergency treatment of dental pain.~~

Rationale for this change: These revisions clarify the reported procedure's nature, scope, and intended outcome. The word "emergency" is ill-defined and unnecessarily limiting. "Minor procedure" is also ill-defined and subject to interpretation. "Per visit" establishes the intended period of service.

There are many other changes in CDT 2023, as seen in the following list, and they will be discussed further in their applicable CDT 2023 Companion category chapter.

Category	Other Change(s)

D0387 **intraoral tomosynthesis – comprehensive series of radiographic images – image capture only**
A radiographic survey of the whole mouth intended to display the crowns and roots of all teeth, periapical areas, interproximal areas and alveolar bone including edentulous areas.

D0388 **intraoral tomosynthesis – bitewing radiographic image – image capture only**

D0389 **intraoral tomosynthesis – periapical radiographic image – image capture only**

D0393 <u>virtual t</u>~~T~~**reatment simulation using 3D image volume** <u>or surface scan</u>
~~The use of 3D image volumes for~~ <u>Virtual</u> simulation of treatment including, but not limited to, dental implant placement<u>, prosthetic reconstruction,</u> orthognathic surgery and orthodontic tooth movement.

Diagnostic

~~D0351~~ ~~3D photographic image~~
~~This procedure is for diagnostic purposes. Not applicable for a CAD/CAM procedure.~~

~~D0704~~ ~~3D photographic image – image capture only~~

D0709 **intraoral – ~~complete~~ <u>comprehensive</u> series of radiographic images – image capture only**
A radiographic survey of the whole mouth~~, usually consisting of 14-22 periapical and posterior bitewing images or~~ intended to display the crowns and roots of all teeth, periapical areas<u>, interproximal areas</u> and alveolar bone <u>including edentulous areas</u>.

Category	Other Change(s)

Endodontics

D3333 **internal root repair of perforation defects**
Non-surgical seal of perforation caused by resorption and/or decay but not iatrogenic by ~~same~~ provider ~~filing claim~~.

D4240 **gingival flap procedure, including root planing – four or more contiguous teeth or tooth bound spaces per quadrant**
A soft tissue flap is reflected or resected to allow debridement of the root surface and the removal of granulation tissue. Osseous recontouring is not accomplished in conjunction with this procedure. May include open flap curettage, reverse bevel flap surgery, modified Kirkland flap procedure, and modified Widman surgery. This procedure is performed in the presence of moderate to deep probing depths, loss of attachment, need to maintain esthetics, need for increased access to the root surface and alveolar bone, or to determine the presence of a cracked tooth~~,~~ or fractured root~~, or external root resorption~~. Other procedures may be required concurrent to D4240 and should be reported separately using their own unique codes.

Periodontics

D4241 **gingival flap procedure, including root planing – one to three contiguous teeth or tooth bound spaces per quadrant**
A soft tissue flap is reflected or resected to allow debridement of the root surface and the removal of granulation tissue. Osseous recontouring is not accomplished in conjunction with this procedure. May include open flap curettage, reverse bevel flap surgery, modified Kirkland flap procedure, and modified Widman surgery. This procedure is performed in the presence of moderate to deep probing depths, loss of attachment, need to maintain esthetics, need for increased access to the root surface and alveolar bone, or to determine the presence of a cracked tooth~~,~~ or fractured root~~, or external root resorption~~. Other procedures may be required concurrent to D4241 and should be reported separately using their own unique codes.

Category	Other Change(s)

D4266 **guided tissue regeneration, natural teeth – resorbable barrier, per site**
This procedure does not include flap entry and closure, or, when indicated, wound debridement, osseous contouring, bone replacement grafts, and placement of biologic materials to aid in osseous regeneration. This procedure can be used for periodontal defects around natural teeth ~~and peri-implant defects~~.

D4267 **guided tissue regeneration, natural teeth – non-resorbable barrier, per site** ~~(includes membrane removal)~~
This procedure does not include flap entry and closure, or, when indicated, wound debridement, osseous contouring, bone replacement grafts, and placement of biologic materials to aid in osseous regeneration. This procedure can be used for periodontal defects around natural teeth ~~and peri-implant defects~~.

D4921 **gingival irrigation with a medicinal agent – per quadrant**
~~Irrigation of gingival pockets with a prescription medicinal agent. Not to be used to report use of over the counter (OTC) mouth rinses or non-invasive chemical debridement~~.

Periodontics

D6105 **removal of implant body not requiring bone removal or flap elevation**

D6106 **guided tissue regeneration – resorbable barrier, per implant**
This procedure does not include flap entry and closure, or, when indicated, wound debridement, osseous contouring, bone replacement grafts, and placement of biologic materials to aid in osseous regeneration. This procedure is used for peri-implant defects and during implant placement.

Implant Services

Category	Other Change(s)	
Implant Services	**D6107**	**guided tissue regeneration – non-resorbable barrier, per implant** This procedure does not include flap entry and closure, or, when indicated, wound debridement, osseous contouring, bone replacement grafts, and placement of biologic materials to aid in osseous regeneration. This procedure is used for peri-implant defects and during implant placement.
	D6197	**replacement of restorative material used to close an access opening of a screw-retained implant supported prosthesis, per implant**
Oral & Maxillofacial Surgery	**D7251**	**coronectomy – intentional partial tooth removal, impacted teeth only** Intentional partial tooth removal is performed when a neurovascular complication is likely if the entire impacted tooth is removed.
	D7509	**marsupialization of odontogenic cyst** Surgical decompression of a large cystic lesion by creating a long-term open pocket or pouch
Adjunctive General Services	**D9953**	**reline custom sleep apnea appliance (indirect)** Resurface dentition side of appliance with new soft or hard base material as required to restore original form and function.
	D9450	**case presentation, subsequent to detailed and extensive treatment planning** Established patient. Not performed on same day as evaluation.

Section 2
Using the CDT Code: Definitions and Key Concepts, Coding Scenarios, and Coding Q&A

Introduction

Individual chapters in this section, including one for each of the CDT Code's 12 categories of service, contain definitions of key terms, information on notable changes, clinical scenarios, and Q&A based on real-life situations. Answers to these questions and scenarios illustrate coding solutions for the situations described. These scenarios and solutions reflect common and accepted practices, but may not reflect the way your office would manage a given situation. The dentist who treats a patient is the person who can best determine appropriate treatment and the CDT codes that best describe it.

The scenarios and Q&A are the products of questions received from ADA members and developed by ADA staff, as well as based on the contributions of chapter authors. They are not to be considered legal advice or a guarantee that individual payer contracts will follow this assistance.

Use this information to get a better understanding of the principles of reporting using the CDT Code. Since it covers subjects from many different perspectives, it is likely that some will be more applicable to your particular situation than others. All the scenarios and Q&A, including those that involve procedures you may not usually report, are of value since the principles demonstrated can often be applied to areas of your practice.

By Ralph A. Cooley, D.D.S.

Introduction

2022 continued to provide challenges nationwide to dental care providers climbing out of the national pandemic climate. Despite these challenges, the dental community was perseverant in providing excellent patient care. As you will see there are code additions and revisions in CDT 2023 in the Diagnostic category. Some definitions of codes that were thought to be foundational have been changed due to technology and greater information.

Hence, it is more important than ever to have a complete and accurate record of dental care provided in today's world. That is why the *Code on Dental Procedures and Nomenclature* (CDT Code) was established, and why knowing those changes occurring in CDT 2023 is crucial. In this chapter, we will discuss key concepts and code changes, some common coding scenarios, and frequently asked questions about coding for diagnostic procedures.

Key Definitions and Concepts

Evaluation: The systematic determination or judgment about a condition, disease, or treatment.

Clinical oral evaluations: As with all ADA procedure codes, there is no distinction made between the evaluations provided by general practitioners and specialists. Report additional diagnostic and/or definitive procedures separately.

Imaging: Creating a visual representation of the interior of a body revealing inner structures that may have been blocked by skin or bone.

Intraoral image: A visual representation of the mouth derived by placing a film, plate, or sensor within the mouth.

Extra-oral image: A visual representation of the mouth derived by placing a film, plate, or sensor outside the mouth.

Tomosynthesis: The creation of a 3D image by digital processing of multiple radiographic images.

Changes to This Category

There are a variety of changes in the Diagnostic category, all involving diagnostic imaging procedures. Some are additions that enable documenting tomosynthesis (see definition on page 29) as a discrete procedure. There are other additions that are replacements for deleted codes and revisions that affect nomenclatures and descriptors of continuing codes.

Additions: (10)

Image Capture with Interpretation

D0372 intraoral tomosynthesis – comprehensive series of radiographic images
A radiographic survey of the whole mouth intended to display the crowns and roots of all teeth, periapical areas, interproximal areas and alveolar bone including edentulous areas.

D0373 intraoral tomosynthesis – bitewing radiographic image

D0374 intraoral tomosynthesis – periapical radiographic image

Note: D0372–D0374 are complemented by the new codes D0387–D0389 listed in the image capture only subcategory.

D0801 3D dental surface scan – direct

D0802 3D dental surface scan – indirect
A surface scan of a diagnostic cast.

D0803 3D facial surface scan – direct

D0804 3D facial surface scan – indirect
A surface scan of constructed facial features.

Note: D0801–D0804 are additions that replace codes D0351 and D0704 listed as deleted below.

Image Capture Only

D0387 intraoral tomosynthesis – comprehensive series of radiographic images – image capture only
A radiographic survey of the whole mouth intended to display the crowns and roots of all teeth, periapical areas, interproximal areas and alveolar bone including edentulous areas.

D0388 intraoral tomosynthesis – bitewing radiographic image – image capture only

D0389 intraoral tomosynthesis – periapical radiographic image – image capture only

Revisions: (3)

Image Capture with Interpretation

D0210 **intraoral – ~~complete~~ comprehensive series of radiographic images**
A radiographic survey of the whole mouth~~, usually consisting of 14–22 periapical and posterior bitewing images or~~ intended to display the crowns and roots of all teeth, periapical areas, interproximal areas and alveolar bone including edentulous areas.

D0393 **virtual t~~T~~reatment simulation using 3D image volume or surface scan**
~~The use of 3D image volumes for~~ Virtual simulation of treatment including, but not limited to, dental implant placement, prosthetic reconstruction, orthognathic surgery and orthodontic tooth movement.

Image Capture Only

D0709 **intraoral – ~~complete~~ comprehensive series of radiographic images – image capture only**
A radiographic survey of the whole mouth~~, usually consisting of 14–22 periapical and posterior bitewing images or~~ intended to display the crowns and roots of all teeth, periapical areas, interproximal areas and alveolar bone including edentulous areas.

Note: The revisions to D0210 and D0709 recognize that it is the dentist who determines the type and number of images required for a comprehensive "full mouth series" (also known as "FMX") as described in the changed nomenclature and descriptor.

Deletions: (2)

Image Capture with Interpretation

~~**D0351**~~ **~~3D photographic image~~**
~~This procedure is for diagnostic purposes. Not applicable for a CAD/CAM procedure.~~

Image Capture Only

~~**D0704**~~ **~~3D photographic image – image capture only~~**

Clinical Coding Scenario #1:
Radiographs – What Constitutes a Full Mouth Series and How Should It Be Coded?

In *CDT 2023*, code D0210's descriptor was changed to clarify the reported procedure's purpose and scope:

D0210 intraoral – comprehensive series of radiographic images
A radiographic survey of the whole mouth intended to display the crowns and roots of all teeth, periapical areas, interproximal areas, and alveolar bone including edentulous area.

Note: There is not a "magical number" or type of radiographs that determine when the D0210 procedure had been delivered. The revised descriptor, which eliminated "…usually consisting of 14–22 periapical and bitewing images…" simplified the criteria for determining when D0210 is the appropriate procedure code.

With this in mind, consider how radiographs for patients A, B, C, D, and E are documented.

Patient A

For a patient with a full complement of 32 teeth, the office takes four posterior bitewing radiograph images to look at the interproximal areas of molars and premolars, four maxillary posterior periapical images (right and left), four mandibular posterior periapical images (right and left), three maxillary anterior periapical images, and three mandibular anterior periapical views. This is a total of 18 individual radiographic images, which captured all of the crowns and roots of the teeth, periapical areas, interproximal areas, and alveolar bone.

How would this be coded?

D0210 intraoral – comprehensive series of radiographic images
A radiographic survey of the whole mouth intended to display the crowns and roots of all teeth, periapical areas, interproximal areas, and alveolar bone including edentulous areas.

Regardless of the number of images, the descriptor's criteria for D0210 is met. If the dental provided elected to also take a panoramic image, it would be coded additionally as:

D0330 panoramic radiographic image

Continued on next page

Patient B

For a patient with a full complement of 32 teeth, the office takes a total of eight periapical x-rays: three upper (maxillary) anterior, three lower (mandibular) anterior and one posterior in each quadrant.

Again, there is not a number of radiographs that define a comprehensive series. However, since the radiographs do not display the crowns and roots of all teeth, periapical areas, and alveolar bone crest, the full mouth series procedure code D0210 would not be appropriate. The correct procedure codes are:

D0220   intraoral – periapical first radiographic image

(Report D0220 one time.)

D0230   intraoral – periapical each additional radiographic image

(Report D0230 once in the claim service line Procedure Code field and the value 09 in the Quantity field.)

Patient C

This patient has 28 fully erupted teeth, with the third molars being removed in the past. The office takes a panoramic x-ray and four posterior bitewings.

D0330   panoramic radiographic image

D0274   bitewings – four radiographic images

Since a panoramic radiographic image is not intraoral, this combination could not correctly be reported as a comprehensive series (D0210).

Note: The ADA Council on Dental Benefit Programs receives many calls stating that claims for D0330 and D0274 are downcoded by third-party payers to D0210 for purposes of reimbursement. This term *downcoding* is defined in the Glossary published on ADA.org as:

> **Downcoding**: A third-party payer claim adjudication process that uses a procedure code that is different from the one reported on the claim so that the reimbursement amount is less than would be allowed for the submitted code.

The ADA frowns upon such downcoding. The dentist should continue to document and report the procedure as described above instead of coding towards any third-party payers' policies.

Continued on next page

The patient presents with many missing teeth. The office takes four periapical radiographic images of the upper edentulous ridge, seven periapicals of the lower arch, and four posterior bitewings, capturing the crowns and roots of all teeth, all edentulous areas, all periapical views, and interproximal areas. This situation, while not the most common scenario, does meet all the criteria for and is correctly coded as a comprehensive series. Again, the definition reads:

D0210 intraoral – comprehensive series of radiographic images
A radiographic survey of the whole mouth intended to display the crowns and roots of all teeth, periapical areas, interproximal areas, and alveolar bone including edentulous areas.

A panoramic radiographic image and seven vertical bitewing radiographic images were taken.

This situation would not be coded as a D0210 because the panoramic image is extraoral, not an intraoral. The following codes are applicable:

D0330 panoramic radiographic image

D0277 vertical bitewings – 7 to 8 radiographic images
This does not constitute a full mouth intraoral radiographic series.

Regardless of the patient's dental benefit plan, the reporting of performed procedures should always reflect what treatment was provided. Alternate payment provisions may apply, but the third-party payer should send statements to patients and providers alike to explain why an alternate benefit was provided.

Dentists who have signed provider agreements with third-party payers should check their contracts to see if there are provisions that apply to this situation.

Clinical Coding Scenario #2:
Office Electing to Use Tomosynthesis for Advanced Radiographic Imaging

A patient of record who had not been seen for seven years returned to the dental office where previous treatment had occurred. The patient had a history of fractured teeth that required restorations with crowns, two teeth needing endodontic therapy, and even an extraction due to an extreme vertical fracture of one tooth. Recently, the office had acquired additional radiographic imaging equipment and software to utilize tomosynthesis or 3D imaging within the oral cavity. The doctor elected to take a comprehensive series of these types of images instead of the standard radiographic comprehensive series.

How should one code for this visit?

D0150 **comprehensive oral evaluation – new or established patient**

D0372 **intraoral tomosynthesis – comprehensive series of radiographic images**
A radiographic survey of the whole mouth intended to display the crowns and roots of all teeth, periapical areas, interproximal areas and alveolar bone including the edentulous areas.

If the dentist had decided to do a comprehensive series of two-dimensional radiographic images, and then additionally take a bitewing radiograph and a periapical radiograph utilizing the tomosynthesis equipment, then the services would be coded as:

D0210 **intraoral – comprehensive series of radiographic images**
A radiographic survey of the whole mouth intended to display the crowns and roots of all teeth, periapical areas, interproximal areas and alveolar bone including the edentulous areas.

D0373 **intraoral tomosynthesis – bitewing radiographic image**

D0374 **intraoral tomosynthesis – periapical radiographic image**

Note: Traditional radiographic images still continue to give good diagnostic images in dental treatment. The decision to use tomosynthesis for the radiographic imaging is the judgment of the dental professional. Tomosynthesis is designed to give a 3D look at oral cavity structures, and can give a different perspective over the traditional two-dimensional radiographic images. Tomosynthetic radiographs require specialized x-ray imaging equipment to digitally capture multiple low-dose base projection radiographs, and specialized software and hardware to process the captured digital images. These provide a layer-by-layer virtual dissection of the targeted anatomy.

Clinical Coding Scenario #3:
Patient Requesting COVID-19 Vaccination in the Dental Office

An adult patient of record was seen for a periodic examination and prophylaxis, but required no radiographic images. During the appointment, the patient's medical history was reviewed, and the patient shared that the COVID-19 vaccine had never been administered to them. The dentist had the Pfizer-BioNTech COVID-19 vaccine in storage at the office and was allowed by state law to administer it to patients. The patient stated that they wanted to receive the vaccine, and their medical history allowed that to occur safely.

How might this visit be coded?

D0120   periodic oral evaluation – established patient

D1110   prophylaxis – adult

Note: When coding for COVID-19 vaccine, it is important to code for the specific vaccine being administered, as well as which dose, for those vaccines requiring a second dose. In this case, the dentist had stored the **Pfizer BioNTech** vaccine, so the appropriate CDT code would be:

D1701   Pfizer-BioNTech Covid-19 vaccine administration – first dose
        SARSCOV2 COVID-19 VAC mRNA 30mcg/0.3mL IM DOSE 1

Again, it is very important to code for the SPECIFIC vaccine being used, as well as whether it is first or second dose for the vaccines requiring two doses.

Note: If a dentist decides to submit a claim for the vaccination procedure to the patient's medical insurance carrier, then the medical claim format (e.g., 1500 paper form/837P electronic claim) and coding systems (e.g., CPT; National Drug Codes) must be used.

Clinical Coding Scenario #4:
Patient Age 11 – Evaluation, Preventive, and Orthodontic Services

A new patient, age 11, was seen for a first exam, cleaning, and fluoride varnish application. During the exam, the dentist noted that the erupting tooth #4 was impinging on the fixed space maintainer that spanned both the right and left side of the mouth. This space maintainer had been placed by another dentist but it was decided that the space maintainer needed to be removed now.

How might this visit be coded?

D0150 **comprehensive oral evaluation – new or established patient**

D1120 **prophylaxis – child**

D1206 **topical application of fluoride varnish**

D1557 **removal of fixed bilateral space maintainer – maxillary**

Note: In this scenario, if the topical fluoride was a rinse or other appropriate in-office fluoride application other than a varnish, D1206 would not be correct. The appropriate CDT code would be:

D1208 **topical application of fluoride – excluding varnish**

But what if the same patient was not new and the doctor had placed the space maintainer two years ago? How would this encounter be coded?

D0120 **periodic oral evaluation – established patient**

D1120 **prophylaxis – child**

D1206 **topical application of fluoride varnish**

D1557 **removal of fixed bilateral space maintainer – maxillary**

The exam, in this case, would be periodic (D0120) because the patient was seen previously, but the prophylaxis and fluoride codes remain the same as would the code to remove the space maintainer. Both codes for removal of a fixed bilateral space maintainer may be reported by either the dentist who placed the appliance, or a different dentist, as placement and removal are discrete procedures that are delivered on different dates of service. D1557 is used when the maintainer is removed from the maxillary arch and D1558 is used for the mandibular arch. In this case, D1557 is the appropriate code.

Clinical Coding Scenario #5:
Patient Seen after Office Hours with a Dental Accident

Andrew was hit in the mouth with a ball while playing catch with his baseball coach. Fortunately, the team coach was also a dentist, so Andrew was seen in the office that night. The dentist did an oral evaluation and noticed that the patient had normal opening and closing, no soft tissue injuries requiring any sutures, slight mobility of #8 and #9, and minimal bleeding of the lip. Two intraoral periapical radiographs were taken to rule out root fractures with the maxillary anterior teeth. The dentist advised Andrew and his parents to return in two weeks for follow-up if there were no complications or discomfort.

How would the dentist code for this visit?

D0140 limited oral evaluation – problem focused
An evaluation limited to a specific oral health problem or complaint. This may require interpretation of information acquired through additional diagnostic procedures. Report additional diagnostic procedures separately. Definitive procedures may be required on the same date as the evaluation.

Typically patients receiving this type of evaluation present with a specific problem and/or dental emergencies, trauma, acute infections, etc.

D0220 intraoral – periapical first radiographic image

D0230 intraoral – periapical each additional radiographic image

Andrew was seen for a follow-up visit two weeks later and reported no problems. The dentist pulp tested teeth #7, #8, #9, and #10 and all tested normally. Andrew was advised to be seen in three months for his regularly scheduled dental visit, and that this area would be re-evaluated at that time.

What CDT codes were utilized for this visit?

D0170 re-evaluation – limited, problem focused (established patient; not post-operative visit)
Assessing the status of a previously existing condition. For example:
- a traumatic injury where no treatment was rendered but patient needs follow-up monitoring
- evaluation for undiagnosed continuing pain
- soft tissue lesions requiring follow-up evaluation

D0460 pulp vitality tests
Includes multiple teeth and contra lateral comparison(s), as indicated.

Clinical Coding Scenario #6:
New Patient with Diagnostic Gathering Challenges and Tobacco Use

A 21-year-old new patient is seen for a first exam. It is noted that he has numerous decayed anterior and posterior teeth, but when an attempt was made to take a full mouth intraoral series of radiographs, the patient has a severe gag response. Only a panoramic image and two extra-oral bitewings are able to be taken.

He is also a heavy chewing tobacco user, so a tissue fluorescence oral cancer exam is performed and about 15 minutes is spent discussing his tobacco use, what it is doing to his mouth, and his options to try to quit.

How would this visit be coded?

D0150 **comprehensive oral evaluation – new or established patient**

D0330 **panoramic radiographic image**

D0251 **extra-oral posterior dental radiographic image**

Choosing the panoramic (D0330) and extra-oral posterior (D0251) radiograph procedures allowed the dentist to get a preliminary understanding of his oral conditions. Note: this is not a "full mouth series" because these are extraoral radiographic images. The dentist may consider utilizing some alternative methods to aid in capturing some intraoral images later.

Codes for the tissue fluorescence oral cancer exam and counseling the patient for his tobacco use are:

D0431 **adjunctive pre-diagnostic test that aids in detection of mucosal abnormalities including premalignant and malignant lesions, not to include cytology or biopsy procedures**

Note: Examples of adjunctive pre-diagnostic tests that aid in detection of mucosal abnormalities may include VELscope, OralID, MicorLux DL, or VizLite Plus. This test is done in addition to your normal visual and palpation exam that is part of a comprehensive evaluation.

D1320 **tobacco counseling for the control and prevention of oral disease**

Clinical Coding Scenario #7:
Child under Three – Evaluation, Parent Counseling, and Preventive Services

Note: The American Academy of Pediatric Dentistry (AAPD) and the ADA both advise that children should have their first dental visit within six months of the eruption of the first primary tooth.

The doctor performed an intraoral examination on a one-year-old patient while the mother restrained the child's forehead in her lap. The dentist determined that the child had maxillary and mandibular primary incisors and that they were caries free. The dentist also removed plaque using an ultra-soft toothbrush and applied fluoride varnish. The doctor explained to the parent how to use a washcloth or soft brush to remove plaque each day and the importance of getting the child to go to sleep without a bottle. They discussed foods that can "lead to decay" (caries) and recommended that she return in a year for an exam after most of the primary teeth have erupted.

Here is what occurred during the child's first dental visit:

- Oral examination
- Toothbrush deplaquing
- Fluoride varnish
- Discussion of diet and preventive care with the parent

How would you code this first visit?

D0145   **oral evaluation for a patient under three years of age and counseling with primary caregiver**

D1120   **prophylaxis – child**

D1206   **topical application of fluoride varnish**

Note: The evaluation and counseling code (D0145):

- has both diagnostic and preventive characteristics
- is specifically for children under three years of age
- includes an evaluation of oral conditions, history, and caries susceptibility
- includes development of an oral hygiene regimen
- always includes counseling the primary caregiver or parent

Continued on next page

What evaluation code could be used on the next visit?

Either the same evaluation and counseling code (D0145) or the periodic evaluation code (D0120) could be used for the next visit. There is nothing in the D0145 nomenclature or descriptor that precludes its use for more than one visit, as long as the patient is still under three years of age and all the components of the procedure are completed. The periodic exam might be appropriate as the primary dentition develops and if the other criteria are not met. The prophylaxis and fluoride would remain the same.

Clinical Coding Scenario #8:
Oral Cancer – An Enhanced Examination

An oral cancer evaluation is included in the descriptors of both the comprehensive oral evaluations (D0150 and D0180) and the periodic oral evaluation (D0120). Visual inspection using operatory lighting and palpation are the techniques that are frequently used in routine oral cancer evaluations. A dentist may decide that patients with increased cancer risk factors should also receive an enhanced oral cancer examination, one that is more extensive than a routine oral cancer screening and may include the use of additional diagnostic aids.

How could the dentist report use of additional diagnostic aids in the oral cancer examination?

There is not an independent code for an enhanced oral cancer examination, but there is a code that can be used when some type of staining or similar procedure is performed:

> **D0431**   **adjunctive pre-diagnostic test that aids in detection of mucosal abnormalities including premalignant and malignant lesions, not to include cytology or biopsy procedures**

This code may be used to report the use of the following:

- Tissue reflectance (e.g., VizLite Plus, MicorLux DL)
- Autofluorescence (e.g., VELscope, OralID)
- Any intraoral vital staining technique (e.g., toluidine blue)

If the additional procedures are not described by D0431 the dentist could use:

> **D0999   unspecified diagnostic procedure, by report**

D0999 can be used to report any diagnostic procedure that does not seem to be included in the CDT Code. A narrative that describes the service must be included on the claim when this code is used.

Clinical Coding Scenario #9:
Impression for an Appliance and Diagnostic Models

A 17-year-old patient of record is seen for a periodic oral exam and prophylaxis. Her radiographic images are up to date and the doctor notes that the patient has nearly perfect occlusion with no evidence of occlusal issues of wear, and had not received any orthodontic care in the past. The patient and her mother inquired about at home tooth whitening. This initial visit was coded as:

D0120 periodic oral evaluation – established patient

D1110 prophylaxis – adult

Two months later, the patient decided to request tooth whitening, and returned for impressions for maxillary and mandibular bleaching trays. She was seen a week later for the trays, and instructions and a follow up visit was scheduled. It was noted that there was no dental benefit reimbursement for bleaching trays, so the patient's mother inquired whether the models on which they were constructed could be considered diagnostic casts (D0470), and submitted as such after the fact.

Could these be considered "diagnostic casts" using code D0470 at this point?

Because these impressions were taken with the purpose of fabricating bleaching trays, the appropriate code is:

D9975 external bleaching for home application, per arch; includes materials and fabrication of custom trays

The dentist could have elected to take impressions for diagnostic models at the periodic exam appointment or any time after, and correctly coded for it, if indeed they were indicated to facilitate diagnosis and treatment planning. Diagnostic casts or models are extremely important for so many patients in diagnosis and treatment planning. However, in this case, the impressions were taken to serve another purpose, i.e., bleaching. Again, the purpose of coding is to show what treatment is actually performed and for what reason.

Clinical Coding Scenario #10:
Orthognathic Surgery Planning

An oral and maxillofacial surgery office recently installed a cone beam radiography machine. It was used to treatment plan some anticipated orthognathic surgery for a patient. Following image capture, several axial and lateral views were consulted to plan the surgery. A panoramic view was also produced to send to the patient's orthodontist.

After consultation with the orthodontist, the surgeon constructed a 3D virtual model, which they viewed together on the computer, to properly locate a temporary implant to anchor the orthodontic appliance. The virtual model could be manipulated on the screen to allow them to visualize other anatomical structures in the area and their relationship to the teeth to determine the ideal location to place the implant.

How could you code the initial treatment planning visit's diagnostic imaging procedures?

D0367   cone beam CT capture and interpretation with field of view of both jaws; with or without cranium

This code is used specifically to report procedures related to cone beam imaging technology. It replaced the separate cone beam data capture (D0360) and two-dimension reconstruction (D0362) codes. The image capture includes two-dimensional sectional (tomographic) views from the axial (coronal or frontal) and lateral (sagittal) planes, as well as the panoramic view.

How could you code the subsequent consultation (3D virtual model)?

D0393   virtual treatment simulation using 3D image volume or surface scan
Virtual simulation of treatment including, but not limited to, dental implant placement, prosthetic reconstruction, orthognathic surgery and orthodontic tooth movement.

Note: D0393's CDT Code entry was revised in 2023 to clarify the processes that are occurring in dentistry today. Virtual has come to mean "existing, seen, or happening online or on a computer screen, rather than in person or in the physical world."

A clinician or technician can manipulate virtual 3D images volumes to perform all manner of dentofacial analysis and appliance construction. A virtual process is becoming a greater and greater aspect of all manner of diagnosis, treatment planning, and appliance and prosthetic construction in dentistry.

Clinical Coding Scenario #11:
Temporomandibular Joint (TMJ) Disorder Treatment

A patient, referred to the dental office by her ear, nose, and throat (ENT) physician, has a history of constant headaches and facial pain. The ENT saw no sinus-related issues after a thorough examination, including radiographic images. After completing a comprehensive oral evaluation (D0150), the dentist recognized the patient's symptoms as a temporomandibular disorder of significant complexity. The patient exhibited limited opening and was in discomfort every morning.

Further evaluation was needed to diagnose this condition, and that examination included listening to the joint with a stethoscope, detailed palpation of all the muscles of mastication, and recording of occlusal relationships, ranges of motion, and areas of musculoskeletal tenderness.

The dentist did an extensive review of the patient's lifestyle, including stress-coping mechanisms. She identified many potential contributing factors to the temporomandibular disorder (TMD) condition. Teeth #18 and #19 were missing, and tooth #15 had super-erupted to the point where the patient could not close without moving her jaw to the right. A tongue thrust habit resulted in a severe anterior open bite, and there was extensive incisal wear on all anterior teeth.

The doctor decided that following extraction of #15, an orthotic TMJ appliance covering the mandibular occlusal surfaces would allow the patient to reposition her jaw to a more comfortable position. It would also protect those teeth from increasing wear due to oral habits. After the patient was more comfortable, the doctor believed that a comprehensive treatment plan could be made.

How would the recent diagnostic visit be coded?

Due to the limited scope, the doctor can choose one of two problem-focused evaluations:

D0140 **limited oral evaluation – problem focused**

or

D0160 **detailed and extensive oral evaluation – problem focused, by report**

In this case, the nature and complexity of the problems suggest that D0160 would be the most appropriate code for this evaluation. Use of this code requires submission of a narrative report.

Clinical Coding Scenario #12:
Treating a Patient Suffering From Swelling, Pain, and Periodontal Disease

A patient presented in pain and complaining about swelling around one particular tooth. The doctor's emergency evaluation focused on the patient's complaint and included two periapical radiographic images and pocket measurements of the teeth in the area. The swelling was clearly adjacent to tooth #3 and there was bleeding and exudate upon probing.

The doctor treated the patient for a periodontal abscess by gross debridement and draining through the sulcus, irrigating the pocket with chlorhexidine, and prescribing the patient an antibiotic.

How could this encounter be coded?

Since the evaluation was both problem-focused and limited to the patient's complaint, the appropriate codes for diagnostic procedures would be:

D0140 **limited oral evaluation – problem focused**

D0220 **intraoral – periapical first radiographic image**

D0230 **intraoral – periapical each additional radiographic image**

In this case, there are several codes that might be used to document the operative services, alone or in combination. The procedure coding options are:

D9110 **palliative treatment of dental pain – per visit**
Treatment that relieves pain but is not curative; services provided do not have distinct procedure codes.

Note: D9110 is a "catch-all" code that covers a broad array of procedures that a dentist may determine are appropriate for the patient.

D7510 **incision and drainage of abscess – intraoral soft tissue**
Involves incision through mucosa, including periodontal origins.

Note: Discussions at the Code Maintenance Committee (CMC) meetings indicated that D7510 was considered to be appropriate even when the incision is made through the gingival sulcus.

Clinical Coding Scenario #13:
A Partially Edentulous Patient with Rampant Calculus and White Oral Lesions – Comprehensive Oral Evaluation Necessary

A patient with permanent dentition who had not seen a dentist in more than ten years presented to the office with concerns about white patches in the mouth, worried that it may be oral cancer. The dentist's initial visual examination revealed that the patient had extensive calculus covering multiple teeth that had to be addressed before the dentist would be able to see oral conditions well enough to begin a D0150 procedure (comprehensive oral evaluation – new or established patient).

An ultrasonic scaler was the doctor's instrument of choice for calculus removal. After calculus removal there were additional diagnostic procedures: radiographs of the entire lower arch, including eight posterior and three anterior periapicals; two bitewings on the left and one on the right side; and a panoramic radiographic image.

Today's treatment included:

- removal of calculus and stains
- radiographs (nine PA, three BW, and one Panoramic)
- disaggregated transepithelial biopsy (brush) of white patch
- dispensing one 16 oz. bottle of chlorhexidine gluconate rinse
- comprehensive oral evaluation

How would the services delivered during today's encounter be coded?

Removal of calculus and stain:

D1110 prophylaxis – adult
Removal of plaque, calculus and stains from the tooth structures and implants in the permanent and transitional dentition. It is intended to control local irritational factors.

or

D1999 unspecified preventive procedure, by report
Used for a procedure that is not adequately described by a code. Describe the procedure.

Continued on next page

Radiographs (nine PA, three BW, and one Panoramic):

Because they did not capture all of the edentulous areas, these 12 radiographs do not match the CDT Code's definition of an intraoral comprehensive series of radiographic images (D0210). Therefore, the radiographs in this scenario would be reported using the panoramic, periapical, and bitewing codes:

D0220   intraoral – periapical first radiographic image

D0230   intraoral – periapical each additional radiographic image

Note: Report D0230 eight times, once for each additional radiographic image.

D0273   bitewings – three radiographic images

D0330   panoramic radiographic image

Note: If these 12 intraoral radiographs (periapicals and bitewings) were taken in such a way to capture all "crowns and roots of all teeth, all periapical areas, interproximal areas, and alveolar bone including edentulous areas," the intraoral imaging procedures could be considered a "FMX" and be coded as **D0210 intraoral – comprehensive series of radiographic images** (instead of the separate D0220, D0230, and D0273 codes). The reported codes for this scenario would then be D0210 and D0330.

Disaggregated transepithelial biopsy of white patch:

D7288   brush biopsy – transepithelial sample collection

Note: The brush biopsy samples disaggregated dermal and epithelial cells. A positive sample usually requires follow-up with an architecturally intact excisional sample.

Dispense one 16 oz. bottle of chlorhexidine gluconate rinse:

D9630   drugs or medicaments dispensed in the office for home use

Comprehensive Oral Examination:

D0150   comprehensive oral evaluation – new or established patient
Used by a general dentist and/or a specialist when evaluating a patient comprehensively. This applies to new patients; established patients who have had a significant change in health conditions or other unusual circumstances, by report, or established patients who have been absent from active treatment for three or more years. It is a thorough evaluation and recording of the extraoral and intraoral hard and soft tissues. *Continued on next page*

It may require interpretation of information acquired through additional diagnostic procedures. Additional diagnostic procedures should be reported separately.

This includes an evaluation for oral cancer, the evaluation and recording of the patient's dental and medical history and a general health assessment. It may include the evaluation and recording of dental caries, missing or unerupted teeth, restorations, existing prostheses, occlusal relationships, periodontal conditions (including periodontal screening and/or charting), hard and soft tissue anomalies, etc.

Clinical Coding Scenario #14:
Preventive Resin Restorations

The patient arrived at the office for a recall visit. On the previous recall visit six months ago, this patient had nutritional counseling as well as several teeth that needed to be restored due to decay.

Before doing anything, the doctor decided that a caries risk assessment should be completed, using the form posted on ADA.org. A look at the answers on the form – especially the combination of frequent consumption of soft drinks and energy drinks, past interproximal restorations, and two incipient carious lesions – led to the conclusion that the patient is at high risk of continuing caries development.

What is the appropriate CDT code to document the caries risk procedure?

D0603   caries risk assessment and documentation, with a finding of high risk
Using recognized assessment tools.

Note: Caries risk assessment information, including the updated tools, is available online at ADA.org/cariesrisk. When a patient receives a caries risk assessment, the procedure is documented and reported with the CDT code whose nomenclature includes the identified level of risk:

D0601   caries risk assessment and documentation, with a finding of low risk

D0602   caries risk assessment and documentation, with a finding of moderate risk

D0603   caries risk assessment and documentation, with a finding of high risk

During the oral exam, the doctor did indeed see what appeared to be small, carious, cavitated lesions on the occlusal surfaces of teeth #30 and #31. After opening the lesions using a handpiece and removing caries, both preparations were very slight, ending in enamel, and did not extend into the dentin.

The doctor concluded that a minimally invasive restorative technique would be appropriate for this situation. A composite resin would be used to restore tooth form and function along with an unfilled resin used afterwards to seal out all the radiating grooves.

Continued on next page

> **D1352** preventive resin restoration in a moderate to high caries risk patient – permanent tooth

Note: The doctor knows that **D2391 resin-based composite – one surface, posterior** is not appropriate since the dentin was untouched. Likewise, **D1351 sealant – per tooth** isn't applicable since decay was present.

D1352 was added to the CDT Code to enable documentation of a conservative restorative procedure where caries, erosion, or other conditions affect the natural form and function of the tooth. This procedure is part of many dental school curricula under names that vary by school and region (e.g., preventive resin restoration; conservative resin restoration; or minimally invasive resin restoration).

Clinical Coding Scenario #15:
Current Patient of Record with Substantial Increase in Carious Lesions on Exam

A 75-year-old patient is currently being seen every six months with preventive visits. This patient has periodontal probing depths of no greater than 3 mm in all four quadrants of the oral cavity, and has had no carious activity or replacement of restorations in the past five years. Upon current examination by the dentist, eight new carious lesions were noted, located on the facial or buccal surfaces of mandibular teeth. The patient shared that he had a change in his medical history, and is taking three new medications known to have "dry mouth" as a side effect. Before preceding further, the dentist decided to perform a caries risk assessment. In addition, the dentist decided to measure the amount of salivary flow for the patient. The patient was instructed to chew on unflavored gum and saliva was collected for five minutes. The patient had a saliva rate flow of 0.4 ml/min.

What are the appropriate CDT codes for this patient visit?

D0120 **periodic oral evaluation – established patient**

D0603 **caries risk assessment and documentation, with a finding of high risk**

D0419 **assessment of salivary flow by measurement**

This procedure is for identification of low salivary flow in patients at risk for hyposalivation and xerostomia, as well as effectiveness of pharmacological agents used to stimulate saliva production.

Note: Salivary assessment technique may vary by diagnosis and available equipment but generally can be evaluated by resting or stimulated saliva assessment.

Resting salivary flow is determined by asking the patient to let saliva accumulate in the floor of the mouth and, with the head tilted forward, let it drool into the collecting cup passively. After five minutes, volume collected is measured and divided by five to obtain the flow rate in mL/min. Rates lower than 0.1 mL/min are considered hyposalivation.

Stimulated salivary flow is determined by chewing paraffin wax or unflavored chewing gum (mechanical stimulation) or by dripping a few drops of citric acid on the tongue (chemical stimulation) and spitting for up to five minutes. Volume obtained is converted into mL/min. Rates lower than 0.7 mL/min are considered hyposalivation.

Clinical Coding Scenario #16:
Oral Evaluation and Prophylaxis with Natural Teeth and Implant Crowns

A 64-year-old patient of record had four implants placed in edentulous areas #18, #19, #30, and #31, and these implants were restored with single zirconia crowns, with all remaining dentition intact. The patient is being seen on a six-month basis for examination and prophylaxis, but now has a "mixed" dentition of both natural teeth and implants that are restored.

How would you code for the visit, which includes an oral evaluation and updated radiographic images?

D0120 **periodic oral evaluation – established patient**
An evaluation performed on a patient of record to determine any changes in the patient's dental and medical health status since a previous comprehensive or periodic evaluation. This includes an oral cancer evaluation, periodontal screening where indicated, and may require interpretation of information acquired through additional diagnostic procedures. The findings are discussed with the patient. Report additional diagnostic procedures separately.

D1110 **prophylaxis – adult**
Removal of plaque, calculus and stains from tooth structures and implants in the permanent and transitional dentition. It is intended to control local factors.

Both prophylaxis procedure codes (D1110 and D1120) include "and implants" in their descriptors to clarify that the prophylaxis procedure and code is properly reported when a patient's dentition includes natural teeth and implant restored areas, and no prosthesis is removed.

Clinical Coding Scenario #17:
Reactivated Recall Patient with Increased Periodontal Disease

A 51-year-old patient finally returns to the dental office after a two-year hiatus. Previously this patient (with a full complement of teeth) had been seen on a six-month basis with generalized 2–3 mm recession, periodontal pocket depths of 2–4 mm, and a propensity to build up supragingival calculus quickly. After performing a full mouth exam, including periodontal readings, most posterior teeth probe at 4–5 mm with some localized 6 mm and nearly 100 percent of the areas exhibit bleeding upon probing.

A full mouth radiographic series was taken two years ago, and the decision is made to take four bitewings. The patient reports increased fatigue and notes that all the nicks and scrapes received from being a mechanic "don't seem to heal as quickly this past year." The patient has not seen their MD in over two years but was previously informed that they were a borderline diabetic and provided nutritional counselling only. The rest of the medical history is unremarkable with no medications being taken, but the patient appears to weigh much more than when last seen.

Today, the dentist performs a finger prick blood glucose test, which reads 180 mg/dl. Due to the elevation of the blood glucose and worsening periodontal condition, the patient is advised to see their physician for diagnosis and management of this chronic condition. The patient schedules two subsequent appointments for scaling and root planing for all four quadrants and is informed that a blood glucose level test will be performed before the procedures are started. A third visit is scheduled for periodontal re-evaluation four to six weeks after the last SRP appointment and another glucose test.

How would you code today's appointment, along with any subsequent treatment and follow up appointment?

Today: Initial Appointment

D0180   **comprehensive periodontal evaluation – new or established patient**

D0274   **bitewings – four radiographic images**

D0412   **blood glucose level test – in-office using a glucose meter**

Continued on next page

Note: A dentist can determine, using the D0412 procedure, how the patient's blood glucose level may affect treatment scheduled for the day's appointment.

- A glucose level below 70 mg/dl is the clinical definition of hypoglycemia alert level, which means the patient is at risk of a hypoglycemic event during the procedure. Therefore, the procedure ought not to be initiated until the patient's blood sugar level is in the acceptable range.

- A glucose level over 300 mg/dl could lead to delayed healing of the surgical site and severe infection. This suggests that elective surgical procedures be rescheduled and delivered when the patient's circulating glucose level is in the acceptable range.

Visit #1: SRP Two Quadrants

D0412 **blood glucose level test – in-office using a glucose meter**

D4341 **periodontal scaling and root planing – four or more teeth per quadrant**

(Report D4341 two times.)

Visit #2: SRP Two Quadrants

D0412 **blood glucose level test – in-office using a glucose meter**

D4341 **periodontal scaling and root planing – four or more teeth per quadrant**

(Report D4341 two times.)

Visit #3: Four to Six Weeks after Completion of SRP and about Three Weeks after the First Visit

D0171 **re-evaluation – post-operative office visit**

D0412 **blood glucose level test – in-office using a glucose meter**

Note: D0412 does not include any guidance on frequency of delivery; third-party payer reimbursement will be based on benefit plan design.

Clinical Coding Scenario #18:
Off-site Radiographic Imaging and Teledentistry

A patient who is unable to travel because of current health concerns calls the dentist's office with symptoms of slight, non-localized dental pain. The patient was seen six months ago in the office for a periodic exam but has not had any radiographic images taken for two years. One of the dentist's hygienists, who frequently visits patients in remote locations or those who are isolated, traveled to the home of the patient. The hygienist took four digital bitewing radiographic images, one periapical image with a portable unit, and two intraoral photographs with the office camera. These images and photos were sent electronically to the dentist in the office to view.

Before leaving, the hygienist advised the patient to expect a call to arrange a follow-up visit in a few days at the practice office after the dentist evaluates the diagnostic images sent today.

How are the procedures completed on this date of service coded?

For services delivered by the hygienist at the patient's home, use the following codes:

D0707   intraoral – periapical radiographic image – image capture only

Report code once with "1" in the claim service line Quantity (Qty.) field since only one periapical image was captured.

D0708   intraoral – bitewing radiographic image – image capture only

Report code once with "4" in the claim service line Quantity (Qty.) field since four separate bitewing images were captured.

D0703   2-D oral/facial photographic image obtained intra-orally or extra-orally – image capture only

Report code once with "2" in the claim service line Quantity (Qty.) field since two separate intra-oral photographic images were captured.

Continued on next page

Note: Since the hygienist captured the images outside the office and transmitted the images for the dentist's interpretation, the applicable codes from the CDT Code's "Image Capture Only" subcategory of service. In this scenario it is not appropriate to report codes from the "Image Capture with Interpretation" subcategory since interpretation of the transmitted images by the dentist occurred at the dentist's practice – and the separate interpretation is reported with its own unique CDT code.

For services delivered by the dentist at the practice office, use the following codes:

D0391 interpretation of diagnostic image by a practitioner not associated with capture of the image, including report

Report code once with "7" in the claim service line Quantity (Qty.) field since four separate bitewing images, two separate photographic images, and one periapical image were interpreted.

D0140 limited oral evaluation – problem focused
An evaluation limited to a specific oral health problem or complaint. This may require interpretation of information acquired through additional diagnostic procedures. Report additional diagnostic procedure separately. Definitive procedures may be required on the same date as the evaluation.

Typically, patients receiving this type of evaluation present with a specific problem and/or dental emergencies, trauma, acute infections, etc.

D9996 teledentistry – asynchronous; information stored and forwarded for subsequent review
Reported in addition to other procedures (e.g., diagnostic) delivered to the patient on the date of service.

Note: For more information about teledentistry events and coding, the ADA publication discussing D9995 and D9996, ADA Guide to Understanding and Documenting Teledentistry Events, is available for download at *ADA.org/CDTEducation*.

Coding Q&A

1. *What is the "right number" of radiographic images that must be taken to be considered a comprehensive series D0210?*

    There is no exact number of radiographs to be taken for the code D0120, whose full CDT Code entry reads:

    D0210   intraoral – comprehensive series of radiographic images
    A radiographic survey of the whole mouth intended to display the crowns and roots of all teeth, periapical areas, interproximal areas and alveolar bone including edentulous areas.

    As long as all of the criteria of the D0210 are met, a "comprehensive series" can consist of different numbers of intraoral radiographic images.

2. *What is the difference between codes* **D0801 3D dental surface scan – direct** *and* **D0802 3D dental surface scan – indirect***?*

    In the current evolution of a digital imaging, an image may be acquired using photographic or video processes that may utilize one or lace many images together to create a 3D image. If the image is acquired by scanning the intraoral structure or structures directly, it would be coded as **D0801 3D dental surface scan – direct**. If the 3D image is acquired indirectly via scanning a model of an intraoral structure or multiple structures, then it would be coded as **D0802 3D dental surface scan – indirect**.

3. *What is the difference between* **D0372 intraoral tomosynthesis – comprehensive series of radiographic images** *and* **D0210 intraoral – comprehensive series of radiographic images***?*

    Although both codes involve radiographic images, they are different in how they are captured and used. Tomosynthetic radiographs require specialized x-ray imaging equipment to digitally capture multiple low-dose base projection radiographs. Specialized software and hardware process the captured digital images to produce a tomosynthetic reconstruction that approximate a 3D volume. These provide a layer-by-layer virtual dissection of the targeted anatomy. Tomosynthetic radiographs are able to provide additional diagnostic information that standard intraoral radiographs are not able to provide.

4. *What are the codes to record in-office Coronavirus test procedures for my patients?*

There are three CDT codes that can be used to document testing patients for the Coronavirus or other public health related pathogens.

One is the test for antigens, which demonstrates that the person currently has the disease and is positive for the virus. This code is:

D0604 antigen testing for a public health related pathogen, including coronavirus

Second is a test for the presence of antibodies, which means that the patient has had the virus in the past, and should not be currently infectious. This code is:

D0605 antibody testing for a public health related pathogen, including coronavirus

The third is a test that detects the presence of the molecular component of an active virus in the patient, showing that the patient is positive for COVID-19. This code is:

D0606 molecular testing for a public health related pathogen, including coronavirus

It is important to know what test you are using when looking for COVID-19 in patients to be able to code accurately. Further guidance is in the online COVID-19 & Lab Testing Requirements Toolkit available at *ADA.org/Virus*.

5. *I see there is a code for an immediate finding of a patient's blood glucose level in the dental office using a glucose meter. Does that mean that this is necessary for every diabetic patient at every visit in my office?*

The decision on whether to administer a glucose test is determined by the judgment of the treating health care provider for each individual circumstance. The code for this test procedure is:

D0412 blood glucose level test – in-office using a glucose meter
This procedure provides an immediate finding of a patient's blood glucose level at the time of sample collection for the point-of-service analysis.

This entry does not make any reference on when the procedure should be delivered, and does not imply that it is necessary in every visit. More information and guidance concerning the D0412 (and D0411) procedure is available on the ADA's Coding Education page linked to *www.ADA.org/cdt*.

6. *Is it possible to use* **D0150 comprehensive oral evaluation – new or established patient** *again within 90 days after the initial visit to our dental office?*

    Reading the full CDT Code entry for D0150 will help determine whether the code is appropriate for documenting and reporting the procedure delivered to a patient. The D0150 descriptor states, in part, that this procedure (comprehensive oral evaluation) is applicable "to new patients, established patients who have a significant change in health conditions or other unusual circumstances, by report, or established patients who have been absent from active treatment for three or more years."

    Reporting the D0150 procedure would be appropriate if the patient had "a significant change in health conditions or other unusual circumstances." In that case, a narrative would accompany the code submission. If that were not the case with the patient, other oral evaluation codes such as **D0140 limited oral evaluation – problem focused** or **D0160 detailed and extensive oral evaluation – problem focused, by report** may be more appropriate.

7. *What is the difference between screening of a patient procedure (D0190) and assessment of a patient procedure (D0191)?*

    Each procedure has a different scope and objective as indicated in their full CDT Code entries:

    D0190 screening of a patient
    > A screening, including state or federally mandated screenings, to determine an individual's need to be seen by a dentist for diagnosis.

    A screening is a quick check to determine if the patient needs a prompt exam and treatment. The oral examination is brief and usually requires only a tongue depressor and light source to check for decay, injury, pain, oral cancer, developmental problems, and other abnormal oral conditions or risk factors. Examples of screenings that can be documented using D0190 include the screening performed as part of the Head Start program.

    D0191 assessment of a patient
    > A limited clinical inspection that is performed to identify possible signs of oral or systemic disease, malformation, or injury, and the potential need for referral for diagnosis and treatment.

    A dental assessment differs from a screening in that it includes a limited clinical examination (recording dental restorations and conditions that should be called to the attention of a dentist), and collection of other oral health data to assist in the development of a professional treatment plan, when the individual has been referred to a dentist.

8. *I sometimes go to assisted living homes to provide dental evaluations for some of the residents. The facility does not have any radiographic imaging equipment or a dental chair, so all of my evaluations take place in the resident's room. I do a visual inspection of the person's oral cavity, share any obvious findings with the family of the patient, and suggest that arrangements be made for transportation to a dental office for more information gathering and possible treatment. How can I code for these "evaluations"?*

Doing this type of service would probably be best addressed under the CDT Code:

D0191   assessment of a patient
A limited clinical inspection that is performed to identify possible signs of oral or systemic disease, malformation, or injury, and the potential need for referral for diagnosis and treatment.

Using any of the clinical oral evaluation codes D0150, D0120, D0140 would not be appropriate due to the lack of a definitive diagnosis resulting from the preliminary visual inspection.

9. *My new panoramic imaging device enables me to acquire a single image that has the same, or more, diagnostic information than I see on multiple posterior bitewing images. I've always considered a bitewing as an intraoral image since the film is placed in the patient's mouth. With my new imaging device, the receptor is outside the oral cavity. What CDT code should I use now?*

The ADA's online Glossary of Dental Clinical and Administrative Terms defines a bitewing radiograph as an "Interproximal radiographic view of the coronal portion of the tooth/teeth. A form of dental radiograph that may be taken with the long axis of the image oriented either horizontally or vertically, that reveals approximately the coronal halves of the maxillary and mandibular teeth and portions of the interdental alveolar septa on the same image." The CDT Code entry that most accurately describes the question's imaging procedure is:

D0251   extra-oral posterior dental radiographic image
Image limited to exposure of complete posterior teeth in both dental arches. This is a unique image that is not derived from another image.

10. *My patient needs several extra-oral images to help diagnose the problem, but I do not see any code for additional images. What do I do?*

When reporting multiple extra-oral images the applicable procedure code is D0250, with the number of images acquired noted in the "Qty." (Quantity) field on the claim form.

D0250   extra-oral – 2D projection radiographic image created using a stationary radiation source, and detector

11. *Are four bitewings and a panoramic radiographic image considered a comprehensive series of radiographs?*

No, this set of images is different from those reported with the **D0210 intraoral – comprehensive series of radiographic images** procedure. A comprehensive series of radiographic images is defined as "a radiographic survey of the whole mouth intended to display the crowns and roots of all teeth, periapical areas, interproximal areas and alveolar bone including edentulous areas."

A panoramic radiographic image is an extra-oral image, and the D0210 code contains the language "intraoral."

This set of images would be coded as **D0274 bitewings – four radiographic images**, and **D0330 panoramic radiographic image** respectively.

12. *Is an oral cancer screening evaluation necessary for every comprehensive (D0150) and periodic (D0120) oral evaluation? The descriptor states that it is performed "where indicated"? What does that mean?*

The descriptors you are reading are from a past CDT Code version. In CDT 2021, the descriptors for both a comprehensive oral evaluation (D0150) and a periodic oral evaluation (D0120) were edited to make it clear that an oral cancer screening examination is not a "where indicated" component of each procedure. A similar revision was made to the descriptor for comprehensive periodic evaluation (D0180) in CDT 2022.

Oral cancer screening is an integral part of all three exams through a visual and hands on examination, and may also include any other diagnostic aids that the dentist may want to utilize.

13. *Our office has begun to use new technology that provides 3D or 2D images of a patient that are generated from a CT-like scan. How do we code this?*

Several procedure codes (e.g., D0364–D0368) are available to document "cone beam CT" diagnostic images taken in the dentist's office. There are separate codes based on the field of view. For example, an initial scan that yields coronal, sagittal, and panoramic views would be documented with:

D0367   cone beam CT capture and interpretation with field of view of both jaws; with or without cranium

The entire "cone beam" nomenclature must be read to determine which describes the diagnostic image.

Chapter 1: D0100–D0999 Diagnostic

14. *I've used D0350 to document oral/facial photographic images, but now I'm able to create both two- and three-dimensional photographic images. How do I document what I do when my diagnosis and treatment planning makes use of one or both types of images?*

"2D" photographic images are reported with the following code:

D0350   2D oral/facial photographic image obtained intra-orally or extra-orally

Reporting 3D images changed with publication of CDT 2023 where the one existing code (D0351 3D photographic image) was deleted and replaced with the following four codes that enable greater specificity:

D0801   3D dental surface scan – direct

D0802   3D dental surface scan – indirect
A surface scan of a diagnostic cast.

D0803   3D facial surface scan – direct

D0804   3D facial surface scan – indirect
A surface scan of constructed facial features.

15. *I took a digital panoramic image and my software was able to manipulate the captured data so that it produced the equivalent of one upper and one lower posterior bitewing on the left side of the patient's oral cavity. Is **D0272 bitewings – two radiographic images** the correct procedure code to report?*

No, the applicable CDT code is **D0330 panoramic radiographic image** as that was the original image capture procedure – and as stated in this scenario the image data was manipulated after capture to create bitewing images.

However, if the panoramic imaging device was set up to capture only a single image whose content is the equivalent of upper and lower bitewing images, the correct coding from the Diagnostic Imaging section is:

D0251   extra-oral posterior dental radiographic image
Image limited to exposure of complete posterior teeth in both dental arches. This is a unique image that is not derived from another image.

Note: Include the number of D0251 images in the claim form's "Qty." field (e.g., "2" if one image captures the left side of the oral cavity and the other captures the right side).

16. *When is it appropriate to report a consultation versus an evaluation procedure?*

Typically, a consultation (D9310) is reported when one dentist refers a patient to another dentist for an opinion or advice on a particular problem encountered by the patient.

17. *Should the dentist who sees a patient referred by another dentist for an evaluation of a specific problem report a problem focused evaluation code (D0140; D0160), or the consultation code (D9310)? Also, does it matter if the dentist initiates treatment for the patient on the same visit?*

Both D0140 and D0160 are both problem focused evaluations and either may be reported if the consulting dentist believes one or the other appropriately describes the service provided. Please note that neither of these evaluation procedures' nomenclatures or descriptors contains language that prohibits the consulting dentist from initiating and reporting additional services. These services are reported separately by their own unique codes.

Code D9310 may be used if the consulting dentist believes it better describes the service provided when a patient is referred by another dentist for evaluation of a specific problem. According to this CDT code's descriptor, the dentist who is consulted may initiate additional diagnostic or therapeutic services for the patient, which are also reported separately by their own unique codes.

18. *When is it appropriate to report oral evaluation codes D0150, D0180, D0120, and D0140?*

These four commonly reported codes are from the CDT Code's series of clinical evaluation codes (D0120–D0180). Each one is thoroughly explained by its respective nomenclature and descriptor. For example:

- The initial evaluation for a new patient may be reported using **D0150 comprehensive oral evaluation – new or established patient** or by **D0180 comprehensive periodontal evaluation – new or established patient**. You would use one of these to code for what you did, but not both simultaneously.
- If this patient becomes a patient of record returning after the initial evaluation, the service would be reported using **D0120 periodic oral evaluation – established patient**.
- An evaluation of a patient who presents with a specific problem or dental emergency may be reported using **D0140 limited oral evaluation – problem focused**.

Again, it is important to read the descriptor to distinguish what type of clinical oral evaluation is being delivered in order to be properly coded for each particular patient visit.

19. *We recently had a patient come in for a periodic oral evaluation. The doctor found signs and symptoms of periodontal disease and performed a complete periodontal evaluation. May I report both the periodic and periodontal evaluations since these are two separate procedures?*

The comprehensive periodontal procedure D0180 includes all the components of a periodic evaluation D0120, and adds additional requirements for periodontal charting and the evaluation of periodontal conditions. When a patient presents with signs or symptoms of periodontal disease, and all these components are performed, only D0180 would be reported.

20. *May I submit a limited oral evaluation (D0140) and another procedure on the same day?*

There is no language in the descriptor of D0140 that precludes the reporting of other procedures on the same date of service. However, some benefit plans have limitations or exclusions about paying for certain combinations of codes performed on the same day.

21. *If seven vertical bitewings and a panoramic image are taken to show the entire oral cavity, can it be coded as a comprehensive series D0210?*

No. The D0210's nomenclature clearly states that this code reports only capture of intra-oral radiographic images. A panoramic image is extra-oral.

The imaging procedures in this encounter would be coded as:

D0330   panoramic radiographic image

D0277   vertical bitewings – 7 to 8 radiographic images
        This does not constitute a full mouth intraoral radiographic series.

22. *Which CDT code could be used to document a periodontal re-evaluation, such as for monitoring post-operative tissue healing?*

The following CDT code, enables documenting and reporting any type of post-operative office visit. Before this code's addition the only option was a "999" code:

D0171   re-evaluation – post-operative office visit

23. *Is reporting the "comprehensive periodontal evaluation – new or established patient" (D0180) limited to periodontists?*

D0180 is not limited to periodontists. All dental procedure codes are available to any practitioner providing service within the scope of her or his license.

24. *I have read the descriptors of the evaluation codes, but am confused as to which code should be reported when a very young child is evaluated in the office. None of them seem to apply. What should be reported?*

If the young child is under age three the procedure code **D0145 oral evaluation for a patient under three years of age and counseling with primary caregiver** should be considered if all aspects of the procedure as described in the nomenclature and descriptor apply. If not (e.g., no counseling of the child's primary caregiver) any of the other evaluation codes may be reported as they are not patient age dependent.

25. *Can code D0145 be reported every time the child comes into the office for an evaluation, or should we report a recall evaluation for subsequent visits?*

This separate evaluation code addresses the unique procedures that are necessary when evaluating a very young child. Depending on the nature of the subsequent evaluation, a periodic evaluation (D0120) or another oral evaluation for a patient under three years of age (D0145) would be appropriate choices to consider.

26. *Must a caries risk assessment procedure be performed and submitted on a third-party claim that includes an oral evaluation code?*

The CDT Code does not specify any joint reporting requirements for caries risk assessment procedures (D0601–D0603) and oral evaluation procedures (e.g., D0120, D0145, or D0150). These are unique procedures documented and reported separately with their own codes. Any requirement for concurrent delivery and reporting of a caries risk assessment procedure and an oral evaluation procedure comes from the payer's reimbursement policies, or benefit plan limitations and exclusions.

27. *Can I submit a code for pulp vitality tests or is this considered to be included in all endodontic procedures?*

Yes, you may submit this as a separate service (D0460) as it is a stand-alone code. This procedure includes multiple teeth and contra lateral comparison(s), as indicated. Note that separate payment for any submitted code is dependent on the benefit plan policies.

28. *Are radiographic images taken during endodontic procedures considered to be part of the procedure as well, or can they be coded for individually?*

Any image taken prior to the start (i.e., prior date of service) of endodontic therapy can be coded individually, but once the endodontic therapy begins, all intra-operative radiographs acquired as part of the treatment are considered part of the endodontic treatment.

29. Are there rules or regulations regarding in office HbA1c testing?

Yes, some states may consider this testing "outside the scope of the state's Dental Practice Act," which could make it unlawful to perform this test. Also, federal rules may limit the type or brand of device that may be used. Lastly, a certificate of waiver may need to be in place prior to use of these tests. For a comprehensive guide on the D0411 procedure and its reporting, visit the ADA's Coding Education web page: *ADA.org/CDTEducation.*

30. I use a laser caries detection device sometimes to help diagnose incipient decay. Is there a code for this?

The following code would be applicable as the laser is considered part of the armamentarium that could be used to deliver the procedure.

D0600 **non-ionizing diagnostic procedure capable of quantifying, monitoring, and recording changes in structure of enamel, dentin, and cementum**

Note: A caries detection procedure is not the same as a caries susceptibility test procedure, which is reported with code "D0425 caries susceptibility tests."

31. A patient was seen for a follow-up visit after a car accident. No treatment was performed on the initial visit other than an evaluation and radiographic images on maxillary anterior teeth. What would be an appropriate code for the follow-up visit?

D0170 **re-evaluation – limited, problem focused (established patient; not post-operative visit)**

This descriptor allows for a patient to be seen for an oral evaluation in certain circumstances, including this one where there was no treatment rendered during the initial visit – as noted in a portion of this code's descriptor.

32. What is the difference between the code for assessment of salivary flow by measurement D0419 and the other codes concerning saliva samples?

D0419 by its descriptor states that the procedure "is for identification of low salivary flow in patients at risk for hyposalivation and xerostomia, as well as effectiveness of pharmacological agents used to stimulate saliva production."

This in-office chairside procedure involves collecting saliva from a patient in a tube or cup for five minutes in either of the following two ways. The first way is to have the patient have a "stimulated salivary flow" by chewing on wax or unflavored gum. The second way is to allow the patient naturally to accumulate in the mouth and "drool" into a cup (resting saliva flow). Volume obtained is converted into mL/min. "Stimulated saliva flow" rates lower than 0.7 mL/min are considered hyposalivation. Also, rates lower than 0.1 mL/min for "resting salivary flow" are considered hyposalivation.

In contrast, codes **D0417 collection and preparation of saliva sample for laboratory diagnostic testing** and **D0418 analysis of saliva sample** require laboratory testing for chemical or biological analysis, not just simply flow rates.

33. *Our office uses "traditional" transillumination with a bright light to check for fractures and caries with anterior teeth. Can D0600 be used to report this?*

The full CDT Code entry for D0600 reads as follows:

D0600   non-ionizing diagnostic procedure capable of quantifying, monitoring, and recording changes in structure of enamel, dentin, and cementum

As stated in the nomenclature, D0600 is specific to calibrated instruments capable of quantifying, monitoring and recording changes in enamel, dentin, and cementum. There are several modalities on the marketplace that use non-ionizing light, such as CariVu, DIAGNOcam, DIAGNOdent, and others. D0600 should not be used to report "traditional" transillumination alone.

34. *What is the difference between an adjunctive pre-diagnostic test procedure (D0431) and a brush biopsy procedure (D7288) for screening of patients for mucosal abnormalities and oral cancer?*

D0431 adjunctive pre-diagnostic test that aids in detection of mucosal abnormalities including premalignant and malignant lesions, not to include cytology or biopsy procedures may be used in addition to basic oral cancer screening that includes a visual and physical examination. This code defines the procedure, not the many products that can be utilized as part of its delivery. Some of these products' names are OralID®, Identafi®, Vizilite® Plus, VELscope®, Microlux™ DL, as well as staining with toluidine blue.

There is a definitive difference between the adjunctive test (D0431) and the oral brush biopsy (D7288). The adjunctive pre-diagnostic test specifically excludes "cytology or biopsy" when describing the procedure. D0431 typically includes steps that illuminate or stain the tissue to check for abnormalities. In contrast, the complete CDT Code entry for D7288, noted below clearly indicates that this is a biopsy procedure where cells are collected.

D7288   brush biopsy – transepithelial sample collection
For collection of oral disaggregated transepithelial cells via rotational brushing of the oral mucosa.

35. *What are the ADA publications that provide coding guidance on virtual patient encounters where different types of examinations (e.g., screenings, problem-focused evaluations) are delivered?*

There is one guidance publication available online, posted on the CDT Coding Education web page:

D9995 and D9996 – ADA Guide to Understanding and Documenting Teledentistry Events

It contains a general discussion of teledentistry encounter documentation.

Summary

The Diagnostic Section of the CDT Code deals with the gathering of data and cognitive skills necessary for patient evaluation. Although small in number, these diagnostic codes in CDT 2023 are the foundation of the CDT Code and are utilized for every patient throughout the course of care. With the increase in teledentistry and the virtual platform in clinical situations, along with the increasing technology in radiographic imaging, knowledge of how to code for diagnostic procedures continues to be a challenge, but extremely important for the health provider. Attention to detail of descriptors allows for correct coding in treatment, as explained in the scenarios and questions presented in this section. "Coding for what you do" does not mean that all procedures will be covered or reimbursed by third-party carriers. However, "coding for what you do" will mean that dental treatment is properly documented in the patient record and reported on a claim.

Contributor Biography

Ralph A. Cooley, D.D.S., is a general dentist who was in private practice for more than 30 years and is currently the Assistant Dean for Admissions and Student Services at the UT Health School of Dentistry in Houston. He still teaches in the clinical setting at the school and works with the future generation of dentists to not only provide excellent dental care but also learn to code for what is performed in the proper way. He is a past member of the ADA Council on Dental Benefits and is currently a member of the Code Maintenance Committee.

By Jim Nickman, D.D.S., M.S.

Introduction

The CDT's Preventive category contains codes for frequently delivered services. Preventive services range from the routine services for disease prevention (e.g., prophylaxis) for adults and children to vaccinations. The type and frequency of preventive services should be based on professional standards of care and the disease risks of the patient. To assist patients in appropriately utilizing their preventive care dental benefits, it is important that the dental office understand the contractual obligations of these benefit plans, especially when the dentist has a participating provider contract with the insurance company. It is not uncommon for dental benefit plans to contain coverage limitations such as annual maximums, age restrictions, and reimbursement for services based on the stage of dentition.

A significant change was made to the Preventive category's Vaccinations subcategory, adding additional CDT codes for administration of emergency use approved COVID-19 vaccination and booster doses in the United States. CDT codes were also added to provide reporting first, second and third doses of Human Papillomavirus (HPV) vaccines.

This chapter will define key concepts of the codes contained within the Preventive category. It also contains the CDT 2023 code changes, examples of coding scenarios, and a question and answer section of common issues.

Key Definitions and Concepts

Prophylaxis: Removal of plaque, calculus, and stains from the tooth structures or implants intended to control local irritational factors. Although the instruments used to remove plaque, calculus, or stains are different for implants (plastic) than natural dentition (metal), the procedure's techniques utilized are the same. CDT codes for prophylaxis are D1110 and D1120.

Prophylaxis is not a therapeutic procedure related to the healing of a disease or condition of the periodontium. These procedures are found under the periodontics codes (D4000–D4999).

The removal of local irritational factors may reduce transitory local gingival inflammation (gingivitis).

Topical application of fluoride varnish and topical application of fluoride excluding varnish: Professionally applied prescription topical fluoride products delivered separately from that contained in prophy paste (the mild abrasive compound used usually with rotary cup instrumentation to remove extrinsic stain and dental plaque from the enamel tooth surface). The CDT codes for topical application of fluoride are D1206 and D1208.

Sealant: Dental sealants (also known as pit and fissure sealants) are materials placed in anatomically caries-susceptible tooth surfaces (usually posterior occlusal pits and fissures, posterior buccal or lingual pits or grooves, or incisor cingulum pits) after the adjacent tooth structure is mechanically or chemically prepared for enamel bonding. The material, after chemical or light curing, forms a mechanical barrier to the penetration of acid-producing cariogenic bacteria, thereby reducing the potential for caries initiation. The procedure is appropriate prior to dentin cavitation and is most effective when applied to enamel that has not undergone significant enamel demineralization. The CDT code for dental sealants is D1351.

Preventive resin restoration in a moderate to high caries risk patient – permanent tooth: Conservative restoration of an active cavitated lesion in a pit or fissure that does not extend into dentin; includes placement of a sealant in any radiating non-carious fissures or pits. This procedure differs from a sealant in that it involves mechanical removal (usually by rotary instrumentation) of demineralized, chalky enamel (enamel caries) and the restoration of the affected tooth surface with a restorative filling material such as a composite resin or glass ionomer cement. Dentin is not penetrated by caries or by instrumentation. The CDT code for this procedure is D1352.

Caries preventive medicament application – per tooth: The application of medicaments to prevent caries formation on high risk surfaces of the dentition. The procedure is different than **application of caries arresting medicament – per tooth** in that the medicament is applied prior to caries formation. The medicaments may be like those used in the caries arrest techniques but do not include the usage of topical fluoride. Examples of high-risk surfaces could include, but are not limited to, exposed root surfaces in elderly patients, deep fissures in primary and permanent teeth, and exposed enamel adjacent to a bonded or cemented orthodontic band or bracket. The CDT code for the caries preventive medicament application procedure is D1355.

Application of caries arresting medicament – per tooth: The treatment of an active, non-symptomatic carious lesion by the topical application of a medicament which arrests or inhibits caries progression. It is often (though not exclusively) intended as an interim measure in the medical management of dental caries in selected situations (such as a tooth nearing exfoliation) or populations (such as the frail elderly, the very young, or patients with special healthcare or developmental needs) to stabilize the tooth until it can later be treated in a conventional restorative manner. It is the appropriate code for the application of silver diamine fluoride or another similar acting medicament. The CDT code for this procedure is D1354.

Distal shoe space maintainer – fixed – unilateral – per quadrant: The fabrication and delivery of a fixed space maintaining appliance extending distally and subgingivally from the first primary molar immediately after extraction of the second primary molar to guide the eruption of the unerupted first permanent molar. While technically a type of fixed unilateral space maintainer (D1510), it differs importantly in that it is intended to be removed and replaced with another space maintenance appliance (usually a D1510) upon eruption of the first permanent molar. The CDT code for this procedure is D1575.

Space maintainer – fixed, unilateral – per quadrant: specifically excludes the distal shoe space maintainer design. The CDT code for this procedure is D1510.

Changes to This Category

The only changes are in Preventive's "Vaccinations" subcategory. CDT 2023 now includes three codes for human papillomavirus (HPV) vaccination:

D1781 **vaccine administration – human papillomavirus – Dose 1**
Gardasil 9 0.5mL intramuscular vaccine injection.

D1782 **vaccine administration – human papillomavirus – Dose 2**
Gardasil 9 0.5mL intramuscular vaccine injection.

D1783 **vaccine administration – human papillomavirus – Dose 3**
Gardasil 9 0.5mL intramuscular vaccine injection.

Similar to last year, seven new codes for COVID-19 vaccinations were approved during the March 2022 CMC meeting for inclusion in the code set's CDT 2022 version. These codes, first published online in the CDT Code "Errata" web page as post publication changes, are now included in the printed CDT 2023 manual:

D1708 **Pfizer-BioNTech Covid-19 vaccine administration – third dose**
SARSCOV2 COVID-19 VAC mRNA 30mcg/0.3mL IM DOSE 3

D1709 **Pfizer-BioNTech Covid-19 vaccine administration – booster dose**
SARSCOV2 COVID-19 VAC mRNA 30mcg/0.3mL IM DOSE BOOSTER

D1710 **Moderna Covid-19 vaccine administration – third dose**
SARSCOV2 COVID-19 VAC mRNA 100mcg/0.5mL IM DOSE 3

D1711 **Moderna Covid-19 vaccine administration – booster dose**
SARSCOV2 COVID-19 VAC mRNA 50mcg/0.25mL IM DOSE BOOSTER

D1712 **Janssen Covid-19 vaccine administration – booster dose**
SARSCOV2 COVID-19 VAC Ad26 5x1010 VP/.5mL IM DOSE BOOSTER

D1713 **Pfizer-BioNTech Covid-19 vaccine administration tris-sucrose pediatric – first dose**
SARSCOV2 COVID-19 VAC mRNA 10mcg/0.2mL tris-sucrose IM DOSE 1

D1714 **Pfizer-BioNTech Covid-19 vaccine administration tris-sucrose pediatric – second dose**
SARSCOV2 COVID-19 VAC mRNA 10mcg/0.2mL tris-sucrose IM DOSE 2

Clinical Coding Scenario #1:
Distal Shoe Space Maintainer

A four-year-old presents to your office in pain. After the emergency examination, you determine that the lower second molars are abscessed and not restorable. The first permanent lower molars are not erupted but can be visualized on the radiographs. After discussing the available treatment options with the child's parents, informed consent is obtained for extraction of the non-restorable molars and placement of two distal shoe space maintainers.

How would the space maintainers be coded?

In addition to the appropriate codes for the services provided at each visit, the appropriate code for the distal shoe space maintainers would be:

D1575 **distal shoe space maintainer – fixed, unilateral – per quadrant**
Fabrication and delivery of fixed appliance extending subgingivally and distally to guide the eruption of the first permanent molar. Does not include ongoing follow-up or adjustments, or replacement appliance, once the tooth had erupted.

Note: D1575 is reported twice on the claim as two separate appliances were placed. The applicable Area of the Oral Cavity code is also reported on each service line.

The same patient reports for a re-care appointment at age seven. You notice that the lower first molars are fully erupted and decide that it is appropriate to remove both of the lower distal shoe space maintainers and replace them with a bilateral lower lingual holding arch space maintainer to avoid potential issues with the development and eruption of the future lower second premolars. The correct code for the new space maintainer would be **D1517 space maintainer – fixed – bilateral, mandibular**.

Would the new bilateral lower lingual arch space maintainer be reimbursable under the patient's dental benefit plan?

Reimbursement by the patient's dental benefits carrier for the new appliance would depend upon the contractual limitations and policies governing covered benefits. Regardless of expected third-party payment, the dentist should record and code for the services provided.

Clinical Coding Scenario #2:
New 11-Year-Old Patient

An 11-year-old female patient presents to your office for a new patient examination. Per the patient's parents, the child's last dental visit was several years ago in a different state. No current radiographs are available for the patient. Based on the clinical findings of a mixed dentition, you decide to capture and interpret two bitewing and one panoramic radiographs. Other services provided at that visit are a prophylaxis and fluoride varnish treatment.

How would you code for this visit?

The appropriate codes that could be used are as follows:

D0150 comprehensive oral evaluation – new or established patient
D0272 bitewings – two radiographic images
D0330 panoramic radiographic image
D1120 prophylaxis – child
D1206 topical application of fluoride varnish

What would change if the patient was 12 years old?

Selection of the prophylaxis code is determined by how the dentist views the patient's dentition. Either the adult (D1110) or the child (D1120) code may be used for patients with transitional dentition regardless of age. Patient age is not a part of either code's nomenclature or descriptor. ADA policy "Age of Child" adopted in 1991 states that dental benefit determinations should be based on dental development rather than patient age:

> **"Resolved**, that when dental plans differentiate coverage of specific procedures based on the child or adult status of the patient, this determination be based on the clinical development of the patient's dentition, and be it further

> **Resolved**, that for the sole purpose of eligibility for coverage, chronological age of at least 21 be used to determine enrollment status."

The prophylaxis codes are dentition-specific rather than age-specific. Some third-party payers have in their contracts' policies that limit available benefits based on patient age, not stage of dentition. Most of these dental benefit plans specify an age between 12 and 21 as to when the patient is considered an adult.

What if the patient had only permanent teeth with eruption completed through the second permanent molars?

Regardless of age, patients with permanent dentition are appropriately coded using D1110.

Clinical Coding Scenario #3:
Silver Diamine Fluoride Palliative Treatment

A long-term patient of your practice has just entered hospice at home. She contacted your office regarding occasional dental pain and sensitivity. Although frail, she is well enough to visit your office for an emergency visit. After a thorough exam and a periapical radiograph of the tender area, you observe recurrent decay on the cervical margin of a crown clinically and radiographically. You discuss your clinical findings with the patient and her current medical status. Unsure of her prognosis and after a review of risks and benefits of possible treatment options, you propose palliative treatment of the recurrent decay using silver diamine fluoride.

What codes might be used to document this visit?

The appropriate codes that could be used are as follows:

D0140 **limited oral evaluation – problem focused**

D0220 **intraoral – periapical first radiographic image**

D1354 **application of caries arresting medicament – per tooth**

Note: **D9110 palliative treatment of dental pain – per visit** is not the appropriate code for documenting SDF delivery as the oral evaluation led the dentist to diagnose an active, non-symptomatic carious lesion (recurrent decay on the cervical margin of a crown).

Clinical Coding Scenario #4:
Silver Diamine Fluoride Application and a Trauma Finding at a Re-care Visit

During a recent re-care visit with a four-year-old male with a complete primary dentition and closed interproximal contacts, you perform a prophylaxis and bitewing radiographs. While taking the radiographs, the parents mention that their son had trauma several weeks ago to his maxillary anterior teeth. Based on the conversation, you decide to also expose and interpret a maxillary periapical radiograph. While interpreting the radiographs, you observe incipient interproximal decay in the lower first molars and widened periodontal ligament space for both central incisors.

After a thorough discussion of your findings and risks and benefits of the possible treatment options, the parents' consent to application of silver diamine fluoride to the incipient interproximal decay on the lower first molars. Based on the patient's caries risk, you also recommend the application of topical fluoride varnish.

How might this be reported using CDT codes?

The appropriate codes that could be used are as follows:

D0120 **periodic oral evaluation – established patient**
D0220 **intraoral – periapical first radiographic image**
D0272 **bitewings – two radiographic images**
D1206 **topical application of fluoride varnish**
D1354 **application of caries arresting medicament – per tooth**

Note: For D1354, report the tooth numbers and number of teeth treated on the claim's service line that lists this procedure.

May the topical fluoride varnish be provided as a separate billable service on the same day as the application of a caries arresting medicament?

Yes. The two services are not mutually exclusive and each discrete procedure is reported with its own CDT code.

Due to the patient's trauma and radiographic findings, you discuss the signs and symptoms of possible future pulpal pathology with the parents. You also recommend that the patient have a follow-up visit in eight weeks to re-evaluate the status of the child's maxillary anterior teeth.

Continued on next page

What codes could be used to report the follow-up visit?

This re-evaluation could be coded as follows:

D0170 **re-evaluation – limited, problem focused (established patient; not post-operative visit)**

D0220 **intraoral – periapical first radiographic image**

Six months later at a subsequent re-care visit, you observe no change in the size of the incipient lesions on the lower first molars. Due to the inconsistent oral hygiene habits and minor dietary changes that have occurred, you determine that the child still has a moderate caries risk. Following established protocols and best practice recommendations, you recommend the re-application of silver diamine fluoride to the affected interproximal areas.

What code would be used on subsequent silver diamine fluoride applications?

D1354 **application of caries arresting medicament – per tooth**

Clinical Coding Scenario #5:
Silver Diamine Fluoride Therapy to Arrest Root Caries

An elderly adult presents to your office with multiple dental root caries and recurrent dental caries along the gingival margins of existing restorations adjacent to receding gingival tissues. You are aware of the efficacy of silver diamine fluoride in treating these lesions, but are unsure how to code for the procedure.

D1354 application of caries arresting medicament – per tooth is the correct code to report application of an agent to arrest or inhibit caries progression on any part of a tooth.

Does the per tooth application of a caries arresting medicament (D1354) apply only to carious lesions occurring on the crown?

This procedure is not limited to carious lesions on the crown. The tooth surface location and etiology of the asymptomatic active carious dental lesion is not relevant.

Clinical Coding Scenario #6:
Silver Diamine Fluoride Therapy for Primary Prevention of Root Caries

A 67-year-old male, presents to your practice for a re-care appointment. During the examination, you note that he has significant recession in the premolar region on his mandibular quadrants. Although he has no decay present today, you determine he has a moderate caries risk due to his poor oral hygiene.

You recently read an evidenced-based dentistry article on the agents available for the primary prevention of root caries using silver diamine fluoride (SDF). In addition to improved oral hygiene at home, Bill is receptive to your recommendation of applying SDF to the at-risk root surfaces. After a thorough informed consent discussion, you apply the SDF and apply fluoride varnish due to his moderate caries risk.

How would the SDF and fluoride application be reported?

The correct code to report the application of a caries preventive medicament in this scenario is:

D1355   caries preventive medicament application – per tooth.

It would be reported for each of the teeth treated.

The topical fluoride varnish would be reported using:

D1206   topical application of fluoride varnish

Is it possible to report the use of the D1355 caries preventive medicament application – per tooth code and the D1206 topical application of fluoride varnish at the same visit?

The two CDT codes (D1206 and D1355) may be utilized on the same day as there is no exclusionary language in either codes nomenclature or descriptor. There may be other reasons for delaying one of the services, including potential compatibility issues between the primary preventive agent and the fluoride varnish. It is up to the dentist to consult the manufacturer to determine if a compatibility issue exists.

Clinical Coding Scenario #7:
Re-cementing Bilateral Space Maintainer

An established ten-year-old patient reports for a re-care appointment. During the clinical examination, you observe that the patient's Nance appliance, a maxillary bilateral space maintainer, is loose in the upper left quadrant. Radiographs exposed at this visit demonstrate that the maxillary second premolars, whose space is being maintained, are not close to eruption. Based on this finding, you remove and immediately re-cement the loose bilateral space maintainer.

How may this be reported using CDT codes?

The appropriate code would be:

D1551   re-cement or re-bond bilateral space maintainer – maxillary

If the missing maxillary second premolars were erupting and the loose space maintainer was no longer indicated, what code could be used to report the removal procedure?

The appropriate code would be **D1557 removal of fixed bilateral space maintainer – maxillary**.

Note: D1557 is the applicable code to report removal by any dentist, who could be the one who originally placed the appliance, or another dentist in the practice where the appliance was placed, or a dentist in a different practice.

Clinical Coding Scenario #8:
Sealant and Preventive Resin Restoration

An established seven-year-old patient reports for a re-care appointment. The first permanent molars are now fully erupted but have deep pits and fissures that contain staining and possible incipient decay. You decide to re-appoint the patient to apply sealants or possible restorations to the occlusal surfaces. At the follow-up visit, you remove the stain in the pits and fissures and find that one of the molars has decay that does not extend into dentin and requires mechanical removal of demineralized enamel. Based on the size of the affected area after the lesion has been removed, a sealant in that area is no longer appropriate. You place a small resin composite and seal the remaining groove structure.

What would be the appropriate CDT code for the tooth with the lesion that did not extend into dentin?

The appropriate code would be:

D1352 **preventive resin restoration in a moderate to high caries risk patient – permanent tooth**

If the lesion on the affected molar extended into the dentin, report the treatment using **D2391 resin-based composite – one surface, posterior.**

D1351 sealant – per tooth would be the appropriate code for the three non-cavitated teeth to report sealant application.

Clinical Coding Scenario #9:
Sealant and Sealant Repair

An established 13-year-old patient reports for a re-care appointment and during the examination, you observe some missing sealant on several of the first permanent molars that had sealant placed in your office more than two years ago. The remaining sealant material on the affected first molars is not easily dislodged with an explorer and you are confident about the integrity of the residual marginal bond. The second permanent molars are now also fully erupted but have deep pits and fissures. Based on these findings, you recommend repair of the defective sealants on the first permanent molars and new sealants on the second permanent molars.

What would be the proper CDT codes for these procedures?

Because you are not removing the remaining sealant material on the first molars and are replacing only that which has been lost, you are accomplishing procedure **D1353 sealant repair – per tooth**. If, instead, you had removed all residual sealant material on the affected first molars and placed a completely new sealant across all occlusal pits, grooves, and fissures you would be performing procedure **D1351 sealant – per tooth**.

Would either procedure be reimbursable service under the patient's dental benefit plan?

As with all other services, this would depend on benefit plan restrictions and limitations, such as time intervals after initial placement or if replacements are a benefit. Regardless, the dentist must code for the specific service provided.

Clinical Coding Scenario #10:
New Patient and Tobacco Counseling

A 12-year-old patient reports for an initial oral evaluation appointment in your practice and no current radiographs are available. The adolescent has a late-mixed dentition with full eruption of the lower second permanent molars. The bitewing radiographs show no signs of interproximal decay, but the lower second primary molars are present and you are unable to visualize the lower second premolars. A panoramic radiograph is exposed and confirms that the lower second premolars are congenitally missing.

During the examination, you detect signs that the patient has been smoking. A conversation with the patient about the potential long-term problems with tobacco use and its impact on the adolescent's oral and systemic health. The patient is receptive to the information and methods of tobacco cessation are discussed in detail. At this visit, the patient receives a prophylaxis, four bitewing radiographs, a panoramic image, and due to patient preference, a fluoride gel treatment.

What would be the proper CDT codes for these procedures?

The appropriate codes to report this visit are:

D0150 **comprehensive oral evaluation – new or established patient**

D0274 **bitewings – four radiographic images**

D0330 **panoramic radiographic image**

D1110 **prophylaxis – adult**

D1208 **topical application of fluoride – excluding varnish**

D1110 prophylaxis – adult is appropriate as the patient's current dentition, although mixed, represents the full and complete natural permanent dentition (e.g., the presence of fully erupted lower second permanent molars).

The oral cancer screening completed during the oral evaluation revealed no changes in tissue structure related to the tobacco usage.

What would be the proper code to report the counseling on tobacco use and cessation?

The appropriate code would be **D1320 tobacco counseling for the control and prevention of oral disease**. Other procedures and referral may be necessary if changes to the tissue were noted during the oral cancer screening.

Clinical Coding Scenario #11:
Periodontal Maintenance Therapy and Prophylaxis Visits

Following either surgical or non-surgical periodontal therapy, the patient is placed by the treating dentist on a program of scheduled periodic periodontal maintenance (D4910) visits, which could be at various intervals (e.g., 2, 3, 4, or 6 months) depending on the patient's clinical condition. The **D4910 periodontal maintenance** procedure includes removal of bacterial plaque and calculus (mineralized deposits) from subgingival and supragingival tooth surfaces, site-specific scaling and root planing, and coronal tooth polishing. Between these scheduled periodontal maintenance visits, the patient is also seen by the dentist for routine dental prophylaxis (tooth cleaning procedures).

May the dentist code and bill for the prophylaxis procedure (D1110 or D1120) or is this prohibited as a duplication of existing services under D4910?

Nothing in the D4910 or the D1110 (or D1120) code nomenclatures or descriptors make these procedures mutually exclusive. If the dentist determines that the patient's periodontal health can be augmented with periodic routine prophylaxis procedures (removal of plaque, calculus, and stains from the tooth structures for the purpose of controlling local irritational factors), then this service should be performed and reported as D1110 or D1120, depending on the state of the dentition.

Does it make any difference if the reporting dentist for prophylaxis (D1110 or D1120) is the same dentist providing periodontal maintenance (D4910)?

No. The dentist should code and report for the services provided regardless of the provision of other services by the same or a different dentist.

Will both procedures be reimbursed by the patient's dental benefit carrier?

Reimbursement will depend upon the dental benefit plan language and the contractual policies governing covered benefits.

Clinical Coding Scenario #12:
Use of Caries Preventive Medicament in an Elderly Patient

A long-term patient of yours has recently transitioned into a long-term care facility from her home. Fortunately, the long-term care facility has a rudimentary dental clinic that allows for limited dental services and you have provided care for other residents in that setting. During a recent visit with the patient, you noted that her oral care has noticeably worsened, placing her at risk for caries formation. After completion of the oral evaluation and caries risk assessment procedures, and a thorough informed consent discussion of the findings with the patient or the patient's legal guardian, you apply a caries preventive medicament to the most at-risk tooth surfaces at that visit.

How would you document and report that patient encounter (e.g., examination, caries risk finding, and medicament application) using CDT procedure codes?

Since the encounter occurred in a long-term care facility and not in the doctor's office, it is appropriate to report **D9410 house/extended care facility call** in addition to any other services provided. The following codes would be used to report and document the other services provided.

> **D0120** **periodic oral evaluation – established patient**
>
> **D0603** **caries risk assessment and documentation, with a finding of high risk**
>
> **D1355** **caries preventive medicament application – per tooth**

Clinical Coding Scenario #13:
High Caries Risk Orthodontic Patient

In your orthodontics practice, you notice several of your patients have extremely poor oral hygiene and poor diet habits that could contribute to caries formation. An avid learner, you have recently read several studies about the effectiveness of using medicaments to prevent dental caries in patients who are in orthodontic appliances. One of your patients, a healthy 12-year-old boy, presented for an orthodontic appointment with extremely poor oral hygiene. This led you to perform a caries risk assessment, which led to a conclusion that the patient is at high risk for caries.

After discussing your findings with the patient and his mother, which included nutritional counseling and oral hygiene instructions, you recommended applying a caries preventive medicament to the at-risk areas adjacent to his brackets and bands. The patient's mother agrees and gives written consent for the procedure. To document the discussion and procedure, you send a letter to the patient's parents and his general dentist.

What CDT procedure codes would be used to report services provided today?

D0140   **limited oral evaluation – problem focused**

D0603   **caries risk assessment and documentation, with a finding of high risk**

D1310   **nutritional counseling for control of dental disease**

D1330   **oral hygiene instructions**

D1355   **caries preventive medicament application – per tooth**

Clinical Coding Scenario #14:
Prophylaxis Usage with a Patient Who Has Dental Implants

A long-term patient of your practice presents for a re-care examination. In the past, she had several dental implants placed to replace congenitally missing mandibular second premolars. During the routine visit, she had four bitewing radiograph images exposed and interpreted. Two periapical radiograph images were also obtained to evaluate the bone structure supporting the implants. Minor supra- and subgingival calculus was removed, and a prophylaxis was completed uneventfully. A routine oral examination was also completed. Although a low caries risk patient, she opted to have a fluoride varnish treatment.

What CDT codes would be reported to document the services provided today?

In addition to the clinical notes, the following CDT codes could be utilized:

D0120 **periodic oral evaluation – established patient**

D0220 **intraoral – periapical first radiographic image**

D0230 **intraoral – periapical each additional radiographic image**

D0274 **bitewings – four radiographic images**

D1110 **prophylaxis – adult**

D1206 **topical application of fluoride varnish**

Clinical Coding Scenario #15:
Teenage Patient Who Is Currently Vaping

A 13-year-old female patient presents to your office for a re-care appointment. During a conversation with her parent/guardian, nothing remarkable was reported during the update of the patient's medical history and chief complaint. The hygienist engaged in a conversation with the patient during the appointment and the patient let it slip that she had started vaping with friends. The patient reported that she has been doing this regularly and now feels that she may have trouble stopping vaping. The conversation also revealed that the patient has been purchasing the off-market vaping refills from her friends as she is unable to legally purchase vaping supplies.

With concern, the hygienist spends a considerable amount of time discussing the dangers of vaping on her oral and physical health. During the examination, the dentist also discusses the long-term danger of vaping and strategies of cessation. Luckily, the teen is interested in stopping due to her vaping experiences and concern over possible addiction. The dentist has the hygienist follow-up with the patient in the upcoming weeks to check on the patient's progress with vaping cessation.

What CDT code would be used to report the counseling that occurred today?

In addition to the clinical notes and coding for other services provided, the following CDT code applies to the vaping discussion and guidance:

D1321 **counseling for the control and prevention of adverse oral, behavioral, and systemic health effects associated with high-risk substance use**

Clinical Coding Scenario #16:
Tobacco Counseling

A long-term patient in your practice started using smokeless tobacco approximately one year ago. During the examination and oral cancer screening, you noticed changes to his gingival tissues and early recession in the areas of frequent use. You discuss your findings and concern that he is flirting with oral cancer in addition to periodontal disease. The patient has been unsuccessful in the past discontinuing the smokeless tobacco. After reviewing his previous attempts, you develop a plan together for cessation and re-appoint him to re-evaluate the affected areas.

In addition to the other services provided, what CDT code would be reported to document the counseling provided today?

The appropriate code would be **D1320 tobacco counseling for the control and prevention of oral disease**. Other procedures and referral may be necessary if changes to the tissue were noted during the oral cancer screening.

Clinical Coding Scenario #17:
Nutritional Counseling

A 20-month-old female and her mother present to your practice with a chief complaint of tooth pain when the child eats. After reviewing her health history, you conduct a thorough lap-to-lap examination of the child and note clinical decay in her maxillary first molars and central incisors. Decalcification is also noted on the labial surfaces of the maxillary canines. After a discussion of the finding with mom and due to the extent of decay, uncooperative behavior of the child, and parental preference, a mutual decision is made to provide treatment under anesthesia in a hospital setting. Due to the child's high caries risk, you and your staff spend time discussing the child's habits and typical diet. You discuss the findings with the mom and go over the impact on the child's oral health, and you mutually agree upon beneficial changes to her oral hygiene and diet routine.

How would the services provided today be reported?

In addition to any other services provided at the visit, the appropriate CDT codes to report would be:

D0150   comprehensive oral evaluation – new or established patient

D1310   nutritional counseling for control of dental disease

Clinical Coding Scenario #18:
Human Papillomavirus (HPV) Vaccine Administration

A nine-year-old male presents with his father to the office for a re-care appointment. During the visit, you review the patient's vaccination schedule and determine that he has not yet received a human papillomavirus (HPV) vaccination. You discuss the findings of the examination with the patient and his father. You also discuss the role of human papillomavirus in the formation of oropharyngeal cancers and the effectiveness of the HPV vaccination. The patient's father has heard about the vaccination and is interested in starting the two-dose series. Having undergone the appropriate training for HPV vaccination administration and verifying that no contraindications are present, you offer to provide the patient with his first HPV dose today and his father agrees.

How would the services provided today be reported?

In addition to any other services provided at the visit, the appropriate CDT code to report in this scenario is:

D1781   vaccine administration – human papillomavirus – Dose 1

The patient and his parent return for a re-care appointment approximately six months after his last visit. In addition to providing his oral care service, you recommend that he receives his second HPV vaccine dose.

The correct code to report the second dose is:

D1782   vaccine administration – human papillomavirus – Dose 2

How is the HPV vaccine administration different for an older patient, and how would the vaccine administration be documented?

The two-dose schedule (0 and 6 months) is indicated for persons initiating vaccination at ages 9 through 14 years, except immunocompromised persons. A minimum of 5 months is recommended between dose one and two.

A three-dose schedule (0, 1–2 months, 6 months) is recommended for persons initiating vaccination at ages 15 through 26 years, and certain immunocompromised persons initiating vaccination at ages 9 through 26 years; three-dose schedule also applies to adults initiating vaccination at ages 27 through 45 years. In a three-dose schedule of HPV vaccine, the minimum intervals are 4 weeks between the first and second dose, 12 weeks between the second and third dose, and 5 months between the first and third dose. Please refer to CDC vaccination guidance (*https://www.cdc. gov/hpv/hcp/schedules-recommendations.html*) for additional and updated HPV vaccine recommendations.   *Continued on next page*

In addition to reporting the initial two doses, the appropriate code to report a third dose is:

D1783 vaccine administration – human papillomavirus – Dose 3

Notes: CDT Preventive's "Vaccination" codes are appropriate for patient record keeping and inclusion on a claim filed with the patient's dental benefit plan. Should the claim be filed against the patient's medical benefit plan (e.g., no dental plan coverage is available), then the medical claim format (e.g., 1500 paper form/837P electronic claim) and coding systems (e.g., CPT; HCPCS; National Drug Codes) must be used. In addition to reporting the vaccine administration procedure to the insurance company, the service should also be reported to the appropriate state vaccine database or health department.

Clinical Coding Scenario #19:
COVID Vaccine Administration

A long-term patient of your practice has presented for a re-care appointment. As part of her medical history update, you noted that she has received the Janssen Covid-19 vaccine in the past and is now eligible for a booster. During the discussion of the findings of your examination today, you mention that she is eligible for a booster vaccine and inquire if she is interested in receiving it today. Due to a recent increase in local Covid infection rates, she agrees to receive a booster today at your office.

How would the vaccine booster provided today be reported?

In addition to any other services provided at the visit, the appropriate CDT code to report the booster is:

D1712 Janssen Covid-19 vaccine administration – booster dose

Information about the vaccine administration codes (including their use, claim submission to the patient's dental or medical benefit plan, and state vaccine database reporting) is in the guidance document posted on the CDT's Coding Education page (*ADA.org/CDTEducation*) titled *COVID-19 Vaccination Procedures* that is available to any member of the dental community.

Notes: CDT Preventive's "Vaccination" codes are appropriate for patient record keeping and inclusion on a claim filed with the patient's dental benefit plan. Should the claim be filed against the patient's medical benefit plan (e.g., no dental plan coverage is available), then the medical claim format (e.g., 1500 paper form/837P electronic claim) and coding systems (e.g., CPT; HCPCS; National Drug Codes) must be used. In addition to reporting the vaccine administration procedure to the insurance company, the service should also be reported to the appropriate state vaccine database or health department.

Coding Q&A

1. *What is the definition of prophylaxis?*

    A prophylaxis is removal of plaque, calculus, and stains from the tooth structures and implants, and is intended to control local irritational factors. It is a preventive and not a therapeutic procedure, and the applicable CDT code is determined by the clinical state of the patient's dentition as determined by the dentist.

2. *Does the patient's age dictate whether a child or adult prophylaxis is reported?*

    Patient age is not the code selection criterion; the clinical state of dentition determines which procedure code is appropriate to report the service. For a patient with permanent or transitional tooth structures or implants, **D1110 prophylaxis – adult** is the correct code. For another patient who has primary and transitional tooth structures and implants, the correct code is **D1120 prophylaxis – child**.

    Although the prophylaxis codes are dentition specific rather than age specific and should be reported in this manner, some third-party payers may have restrictions in their contracts that limit available benefits or benefit levels based on age and not stage of the dentition.

    According to the ADA Policy "Age of 'Child'" adopted in 1991, benefits should be based on stage of dentition:

    > "**Resolved**, *that when dental plans differentiate coverage of specific procedures based on the child or adult status of the patient, this determination be based on the clinical development of the patient's dentition…*"

    Nonetheless, prophylaxis claims may be rejected by third-party carriers as not meeting plan age specifications for this service. It is appropriate to appeal such claim rejection. It is not appropriate for a dental benefit plan to ask that the claim be resubmitted with a different prophylaxis code solely for reimbursement.

3. *What code is appropriate for a difficult prophylaxis?*

    There is no separate procedure code that reflects a greater degree of difficulty of a dental prophylaxis. The available prophylaxis codes are **D1110 prophylaxis – adult and D1120 prophylaxis – child**.

    However, if the patient's clinical condition reveals moderate to severe gingival inflammation without bone loss, it may be that the patient's condition may more appropriately be treated by the **D4346 scaling in the presence of generalized moderate or severe gingival inflammation – full mouth, after oral evaluation** procedure.

4.   *When might a patient have benefits coverage for more than the usual two prophylaxis procedures in a 12-month period or in a calendar year?*

Some dental benefit plans may allow more frequent prophylaxis procedures based on medical risk or other factors (e.g., diabetic; immunosuppressed; pregnancy).

Other patients in the same plan who are not deemed "at risk" would be subject to standard frequency limitations. If the dentist determines medical necessity for more frequent cleanings not provided under plan parameters, the dentist or the patient may explore the plan's appeal process or that appeal process provided under state regulation.

5.   *What code is used to report a scaling and root planing in the presence of generalized moderate or severe gingival inflammation?*

When the dentist's oral evaluation reveals generalized moderate to severe gingival inflammation with no loss of attachment or bone, the appropriate procedure is **D4346 scaling in the presence of generalized moderate or severe gingival inflammation – full mouth, after oral evaluation**. D4346 is delivered and reported as a separate procedure and not in conjunction with a prophylaxis.

When any inflammation present is localized and there is no loss of attachment or bone, a prophylaxis procedure is appropriate and would be reported with the applicable CDT code (D1110 or D1120).

6.   *After a full mouth debridement (D4355) for the purpose of enabling a later comprehensive periodontal evaluation is delivered, may the patient receive a prophylaxis procedure on the next visit? Also, can an oral examination be performed on the same day as the full mouth debridement?*

A prophylaxis (e.g., D1110) procedure may be reported when the dentist determines that the need is indicated. There is no wording in the full CDT Code entries for D1110 and D4355 that establishes any relationship between the two procedures.

An oral evaluation (e.g., D0120; D0150) may be delivered at any time, including the same day as a prophylaxis, when the need for one is determined by the dentist. The one exception on timing is delivering a comprehensive periodontal evaluation reported with CDT code D0180.

Note: Third-party reimbursement for these procedures is dependent on the specific dental benefit plan provisions. Some plans may pay for both services when delivered at the same time, while others might impose a specified interval.

7. *Can* **D1110 prophylaxis – adult and D4342 scaling and root planing – one to three teeth per quadrant** *be reported on the same date of service?*

   There is no language in the descriptor of an adult prophylaxis that precludes the reporting of any other procedure on the same date of service and no language in the descriptor of D4342 that precludes at the same visit the provision of a dental prophylaxis. However, third-party reimbursement for these procedures is dependent on the specific dental benefit plan provisions. Some plans may pay for both services when delivered at the same time, while others might impose a specified interval.

8. *Could the CDT code* **D1206 topical application of fluoride varnish** *be used when applying fluoride varnish to desensitize a tooth?*

   No. When fluoride varnish is utilized to desensitize a tooth, the appropriate CDT code is **D9910 application of desensitizing medicament**. CDT code **D1206 application of topical fluoride varnish** is exclusive to the use for caries prevention.

9. *When resin is applied to a tooth's pit and fissure area, what distinguishes a sealant (D1351) from a preventive resin restoration (D1352)?*

   Application of an unfiled resin or glass ionomer cement limited to the enamel surface is a sealant procedure and would be documented using D1351. When a filled resin or glass ionomer cement is applied to an area of an active cavitated lesion that does not extend into the dentin, this procedure is a preventive resin restoration and the applicable procedure code is D1352.

   Note: Should the lesion extend into the dentin, the procedure code for a one surface composite resin restoration (D2391) would be used to document the service.

10. *I have several questions concerning the caries arresting medicament application procedure reported with CDT code D1354:*

    a. *I've heard this code referred to as the Silver Diamine Fluoride application procedure; is this implied limitation correct?*

       No. D1354's CDT Code entry describes a discrete procedure for delivery "of a caries arresting or inhibiting medicament." The dentist providing this service would determine the appropriate medicament to be applied, and the choice is not limited to Silver Diamine Fluoride.

    b. *Is the procedure reported with this code limited to primary teeth?*

       No. There are no words in either the nomenclature or descriptor that limits the procedure to primary dentition. This is a per-tooth procedure that may be delivered to any type of dentition – primary, succedaneous, and permanent.

c. *Does the delivery of the D1354 procedure preclude a subsequent restorative procedure at a later time?*

No. A subsequent restorative procedure may be needed some time after application of a caries arresting medicament. Caries is a disease that is treated with the medicament. The lesion in the tooth resulting from the disease (i.e., the cavity) may need a subsequent restoration to restore function.

d. *Must there be a specific interval between the D1354 procedure and a restorative procedure on the same tooth?*

No. As noted in 10.c, the clinical condition of a patient's tooth is affected by a variety of factors and can change over time. The patient's dentist is in the best position to evaluate the need for restorative services, and when such services should be delivered.

e. *May other preventive procedures be delivered to the tooth on the same day it receives the D1354 treatment?*

Yes. Other preventive procedures may be delivered as there is no such exclusionary language in D1354's nomenclature or descriptor. Individual circumstances would affect the order in which preventive services are delivered (e.g., prophylaxis before medicament application).

11. *Sometimes dental sealants fail completely (i.e., no sealant material remains bonded to the tooth surface), but most often failure is incremental with a partial loss of sealant material. The fix is to reapply sealant material only to the unprotected caries-susceptible pits and fissures. This is a much more limited procedure than D1351, which applies when the entire tooth surface is re-sealed. What CDT code applies to a sealant repair?*

The correct CDT code for this application is **D1353 sealant repair – per tooth**.

12. *What code should be used to report the removal of a fixed space maintainer?*

When the dentist determines that the space maintainer has served its useful purpose, the appropriate codes depending on type are as follows:

For unilateral space maintainers, the appropriate code is:

D1556   removal of fixed unilateral space maintainer – per quadrant

For bilateral space maintainers, the appropriate codes are:

D1557   removal of fixed bilateral space maintainer – maxillary

D1558   removal of fixed bilateral space maintainer – mandibular

Dental health care professionals should use the CDT code set to report what was done, not what would be reimbursed. Reimbursement will depend upon the dental benefit plan language and the contractual policies governing covered benefits. Regardless of any expected benefit payment, the dentist should provide and code for medically necessary services that are determined by community standards and the patient's informed consent for these services.

13. *Can a practice post a fee for a space maintainer appliance at the time that the impression is taken and sent to a dental lab for appliance fabrication?*

   Historically, the dentist has preferred to post the cost of the service at the time of tooth preparation in the case of indirect restorations or at the time of impression in the case of dental appliances. Likewise, third-party payers adjudicate claims and make reimbursements based on the dental benefit plan coverage provisions. What prevail are the legally enforceable provisions of the dental benefit plan and the provisions of an applicable participating provider agreement.

14. *What is the difference between the* **D1355 caries preventive medicament application – per tooth** *and* **D1354 application of caries arresting medicament – per tooth***? It appears that some of the same medicaments are recommended for both applications.*

   The difference is in the intent of the usage of the medicament. D1355 is intended to prevent the development of a caries lesion in a high-risk area. D1354 is appropriate with the intent of arresting an active carious lesion. Primary prevention (D1355) is intended to prevent the formation of disease in a healthy population. Secondary prevention (D1354) emphasizes early detection and is intended to prevent the progression of subclinical forms of the disease (e.g., decalcification, incipient lesions). Tertiary prevention aims to reduce the severity of the disease (e.g., large cavity without pulpal involvement). D1354 may be an appropriate code to report the use of a caries arresting medicament in an attempt to prevent further progression until a definitive restoration can be placed.

15. *There currently are two CDT codes that could be used for patients that are using tobacco products. Which code is recommended?*

   D1320 tobacco counseling for the control and prevention of oral disease is used when counseling a patient on the adverse oral health effects of tobacco products and the value of cessation.

   Patients that we serve may use other harmful substances in addition to tobacco. **D1321 counseling for the control and prevention of adverse oral, behavioral, and systemic effects associated with high-risk substance use** has a broader application potential for those individuals.

16. *There are several counseling codes within the CDT Code's Preventive category of service. What determines whether the usage of these codes will be reimbursed?*

Dental health care professionals are constantly striving to improve the oral and overall health of the patients that they serve. The CDT code set is available to assist the practitioner in documenting what services are provided. Reimbursement by the patient's dental benefits carrier for these services would depend upon the contractual limitations and policies governing covered benefits. Regardless of expected third-party payment, the dentist should record and code for the services provided.

17. *I noticed that the CDT now contains code for vaccinations for COVID-19 and human papillomavirus (HPV). I have several questions regarding their use.*

a. *Will the vaccinations require approval and training?*

Dentists are encouraged to contact their state Board of Dentistry (or equivalent) to determine if they are authorized to administer the COVID-19 and/or HPV vaccinations. Additionally, the Board of Dentistry may be able to provide information on required training, registration, and reporting.

b. *Will the patient's insurance company reimburse me for the vaccination provided?*

The dental office is encouraged to contact the patient's medical and dental insurance companies for guidance on vaccine reimbursement. The State's Department of Health or equivalent may also be a helpful resource on reporting and potential reimbursement. Reimbursement by the patient's medical and or dental benefits carrier for these services would depend upon the contractual limitations and policies governing covered benefits. Regardless of expected third-party payment, the dentist should record and code for the services provided.

18. *I have been using fluoride varnish for primary caries preventative reasons in high caries risk patients. Is it possible to use the* **D1355 caries preventive medicament application – per tooth** *code to report the application?*

No, the **D1355 caries preventative application – per tooth** code nomenclature specifically prohibits the use of fluoride products with this code. Although fluoride varnish is an effective agent for the primary prevention of dental caries, its use would need to be reported using **D1206 topical application of fluoride varnish**.

19. *I had a 10-year-old new patient present for a new patient exam, and he had a distal shoe space maintainer in his lower right quadrant. His first molars are fully erupted, but the radiographic images demonstrate delayed development of his lower second premolar. Also, his second permanent molar is near eruption. A bilateral space maintainer is indicated as his anchorage tooth for the distal shoe is near exfoliation. How would I report the removal of the distal shoe space maintainer and placement of the bilateral space maintainer?*

The dentist would report the removal of the distal shoe appliance using **D1556 removal of fixed unilateral space maintainer – per quadrant** and documenting the applicable quadrant of the appliance on the service line. The new bilateral space maintainer would be reported using **D1517 space maintainer – fixed – bilateral, mandibular**.

20. *I was planning on repairing an existing sealant on a permanent molar that a portion was missing. Upon removal of the unsound portion of the failed sealant, I found decalcified enamel that required removal. Fortunately, the decay was confined to the enamel layer and was able to repair with a small composite restoration. How would I report the sealant repair?*

If no decalcification was present, the repair would be reported using **D1353 sealant repair – per tooth**. As decalcified enamel was found requiring mechanical removal and was confined to the enamel layer, the dentist should utilize the code **D1352 preventative resin restoration in a moderate to high caries risk patient – permanent tooth**. If the lesion extended into the dentin layer, the appropriate code would be **D2391 resin-based composite – one surface, posterior**.

21. *I have a 5-year-old patient whose oral hygiene has worsened after a prolonged absence from my practice. She now has numerous areas of decalcification on her primary dentition. I am concerned as her diet is also poor, and my staff and I have discussed the impact of her oral hygiene habits and poor diet on her overall dental health with the her parents. How would I report the time spent analyzing her diet and demonstrating proper oral hygiene techniques?*

The appropriate codes to report the diet analysis and demonstration of proper hygiene technique are **D1310 nutritional counseling for control of dental disease** and **D1330 oral hygiene instructions**. Reimbursement for the services provided by the patient's dental benefits carrier for these services would depend upon the contractual limitations and policies governing covered benefits. Regardless of expected third-party payment, the dentist should record and code for the services provided.

Chapter 2: D1000–D1999 Preventive

Summary

The 44 codes which comprise the preventive category are straightforward and easy to understand because some of these procedures are among the most common services in dental practice, especially in the care of infants and children. Prevention of dental disease is the cornerstone of the profession and procedures such as professional removal plaque and calculus, application of prescription strength topical fluoride, nutritional counseling, oral hygiene instruction, and sealant placement help ensure optimal oral health.

Contributor Biography

Jim Nickman, D.D.S., M.S., is a practicing pediatric dentist in St. Paul, Minnesota, and a Clinical Associate Professor of the Division of Pediatric Dentistry at the University of Minnesota School of Dentistry. He serves as chair of the American Academy of Pediatric Dentistry Committee on Dental Benefit Programs and is a voting member of the American Dental Association's Code Maintenance Committee, representing the AAPD.

Chapter 3: D2000–D2999 Restorative

By Fred L. Horowitz, D.M.D.

Introduction

Restorative codes continue to represent the majority of dental procedures done in a general dental practice on a day-to-day basis. Selection of the applicable code, or codes, for restorative services is generally straightforward when the user understands the CDT Code's underlying organization and concepts. However, the advent of new technology can present some challenges.

Key Definitions and Concepts

Direct Restorations

Direct refers to a restoration that is fabricated completely in the mouth without the use of an impression, physical or digital, to create a model outside the mouth for fabrication.

> The ADA Glossary definition of **direct** is "A procedure where the service is delivered completely in the patient's oral cavity and without use of a dental laboratory."

Amalgam restorations include the tooth preparation, all adhesives (including amalgam bonding agents), as well as liners and bases. If pins are used, they are reported separately using the applicable procedure code (see D2951).

The amalgam codes are used to report procedures performed on primary or permanent dentition, with no differentiation between anterior and posterior teeth.

> The ADA Glossary definition of **amalgam** is "An alloy used in direct dental restorations. Typically composed of mercury, silver, tin and copper along with other metallic elements added to improve physical and mechanical properties."

Resin-based composite restorations include tooth preparation, acid etching, adhesives, liners and bases and curing of the material. There is no differentiation based on the various composite resin materials utilized. If pins are used, they are reported separately (see D2951).

The resin-based composite codes are used for reporting procedures performed on the primary or permanent dentition. However, unlike amalgam codes, the resin-based codes differentiate between procedures performed on anterior and posterior dentition.

The ADA Glossary definition of **resin-based composite** is "A dental restorative material made up of disparate or separate parts (e.g., resin and quartz particles)."

All glass ionomers, when used as restorations, are reported using the resin-based composite codes.

The ADA Glossary definition of **glass ionomer** is "A restorative material listed as a 'resin' in the CDT manual's "Classification of Materials" that may be used to restore teeth, fill pits and fissures, lute and line cavities."

Indirect Restorations

Indirect refers to a restoration that is fabricated outside of the mouth through use of impressions, physical or digital, and creation of the either physical or digital reproductions of the mouth or area of the mouth to be restored.

The ADA Glossary definition of **indirect** is "A procedure that involves activity that occurs away from the patient, such as creating a restorative prosthesis. An indirect procedure is also known as a **laboratory** procedure, and the laboratory's location can be within or separate from the dentist's practice."

Inlay restorations are intra-coronal restorations made outside the mouth. They conform to a prepared cavity and do not restore any cusp tips.

The ADA Glossary definition of **inlay** is "A fixed intracoronal restoration; a fixed dental restoration made outside of a tooth to correspond to the form of the prepared cavity, which is then luted to the tooth (*Glossary of Prosthodontic Terms*, 9th Edition; ©2019 Academy of Prosthodontics)."

Onlay restorations are made outside the mouth. They cover one or more cusp tips and adjoining occlusal surfaces, but not the entire external surface.

The ADA Glossary definition of **onlay** is "A partial coverage restoration that restores one or more cusps and adjoining occlusal surfaces or the entire external surface and is retained by mechanical or adhesive means (Glossary of Prosthodontic Terms, 9th Edition; ©2019 Academy of Prosthodontics)."

Crown restorations are made outside the mouth. They cover all of the cusps on posterior teeth, extend beyond the height of contour on all covered surfaces and restore all four proximal surfaces.

The ADA Glossary definition of **crown** is "An artificial replacement that restores missing tooth structure by surrounding the remaining coronal tooth structure, or is placed on a dental implant. It is made of metal, ceramic or polymer materials or a combination of such materials. It is retained by luting cement or mechanical means (American College of Prosthodontics; The *Glossary of Prosthodontic Terms*)."

¾ crown restorations are made outside the mouth. They cover all of the cusps on posterior teeth, extend beyond the height of contour on the covered surfaces and restore three of the four proximal surfaces.

Explanation of Restorations

Please note that "Facial" and "Labial" as used in this table are synonymous terms when describing surfaces involved in a restoration.

Location	Number of Surfaces	Characteristics
Anterior	1	Placed on one of the following five surface classifications – Mesial, Distal, Incisal, Lingual, or Facial (or Labial)
	2	Placed, without interruption, on two of the five surface classifications – e.g., Mesial-Lingual
	3	Placed, without interruption, on three of the five surface classifications – e.g., Lingual-Mesial-Facial (or Labial)
	4 or more	Placed, without interruption, on four or more of the five surface classifications – e.g., Mesial-Incisal-Lingual-Facial (or Labial)
Posterior	1	Placed on one of the following five surface classifications – Mesial, Distal, Occlusal, Lingual, or Buccal
	2	Placed, without interruption, on two of the five surface classifications – e.g., Mesial-Occlusal
	3	Placed, without interruption, on three of the five surface classifications – e.g., Lingual-Occlusal-Distal
	4 or more	Placed, without interruption, on four or more of the five surface classifications – e.g., Mesial-Occlusal-Lingual-Distal

Note: Tooth surfaces are reported on the HIPAA standard electronic dental transaction and the ADA Dental Claim Form using the letters in the table on the right.

Surface	Code
Buccal	B
Distal	D
Facial (or Labial)	F
Incisal	I
Lingual	L
Mesial	M
Occlusal	O

Chapter 3: D2000–D2999 Restorative

Changes to This Category

There are no CDT code additions, revisions, or deletions in this category for 2023.

Clinical Coding Scenario #1:
Fractured Tooth – After Hours Visit and the Final Restoration

The patient presents with a broken front tooth on Saturday, a day the office was usually closed. On examination, tooth #8 appeared to have a fractured mesial-incisal angle and lost a mesial composite restoration, with no pain reported. The doctor removed enough tooth structure to fit and cement a polycarbonate crown. The patient was told that the tooth would need a porcelain-fused-to-metal crown (PFM), but this could be done at a scheduled appointment during regular office hours.

How could you code for this after hours visit?

D0140   **limited oral evaluation – problem focused**

D2799   **interim crown – further treatment or completion of diagnosis necessary prior to final impression**

D9440   **office visit – after regularly scheduled hours**

Note: The after-hours office visit code (D9440) is from the CDT Code's Adjunctive General Services category and can be reported in addition to the other services performed at that appointment. This service may not be covered or reimbursed by some dental benefits plans.

When the patient returned to the office, the doctor removes the polycarbonate crown. Following caries excavation, the doctor determines that the tooth required some replacement of lost structure to achieve proper strength and retention for the crown. One threaded titanium pin and a bonded resin core material were used to restore the tooth, followed by a preparation and an impression for a PFM. The PFM was fabricated using an alloy containing gold 15%, Palladium 25%, and Platinum 10%.

How would this visit during regular office hours be coded?

D2950   **core buildup, including any pins, when required**

Replacement of tooth structure that is more than simply filling undercuts is appropriately reported using the core buildup procedure code. The retentive pin that was placed is included in the procedure documented with this code.

Note: D2950 would not be appropriate if the material is used only to eliminate undercuts or to yield a more ideal form for a subsequent indirect restoration.

Continued on next page

In this situation, the procedure would be documented as **D2949 restorative foundation for an indirect restoration**.

D2752   crown – porcelain fused to noble metal

The code for a PFM crown utilizing a noble metal (D2752) was selected instead of the high noble metal PFM code (D2750) because of the alloys used in fabrication. The noble metal percentage of the alloy was 50%, which is under the 60% high noble metal (gold + palladium + platinum) threshold specified in the CDT Code's Classification of Metals table that is published in the CDT manual.

Note: A porcelain fused to titanium crown procedure is reported with its own unique code – **D2753 crown – porcelain fused to titanium and titanium alloys**. According to the Classification of Metals, titanium and titanium alloys are not considered noble or high noble metals from the coding perspective.

Clinical Coding Scenario #2:
Restorative Material to Protect a Tooth

The doctor placed a CaOH liner under an amalgam restoration.

Should CDT code D2940 protective restoration be utilized to report this?

No. The following subcategory descriptors printed in the CDT manual state that bases and liners are part of the restorative procedure and should not be reported separately.

Amalgam Restorations (Including Polishing)
Tooth preparation, all adhesives (including amalgam bonding agents), liners and bases are included as part of the restoration.

Resin-Based Composite Restorations – Direct
Tooth preparation, acid etching, adhesives (including resin bonding agents), liners and bases, and curing are included as part of the restoration.

The D2940 descriptor clearly states that a protective restoration procedure is not reported when a base or liner is placed under any type of restoration.

D2940   protective restoration
Direct placement of a restorative material to protect tooth and/or tissue form. This procedure may be used to relieve pain, promote healing, or prevent further deterioration. Not to be used for endodontic access closure, or as a base or liner under restoration.

Clinical Coding Scenario #3:
Labial Veneer (Resin Laminate)

Patient #1

The patient presents for the fabrication of a resin labial veneer on tooth #9. The doctor prepares the tooth and fabricates the restoration directly on the tooth on the same day. The veneer is then bonded in place.

Patient #2

The patient presents for the fabrication of a resin labial veneer on tooth #9. The doctor prepares the tooth and makes an impression utilizing a 3D scanner. The scanned image is then transferred to a milling machine wherein the veneer is created. The doctor then fits and bonds the veneer in place on the same day as the tooth was prepared.

What CDT codes are appropriate for these procedures?

For Patient #1, the doctor will record the procedure as **D2960 labial veneer (resin laminate) – direct**, and for patient #2 the doctor will record the procedure as **D2961 labial veneer (resin laminate) – indirect**.

Although both restorations were created on the same day and in the office, they are recorded differently as the veneer fabrication locations differed – Patient #1 inside the oral cavity and Patient #2 outside the oral cavity.

Clinical Coding Scenario #4:
Modifying an Existing Partial Denture after an Extraction

The patient presented complaining that he could not wear his upper partial because of some loose, painful teeth. After clinical evaluation, the doctor determined that a well-designed maxillary removable partial denture had been placed and that it could be reused. This partial denture replaced teeth #2, #3, #4, and #14, with clasps on teeth #5, #13, and #15. The doctor's examination indicated that tooth #13 had Class III mobility due to advanced periodontal bone loss; #12 was fractured and decayed so that only a small piece of root remained exposed; and #15 had a fractured MOBL silver amalgam restoration with a fair amount of recurrent decay.

These findings led to a treatment plan that contained several separate procedures, coded as follows:

Extractions involving teeth #12 (residual root) and #13 (entire tooth)

D7140 extraction, erupted tooth or exposed root (elevation and/or forceps removal)

Both the routine extraction of #13 and the root tip removal of #12 are coded using D7140. If #12's root tip removal required the laying of a mucoperiosteal flap and bone removal, the appropriate code for surgical extractions is D7210.

Addition of teeth #12 and #13 to the partial

D5650 add tooth to existing partial denture

This procedure is reported twice in this scenario, one time for each tooth added, and generally requires reporting the tooth number added (based on its anatomy).

Additional clasp to the partial for retention on tooth #11

D5660 add clasp to existing partial denture – per tooth

There is a single code for the addition of a clasp to a partial, whether it is wrought wire and processed or cast and soldered.

Full cast noble metal crown (tooth #15) to fit the existing clasp

D2792 crown – full cast noble metal

D2971 additional procedures to customize a crown to fit under an existing partial denture framework

When a crown is constructed to fit an existing partial denture, the code for a regular crown is selected based on the material from which it is fabricated. The additional procedures required to allow the crown to accommodate the existing clasp are coded using D2971.

Clinical Coding Scenario #5:
A Child Who Needs Endodontic Treatment and a Crown

It was a sad story that the doctor had heard too often. The three-year-old patient had early childhood caries and was in pain. Treatment consisted of three pulpectomies followed by a resorbable filling and four esthetic-coated stainless steel crowns cemented on the maxillary incisors.

How would you code for this encounter?

Endodontic procedure

> **D3230** **pulpal therapy (resorbable filling) – anterior, primary tooth (excluding final restoration)**

"Pulpal therapy" with a resorbable filling is a typical pulp treatment for primary teeth that have carious pulp exposure. It is <u>reported three times</u> in this case, once for each treated tooth.

Primary crowns

> **D2934** **prefabricated esthetic coated stainless steel crown – primary tooth**

There are three types of stainless steel crowns for primary teeth: the standard stainless steel crown, one with a resin window, and the esthetic coated stainless steel crown. The esthetic coated crown was used in this case, and it is reported four times on the claim.

Clinical Coding Scenario #6:
Repair Existing Crown

The patient presents with a small chip from the porcelain on a crown for tooth #29. The dentist verified that the missing piece is not in occlusion and is only cosmetic. The dentist was able to bond a composite resin to the crown to achieve satisfactory results.

What CDT code should be used to report the procedure performed?

The dentist should record the procedure as **D2980 crown repair necessitated by restorative material failure**.

Clinical Coding Scenario #7:
Failed Endodontically Treated Tooth with Post, Core, and Crown

The patient complained of "a bad taste" in their mouth at a routine recall exam and prophylaxis. Upon examination, the doctor found a draining fistula between teeth #28 and #29. After reviewing the chart and taking a periapical radiographic image, the doctor determined that #28's root canal therapy was failing and there was decay evident at the distal margin of the tooth's existing PFM crown. In addition to treating the failed root canal therapy, the dentist replaced the PFM crown with a prefabricated post and core followed by placement of a new titanium crown.

How would you code to treat this situation?

 D1110 **prophylaxis – adult**

 D0120 **periodic oral evaluation – established patient**

 D0220 **intraoral – periapical first radiographic image**

 D3347 **retreatment of previous root canal therapy – premolar**

 D2954 **prefabricated post and core in addition to crown**

 D2794 **crown – titanium and titanium alloys**

Clinical Coding Scenario #8:
Removal of Post from Tooth to Enable Endodontic Retreatment

A patient presents with endodontically treated tooth #7 that was restored with a prefabricated post and core. The dentist determines that she must remove the post and core to have access for the tooth's endodontic retreatment.

How would the dentist record the removal of the prefabricated post?

D2955   post removal

Clinical Coding Scenario #9:
Porcelain Crown Type Choices

The patient requires a crown to restore tooth #12. Based on occlusal analysis and the patient's concern about esthetics, the dentist chooses to fabricate an all ceramic crown versus a porcelain fused to metal crown. The dentist also decides to use a Bruxzir® crown versus a CEREC milled crown.

How would you code this particular restoration?

D2740   crown – porcelain/ceramic

There is no coding difference among various ceramic manufactured crowns, no matter the process utilized in fabrication.

Coding Q&A

1. *How may I document and report local anesthesia as a separate procedure when restorative (or any other operative or surgical) services are being delivered?*

   D9215 local anesthesia in conjunction with operative or surgical procedures is the available code to document this procedure and, if you wish, to report it separately on a claim. Benefit plan limitations may preclude separate reimbursement for local anesthesia.

2. *I prepared tooth #7 for a porcelain laminate veneer, made a digital impression, and sent it to my lab for fabrication. Do I code that as a lab created veneer?*

   Yes, using CDT code **D2962 labial veneer (porcelain laminate) – indirect**.

   In CDT 2021, the last word of the nomenclature was changed from "laboratory" to "indirect" – a change that does not affect the nature or scope of the procedure.

3. *How do I report two separate two-surface restorations on the same tooth? Carriers advise me to report a MO amalgam and a DO amalgam as a MOD restoration. Is this correct?*

   The carriers' advice is incorrect. Dentists must document the procedures performed and in this scenario, there are two separate two-surface restorations, an MO and a DO. Guidance applicable to reporting procedures on a single tooth is found in the CDT manual's "Explanation of Restorations."

   Following the carriers' advice and reporting a single MOD procedure instead of properly reporting the two separate procedures will lead to a discrepancy between your accurate patient records and the carrier's claim records. Such a difference may become a problem during any audit or other review of services rendered.

   Note: Some dental plans may have clauses that restrict coverage on the same surface twice on the same date of service. This is why the carriers may apply an alternate benefit provision that leads to reimbursement of the two separate two-surface restorations as a single three-surface restoration.

4. *I recently purchased a laser and have been unable to find any "laser" codes in the CDT manual. Where are the "laser" codes?*

   CDT codes are procedure based rather than instrument based. You would report the appropriate code based on the actual procedure that was performed without regard to the armamentarium used to deliver the procedure.

5. *A 17-year-old patient required the placement of a crown on tooth #18. Clinically, the tooth has not quite fully erupted. I wanted to place a crown on the tooth that would last a few years, but understood it will need to be replaced. I did not feel that either an acrylic or stainless steel crown would have a good prognosis. Instead I used prefabricated ceramic crown. How do I code this?*

There is a discrete CDT code for this type of crown procedure: **D2928 prefabricated porcelain/ceramic crown – permanent tooth**.

6. *Should single crowns that are splinted together be coded as single crowns (in the D2700 series of codes) or as a bridge (in the D6700 series)?*

Single crowns that are splinted together are appropriately reported as single crowns using the applicable code(s) from the "Crowns – Single Restorations Only" (D2700) series of codes.

7. *What procedure code should I report for a porcelain fused to a zirconium substrate crown?*

This question contains a commonly made error, using the word zirconium when describing the crown's material. Dental crowns use zirconia, which is an oxide and considered chemically to be a ceramic.

With this in mind, the applicable procedure code is **D2740 crown – porcelain/ceramic**.

8. *How do I code a porcelain fused to titanium crown? I only see a metallic titanium crown code **D2794 crown – titanium and titanium alloys**.*

Code **D2753 crown – porcelain fused to titanium and titanium alloys** is the available code to report the single crown procedure described.

Note: At one time, D2794 was the only code with "titanium" in its nomenclature. Now, as a result of the CDT Code's evolution into a more robust code set there are more. The CDT Code's growth sometimes results in code entries with similar key words, such as titanium, having code numbers that are not sequential—as seen here. Identification of an appropriate code is aided by looking through the CDT manual's alphabetical index of key words, or by a key word search in the CDT App.

9. *Is there a code for retrofitting a new crown to an existing partial denture?*

The code is **D2971 additional procedures to customize a crown to fit under an existing partial denture framework** and should be reported in addition to the crown.

10. *Is there a procedure code for re-cementing an onlay?*

   D2910 re-cement or re-bond inlay, onlay, veneer or partial coverage restoration includes the re-cementation of an onlay, as well as inlays and any other partial coverage restorations such as a veneer.

11. *If I place an IRM (intermediate restorative material) restoration, do I report this as protective (aka "sedative") restoration or a palliative procedure?*

   Delivery and reporting placement of IRM may be reported as palliative (e.g., emergency) treatment of dental pain (D9110) if placement is temporary (e.g., to immediately address discomfort associated with heat or cold) and the patient will subsequently receive an oral evaluation that leads to definitive treatment. In other circumstances, the dentist may determine that the service should be reported as a protective restoration procedure (D2940).

12. *With all the restorative codes published in the CDT manual, when may it be necessary to consider using* **D2999 unspecified restorative procedure, by report** *to document and report services rendered?*

   No matter how many definitive CDT codes exist, exceptional situations arise. Sometimes, due to widespread adoption of a new procedure, the CDT Code's maintenance timetable, or limited frequency or scope of occurrence, there is a need to use D2999. Some examples of situations where D2999 would be applicable follow:

   - The restorative procedure was started but was not completed due to clinical complications requiring a referral (e.g., extensive decay necessitating surgical extraction instead of direct restoration) or patient compliance (e.g., patient does not return for placement of permanent crown).

   - The patient's treatment plan includes placement of a prefabricated post and core under an existing crown.

   - The patient's treatment plan includes placement of a prefabricated post without a core.

13. *An access cavity was made through a crown for endodontic treatment. What procedure code is appropriate to report sealing an endodontic access cavity?*

   There is no code that specifically addresses the procedure for sealing an endodontic access cavity. Sealing the access cavity is a procedure reported with the appropriate single surface direct restoration code e.g., **D2391 resin-based composite – one surface, posterior**.

14. *My patient had a fractured tooth, and I placed a temporary crown solely to protect the remaining tooth structure and space. What procedure code should I use to report this service?*

The available code to report the procedure delivered is:

D2940 **protective restoration**
Direct placement of a restorative material to protect tooth and/or tissue form. This procedure may be used to relieve pain, promote healing, or prevent further deterioration. Not to be used for endodontic access closure, or as a base or liner under restoration.

This is a procedure that protects the tooth and surrounding tissues.

15. *There are post and core codes only in the restorative category, but not in the fixed prosthodontics category. What is the correct code to use when the final restoration will be a multiple unit fixed bridge?*

The codes in the restorative category may be used when a single crown or a multiple unit fixed prosthesis is the final restoration. Remember the placement of codes within categories is to enable ease of navigation through the CDT Code and does not limit use of codes across specialties:

D2952 **post and core in addition to crown, indirectly fabricated**

D2954 **prefabricated post and core in addition to crown**

16. *What code should be reported for placement of a composite restoration in a non-carious cervical lesion or an erosive lesion in a cusp tip or other surface of a tooth?*

Such lesions are treated with resin materials, which include glass ionomers, and the appropriate code depends on tooth position: anterior or posterior. The applicable code for an anterior tooth is:

D2330 **resin-based composite – one surface, anterior**

For a posterior tooth the applicable code is:

D2391 **resin-based composite – one surface, posterior**
Used to restore a carious lesion into the dentin or a deeply eroded area into the dentin. Not a preventive procedure.

Note: Non-carious cervical lesions commonly extend into the dentin due to thin enamel at this portion of a tooth's anatomy. In an exceptional situation where the lesion does not extend into a posterior tooth's dentin, the available procedure code is:

D2999 **unspecified restorative procedure, by report**

17. *I repaired a porcelain "chip" on a PFM crown. What procedure code would I use?*

   D2980   crown repair necessitated by restorative material failure

18. *A college student presented with a "chip" on #10. The patient had an enamel fracture of the distoincisal of #10. She had the chipped piece of enamel. I bonded the fractured enamel piece back on the tooth until the patient could get back to her hometown dentist. What procedure code should I use?*

   D2921   reattachment of tooth fragment, incisal edge or cusp

19. *A child became uncooperative as I was removing the decay on a primary molar. I was able to remove all the decay but unable to place a permanent restoration due to the patient's behavior. Eventually the primary molar will need a stainless steel crown. However, I placed glass ionomer in the cavity to aid in healing prior to definitive treatment. How should I code this?*

   D2941   interim therapeutic restoration – primary dentition

20. *I had to remove a post and core on tooth #9. What code should I use to document this?*

   D2955   post removal

21. *The periodontal diagnosis suggests the fabrication of two adjacent PFM single crowns that are splinted for additional strength to oppose masticatory forces. Appropriate individual crown codes should be utilized, as there is no CDT coding mechanism to indicate the crowns are splinted. How should I code this?*

   D2750   crown – porcelain fused to high noble metal

   This procedure is reported twice, and the patient's record should note that the individual crowns were splinted for additional strength. The splint may be reported with **D2999 unspecified restorative procedure, by report**.

22. *A patient presented with a fractured gold inlay. The doctor placed a provisional inlay, anticipating a final restoration. What code should be used to report this treatment?*

   D2999   unspecified restorative procedure, by report

23. *A patient presented with a partial fracture of a fixed partial denture. The doctor believes this can be repaired without complete replacement. What code should be used to report the repair?*

   D6980   fixed partial denture repair necessitated by restorative material failure

24. What is a strip crown, and how do I record it?

A "strip crown" is a direct procedure that involves: 1) placing a form on the tooth; 2) filling the form with composite resin that bonds directly to the tooth in the shape of a crown; 3) removing the form from the tooth after the composite resin cures (i.e., the form is "stripped away" from the tooth and composite resin crown); and 4) finishing and final polishing as necessary.

The ADA's position is that a "strip crown" procedure would be reported with a CDT code listed within the "Resin-Based Composite Restorations – Direct" subcategory of service. Further, the dentist who delivers this procedure would consider the full CDT code entry when determining the code that appropriately describes the service she or he delivered. Should a dentist be delivering a direct composite resin restoration, selection of the appropriate CDT code is affected by the preparation.

If the restoration is full coverage with no visible original enamel, this is a crown procedure documented with the following CDT code.

D2390 resin-based composite crown, anterior
> Full resin-based composite coverage of tooth.

Note: Should a dentist elect to deliver such a direct crown to a posterior tooth, the applicable CDT code is **D2999 unspecified restorative procedure, by report**.

If some of the original enamel is preserved on any of the surfaces, this is a multi-surface restoration procedure documented with one of the following CDT codes.

D2335 resin-based composite – four or more surfaces or involving incisal angle (anterior)
> Incisal angle to be defined as one of the angles formed by the junction of the incisal and the mesial or distal surface of an anterior tooth.

D2394 resin-based composite – four or more surfaces, posterior

There is no question that a "strip crown" procedure is a direct resin-based composite restoration procedure. All the clinical steps occur inside the patient's mouth, which meets the ADA Glossary of Dental Clinical and Administrative Terms definition of direct restorations ("a restoration fabricated inside the mouth"). The "strip" is simply a form that enables creation of the artificial crown in-situ.

Summary

Restorative procedures are an integral part of treatment that patients receive every day. Because we use the restorative codes so frequently, we must make sure that over time we are indeed using the correct code. It is important for the dentist and the coder to be familiar with any CDT Code changes that enable them to more accurately document and report the procedure delivered to a patient.

Remember, "Code for what you do."

Contributor Biography

Fred L. Horowitz, D.M.D., is president and on the board of directors of Primecare Benefits Group, Inc., a dental insurance holding company based in Nevada. Following graduation from Washington University School of Dental Medicine, Dr. Horowitz completed a general practice residency at Sinai Hospital of Detroit. He practiced full time for ten years and has since had executive level positions with dental benefits companies across the country. He is also a three-term board member of the National Association of Dental Plans (NADP) and served on the Board of the National Dental EDI Council, Access Health Dental (a Nevada-based DSO), and the National Association of Specialty Health Organizations. He represented the United States dental payer industry to the International Health Terminology Standards Development Organization (now SNOMED), serving as the Vice-Chairman of the International Dental SIG component. He also currently serves on the Executive Steering Committee of the Culinary Health Center Las Vegas, and on the board of directors of Mobile Management Group, Primecare Administrators, Inc., and Nevada Dental Benefits, Ltd.

By Elizabeth Shin Perry, D.M.D.

Introduction

The specialty of Endodontics has progressed to allow dentists the ability to predictably save more teeth than ever. The advent of sophisticated diagnostic capabilities as well as the continued improvement of techniques to preserve a patient's dentition has expanded the Endodontics CDT codes.

The Endodontics category of service describes procedures that involve treatment of the dental pulp, root canals, and the tissues surrounding the roots of the tooth. These codes describe nonsurgical procedures related to debridement and disinfection of the root canal space, maintenance and regeneration of the pulp, removal of previously placed materials within the root canal space (including root canal filling, posts, and broken instruments), and obturation of the root canal space. In addition, endodontic surgical codes describe periradicular surgical procedures such as apicoectomy and root amputation, root repair due to perforation or resorptive defects, exploratory curettage to examine for root damage, placement of retrograde filling materials, intentional reimplantation, and placement of bone grafting and regeneration materials.

Some of the main challenges typical to endodontics involve coding for procedures that require multiple appointments. Other concerns relate to what should be coded separately from an endodontic therapy procedure, such as D3331 (treatment of root canal obstruction; non-surgical access) or D2955 (post removal). Another question often encountered is which radiographs are considered part of the endodontic therapy procedure. Separately, CDT Code entries for other endodontic procedures that involve surgery, pulpal regeneration, and vital pulp therapy are less commonly used and can be confusing unless the process has been studied by the office coding specialist.

It is important to understand that procedure codes are meant to describe the treatment rendered, not the means that are used to accomplish the treatment. For example, disinfection of a root canal during endodontic therapy can be accomplished using different techniques, including irrigation with multiple irrigating solutions and devices. The code used for the procedure, however, is the same.

Key Definitions and Concepts

Apexification: A method to induce a calcified barrier in a root with an open apex or the continued apical development of an incompletely formed root in teeth with necrotic pulps.

> The ADA Glossary definition of **apexification** is "The process of induced root development to encourage the formation of a calcified barrier in a tooth with immature root formation or an open apex. May involve the placement of an artificial apical barrier prior to nonsurgical endodontic obturation."

Apexogenesis: A vital pulp therapy procedure performed to encourage continued physiological development and formation of the root end.

> The ADA Glossary definition of **apexogenesis** is "Vital pulp therapy performed to encourage continued physiological formation and development of the tooth root."

Dental dam: Also known as "rubber dam," the dental dam is a rubber-like sheet used to isolate a tooth from the oral environment and to prevent migration of fluids or foreign objects into or out of the operative field. Dental dams are considered standard operating procedure per the American Association of Endodontists's Position Statement, "Dental Dams" available at *www.aae.org/specialty/wp-content/uploads/sites/2/2017/06/dentaldamstatement.pdf*

Decoronation: The intentional removal of the coronal portion of a tooth, with retention of its root(s) in order to preserve the width and vertical height of the alveolar bone.

Endodontic therapy: The procedure that involves the cleaning, shaping, and obturating the root canals of a tooth. Also known as root canal therapy.

Intraorifice barrier: The placement of a flowable composite, resin-modified glass ionomer cement or bioceramic restorative material directly over the canal obturation material within the canal orifice to allow for a bonded seal when placement of a core buildup or definitive access opening restoration cannot be placed immediately following completion of root canal therapy. A temporary restoration is placed over the intraorifice barrier as an interim restoration.

Irrigation: Part of the endodontic therapy procedure in which a disinfectant fluid is used to flush and disinfect the root canals.

Obturation: The process of filling the root canal space (where the dental pulp normally resides) with some type of dental material. This process must be performed for endodontic therapy to be complete. After obturation, a tooth must be permanently restored with a coronal restoration.

The ADA Glossary definition of **obturate** is "With reference to endodontics, refers to the sealing of the canal(s) of tooth roots during root canal therapy procedure with an appropriately prescribed material such as gutta percha in combination with a suitable luting agent."

Pulpectomy: The process of removal of the pulp entirely from the root canal space.

The ADA Glossary definition of **pulpectomy** is "Complete removal of vital and non-vital pulp tissue from the root canal space."

Pulpal debridement: Elimination of organic and inorganic substances as well as microorganisms from the root canal by mechanical and/or chemical means.

Pulpal regeneration: A biologically based procedure designed to physiologically replace damaged tooth structures, including dentin and root structures, as well as cells of the pulp-dentin complex of an incompletely formed root in teeth with necrotic pulps (also known as Regenerative Endodontics).

Pulpotomy: The process of removal of the pulp from the pulp chamber only, but not the root canal spaces within a tooth. A pulpotomy may be used as a temporary solution to relieve symptoms or as a permanent solution for a tooth which may be able to maintain pulp vitality despite exposure of the pulp.

The ADA Glossary definition of **pulpotomy** is "Removal of a portion of the pulp, including the diseased aspect, with the intent of maintaining the vitality of the remaining pulpal tissue by means of a therapeutic dressing."

Resorption: A condition associated with either a physiologic or a pathologic process resulting in a loss of dentin, cementum, and/or bone.

Root canal: This term is used both for the passage or channel in the root of the tooth extending from the pulp chamber to the apical foramen, and to describe the endodontic therapy procedure that involves cleaning, shaping and obturating the canals with a dental material. Thus, it has two different definitions, as a noun and also as a verb, as in "to root canal." Some teeth have a single root canal space, while others have multiple. A root canal procedure for a given tooth treats all of the root canal spaces within the tooth. The root canal therapy procedure is referred to as "endodontic therapy" in the CDT Code set.

The ADA Glossary definition of **root canal** is "The portion of the pulp cavity inside the root of a tooth; the chamber within the root of the tooth that contains the pulp."

The ADA Glossary definition of **root canal therapy** is "The treatment of disease and injuries of the pulp and associated periradicular conditions."

Vital pulp therapy: Treatment performed with the intention of preservation of the vitality of the pulp tissue after compromise by trauma, caries, or restorative procedures.

Changes to This Category

There was one revision in this category in CDT 2023.

D3333   **internal root repair of perforation defects**
Non-surgical seal of perforation caused by resorption and/or decay but not iatrogenic by <u>same</u> provider ~~filing claim~~.

Clinical Coding Scenarios

Clinical Coding Scenario #1:
Endodontic Consultation with CBCT

A general dentist refers a patient for evaluation of ongoing pain in the upper right quadrant. The patient had multiple restorations in the quadrant and had developed increasing pain in the area. The dentist and patient were unsure which tooth was causing the pain. A problem-focused oral examination is performed, including pulp vitality testing. Two periapical radiographs and one bitewing radiograph are taken as well as a limited view CBCT. Periapical radiographs are not conclusive due to the proximity to the sinus and zygomatic arch. The limited view CBCT reveals an area of apical and lateral loss of bone extending the level of the osseous crest on the mesial, associated with the upper second molar. A diagnosis of pulpal necrosis with symptomatic apical and lateral periodontitis is made and the patient is informed that a crown to root fracture is present. Due to the guarded prognosis, extraction is recommended.

What procedure codes would be used to document and report the services provided?

D0140   **limited oral evaluation – problem focused**

D0460   **pulp vitality tests**

D0220   **intraoral – periapical first radiographic image**

D0230   **intraoral – periapical each additional radiographic image**

D0270   **bitewing – single radiographic image**

D0364   **cone beam CT capture and interpretation with limited field of view – less than one whole jaw**

Clinical Coding Scenario #2:
Endodontic Evaluation and Root Canal Therapy

A patient is referred for root canal therapy of tooth #31 with the chief complaint of ongoing pain to hot, cold, and biting, as well as a spontaneous low grade toothache. Prior dental history of the tooth includes placement of a full coverage crown six months previously. A problem-focused examination including pulp vitality testing is performed, and diagnostic, preoperative radiographs (two periapicals and a bitewing) are taken and evaluated. The radiographs show evidence of widening of the periodontal ligament space at the root apices and close proximity to the inferior alveolar nerve canal. A limited view CBCT is taken, the presence of pathology is confirmed, and the root apices are seen to be directly over the mandibular canal. A diagnosis of symptomatic irreversible pulpitis with symptomatic apical periodontitis is made, and a treatment plan for root canal therapy is recommended. The referring dentist requested that a temporary restoration be placed so that he could restore the access opening in the crown.

Root canal therapy was completed in a single visit, using the pre-operative CBCT as a guide to avoid any violation of the inferior alveolar nerve canal. Upon completion of obturation of the canals, 3 mm of a flowable bioceramic restorative material was placed over each canal orifice and over the pulpal floor to prevent microleakage and contamination of the completed root canal therapy. A temporary restoration was placed in the access opening, and the patient was advised to return to her dentist for restoration and repair of the crown.

What procedure codes would be used to document and report the services provided?

D0140   **limited oral evaluation – problem focused**

D0460   **pulp vitality tests**

D0220   **intraoral – periapical first radiographic image**

D0230   **intraoral – periapical each additional radiographic image**

D0270   **bitewing – single radiographic image**

D0364   **cone beam CT capture and interpretation with limited field of view – less than one whole jaw**

D3330   **endodontic therapy, molar tooth (excluding final restoration)**

D3911   **intraorifice barrier**

Note: D3911 is a code used to report placement of an intraorifice barrier over the obturated canals when the permanent restoration is not placed at the time of completion of root canal therapy. The barrier is not a final restoration.

Clinical Coding Scenario #3:
Root Canal Started by Another Practitioner

A patient presents for endodontic treatment of tooth #29, having had a root canal started on this single rooted tooth in another state while on vacation. The patient is not in any pain. An exam is performed and diagnostic, preoperative radiographs (a periapical and a bitewing) and CBCT are taken and evaluated. The radiographic images show evidence of a large periapical radiolucency as well as radiopaque evidence that calcium hydroxide has likely been placed in the root canal space. A treatment plan is made to complete root canal therapy and restore the tooth with a buildup and crown.

During the patient's second visit, the appointment during which the root canal was intended to be completed, it is found that ninety minutes was insufficient to complete the case. A significant amount of purulence was seen actively exuding into the tooth from the periapical tissues. The tooth was dressed with calcium hydroxide and temporized. A third treatment visit was scheduled.

During the third visit the root canal was completed and a core buildup was placed. An intraoperative radiograph and two post-operative radiographs were taken during this appointment. A crown preparation appointment was scheduled for a later date.

What procedure codes would be used to document and report the services provided during each of the three encounters?

Visit #1: Initial Appointment

> **D0140** limited oral evaluation – problem focused
>
> **D0220** intraoral – periapical first radiographic image
>
> **D0270** bitewing – single radiographic image
>
> **D0364** cone beam CT capture and interpretation with limited field of view – less than one whole jaw

Visit #2: Root Canal Begun, but Not Completed

> **D3221** pulpal debridement, primary and permanent teeth
>
> [root canal was not completed]

Continued on next page

Visit #3: Root Canal Completed and Core Buildup Placed

    D3320   **endodontic therapy, premolar tooth (excluding final restoration)**

    D2950   **core buildup, including any pins when required**

Note: The third visit radiographs would be documented in the patient's record but not included in the claim submission. "Endodontic Therapy" subcategory descriptor states that the procedures "…includes intra-operative radiographs…" Any radiographs taken for diagnostic purposes, during visit #1 in this scenario, are appropriately included separately on the claim for that date of service.

Clinical Coding Scenario #4:
Pulpectomy

A patient of record calls the office with a severe toothache. He did not sleep well the previous night and needs to be seen by a dentist immediately. The schedule is already fully committed, but accommodations are made to see the patient during the office lunch hour.

The patient presents to the office and periapical and bitewing radiographs and CBCT are taken. A problem-focused examination is performed and the patient is diagnosed with symptomatic irreversible pulpitis and symptomatic apical periodontitis of tooth #30. Definitive treatment is recommended to relieve the patient's pain.

A complete pulpectomy was performed and a temporary restoration was placed as emergency treatment. Three weeks later, the patient returns for completion of the root canal and the access opening closed by placement of composite resin restorative material.

What procedure codes would be used to document and report the services provided during each of the two encounters?

Visit #1

D0140	**limited oral evaluation – problem focused**
D0220	**intraoral – periapical first radiographic image**
D0270	**bitewing – single radiographic image**
D0364	**cone beam CT capture and interpretation with limited field of view – less than one whole jaw**
D3221	**pulpal debridement, primary and permanent teeth**

Visit #2

D3330	**endodontic therapy, molar tooth (excluding final restoration)**
D2391	**resin-based composite – one surface, posterior**

Note: D2391 is the procedure often used when sealing the access opening in the tooth's crown requires a relatively uncomplicated restoration. When sealing the access opening is more complicated, core buildup (D2950) is more likely to be delivered and reported.

Clinical Coding Scenario #5:
Emergency Root Canal Patient

A patient of record presents with a dental emergency of severe pain in tooth #9. Clinical examination is performed and radiographs are taken. A CBCT is taken due to the patient's history of trauma. A diagnosis of symptomatic irreversible pulpitis with symptomatic apical periodontitis is made, and root canal therapy is recommended as emergency treatment.

The following codes would be utilized for what would be a typical and straight forward procedure that is completed in the same day, with the access opening restored with composite resin material:

D0140 limited oral evaluation – problem focused

D0220 intraoral – periapical first radiographic image

D0364 cone beam CT capture and interpretation with limited field of view – less than one whole jaw

Note: If more than one periapical is taken, cite the number of additional images with: **D0230 intraoral – periapical each additional radiographic image**. If a bitewing radiograph is also taken: **D0270 bitewing – single radiographic image**.

D3310 endodontic therapy, anterior tooth (excluding final restoration)

D2330 resin-based composite – one surface, anterior

What if I see them for a root canal appointment on emergency basis, then have to refer it out to a specialist?

In this case, if a general dentist opens a tooth on an emergency basis due to pain and then feels the need to refer the case, the following codes could be utilized to document the situation:

D0140 limited oral evaluation – problem focused

D0220 intraoral – periapical first radiographic image

D3221 pulpal debridement, primary and permanent teeth

Notes: The pulpal debridement (D3221), also known as pulpectomy, is done to debride the root canal for the purpose of alleviating pain or preparing the root canal for placement of an intracanal medication when indicated.

A referral is then made to an endodontist for specialty care. The endodontist would then perform and code for the following procedures: a limited oral evaluation; new diagnostic preoperative radiographs to establish the present condition; endodontic therapy; restoration of the access opening if a permanent restoration is placed. (The procedures and coding for access opening restoration would depend upon the restorative situation.)

Clinical Coding Scenario #6:

Emergency Incision and Drainage and Endodontic Therapy

A patient presents with significant facial swelling and pain in the upper right quadrant. She reports that she had multiple crowns placed in this quadrant and that her dentist told her that she may need a root canal in the future. Clinical examination is performed and a periapical and bitewing radiographs are taken. In addition, a CBCT scan is taken to aid in the diagnosis. A diagnosis of pulpal necrosis with acute apical abscess of tooth #2 is made, and a treatment plan for incision and drainage of the facial swelling followed by endodontic therapy of tooth is discussed.

Incision and drainage is performed with significant purulent drainage. Root canal therapy of tooth #2 is initiated at the same visit; the root canals are instrumented completely and the tooth is medicated with calcium hydroxide followed by the placement of a temporary restoration.

The patient returns two weeks later and the swelling and discomfort has resolved completely. Root canal therapy of tooth #2 is completed with re-instrumentation followed by obturation of the canals. The access opening is permanently restored with composite.

How would you code for this scenario?

Visit #1

D0140 limited oral evaluation – problem focused

D0220 intraoral – periapical first radiographic image

D0270 bitewing – single radiographic image

D0364 cone beam CT capture and interpretation with limited field of view – less than one whole jaw

D7510 incision and drainage of abscess – intraoral soft tissue

D3221 pulpal debridement, primary and permanent teeth

Note: Root canal procedure was initiated but not completed. Record should note that pulpal debridement was performed on this date of service.

Visit #2

D3330 endodontic therapy, molar tooth (excluding final restoration)

D2391 resin-based composite – one surface, posterior

Clinical Coding Scenario #7:
Patient Referral for Apicoectomy

A patient is referred by a friend who is a general dentist. The general dentist referred this patient for an "apico" of tooth #3 since the referring dentist prefers not to do this type of procedure in her practice. It is determined that periapical radiographs and a cone beam computed tomography (CBCT) image are needed to evaluate the complex case prior to determining the treatment plan.

A problem-focused examination was performed, along with capture and evaluation of a CBCT image of a portion of the upper jaw and two periapical radiographs. A diagnosis of chronic apical periodontitis was made and a treatment plan for apicoectomy was confirmed. Included in the plan is a bone graft, which will be used due to the presence of the large lesion that appears to have eroded both the buccal and palatal cortical plates of bone. Consent is received and an appointment is scheduled.

Note: A surgery of this nature is not usually done on an emergency basis and often the examination is done on a day separate from the procedure.

The surgery is performed for tooth #3 on both the MB and DB roots. 3 mm of each root end was resected and a root-end filling was placed in each root end. A confirmation periapical radiograph was taken. An absorbable collagen wound dressing was placed.

Sutures were placed and post-operative instructions given. The patient returned for suture removal after a few days. This follow-up appointment was uneventful and sutures were removed.

What procedure codes would be used to document and report the services provided during each of the three encounters?

Visit #1: Initial Appointment

> **D0140** **limited oral evaluation – problem focused**
>
> **D0220** **intraoral – periapical first radiographic image**
>
> **D0230** **intraoral – periapical each additional radiographic image**
>
> **D0364** **cone beam CT capture and interpretation with limited field of view – less than one whole jaw**

Continued on next page

Visit #2: Endodontic Procedures Delivered

D3425 apicoectomy – molar (first root)

D3426 apicoectomy (each additional root)

D3430 retrograde filling – per root

D3430 retrograde filling – per root

D3431 biologic materials to aid in soft and osseous tissue regeneration in conjunction with periradicular surgery

Note: Root-end fillings are coded per root. For a tooth #3, often there are two roots, which is why D3430 is reported twice.

Visit #3: Post-Operative Follow Up, Sutures Removed

D0171 re-evaluation – post-operative office visit

Note: Visit #3 is the suture removal appointment that is considered part of the patient's routine follow-up care. There is no CDT code for the post-operative suture removal procedure.

Clinical Coding Scenario #8:
Apicoectomy with Bony Defect

A 36-year-old patient presents complaining of pain on tooth #9. The tooth is very dark and the soft tissues buccal to the tooth exhibit swelling and fluctuance. Radiographic examination (two periapical images and a CBCT image of a portion of the lower jaw were captured and interpreted) reveals a very large periapical radiolucency associated with tooth #9. The patient reports a history of a traumatic injury involving the tooth when he was a child. An antibiotic was prescribed.

The next morning, the patient returns and endodontic therapy of tooth #9 is performed. Later that same day, surgical exposure of the area is performed, with an incision extending from the distal of #8 to the distal of #10 to reveal a large area of perforation of the buccal cortical plate. Curettage of the bony defect was performed to reveal the lesion extends to the palatal cortical plate, with a through and through lesion. Apicoectomy of tooth #9 was completed, the bony defect was irrigated, and 2 gm of bone graft material was placed, followed by a resorbable collagen membrane.

How would these procedures be documented?

Visit #1: Initial Appointment

Radiographs

> **D0220**   **intraoral – periapical first radiographic image**
>
> **D0230**   **intraoral – periapical each additional radiographic image**
>
> **D0364**   **cone beam CT capture and interpretation with limited field of view – less than one whole jaw**

Oral Evaluation

> **D0140**   **limited oral evaluation – problem focused**

Prescribe antibiotic – No applicable CDT code

Note: D9630 drugs or medicaments dispensed in office for home use is not applicable since the nomenclature states this procedure applies to drugs or medicaments dispensed in the office for home use, and its descriptor specifically excludes writing prescriptions.

Continued on next page

Visit #2

Root canal on #9

D3310   endodontic therapy, anterior tooth (excluding final restoration)

Visit #3

Apicoectomy on #9

D3410   apicoectomy – anterior

Note: Curettage and irrigation of the bony defect require no separate CDT code; these actions are considered a component of the D3410 procedure.

Placement of 2 gm of bone graft material to preserve the bone around teeth #8 and #9.

D3428   bone graft in conjunction with periradicular surgery – per tooth, single site

D3429   bone graft in conjunction with periradicular surgery – each additional contiguous tooth in the same surgical site

D3432   guided tissue regeneration, resorbable barrier, per site, in conjunction with periradicular surgery

Note: **D7955 repair of maxillofacial soft and/or hard tissue defect** could apply depending on how much the defect that requires bone grafting extends beyond the treated tooth. But, D7955 should not be reported in addition to D3428 or D3429.

Clinical Coding Scenario #9:
Non-carious Cervical Resorption Lesion

A patient presents with invasive cervical resorption on the buccal of tooth #18. It was discovered during a routine hygiene appointment when a periapical and a bitewing radiograph were taken. The tooth has no symptoms. It is clear that this lesion is not caries, as a cavitated lesion cannot be detected with any type of explorer. There is no periapical radiolucency.

When areas of resorption are suspected, the American Association of Endodontics and the American Association of Oral and Maxillofacial Radiography recommend the following: "Limited field of view CBCT is the imaging modality of choice in the localization and differentiation of external and internal resorptive defects and the determination of appropriate treatment and prognosis."

The CBCT scan is taken and a diagnosis of a Heithersay Class I external cervical invasive resorption on the buccal surface of the tooth #18 is made. The treatment plan includes surgical exposure of the resorptive defect followed by external repair of the resorptive lesion.

A full thickness mucoperiosteal flap is reflected and the area of resorption is identified and excavated. There is no exposure of the pulp in the excavation of the resorptive defect. The area of resorption is then treated with 90% trichloracetic acid to arrest the progression of the resorption. The defect is restored with a resin-modified glass ionomer. The area is surgically closed and sutures are placed. The patient is instructed to return for suture removal and continued follow up to monitor the pulpal status and to identify any onset of pulpitis.

How would you code for this scenario?

> **D0140** limited oral evaluation – problem focused
>
> **D0220** intraoral – periapical first radiographic image
>
> **D0270** bitewing – single radiographic image
>
> **D0364** cone beam CT capture and interpretation with limited field of view – less than one whole jaw
>
> **D3473** surgical repair of root resorption – molar
>
> **D2391** resin-based composite – one surface, posterior

Clinical Coding Scenario #10:
Surgical Exposure of Root Surface for Exploration

A patient presents for evaluation and treatment of tooth #10, which has a persistent sinus tract. The tooth has a history of root canal therapy two years previously. Radiographic examination with a periapical radiograph reveals a small periapical radiolucency. Clinically, no significant periodontal probing defects are seen, and the sinus tract can be traced to the apex of tooth #10.

When evaluating a previously endodontically treated tooth with a non-healing lesion, the American Association of Endodontics and the American Association of Oral and Maxillofacial Radiography recommend the following:

> "Limited field of view CBCT should be the imaging modality of choice when evaluating the non-healing of previous endodontic treatment to help determine the need for further treatment, such as nonsurgical, surgical or extraction."

A CBCT scan is taken, and a diagnosis of chronic apical abscess of previously endodontically treated tooth #10 is made. The treatment plan includes surgical exposure of the periapex of tooth #10 followed by apicoectomy, if indicated.

A submarginal mucoperiosteal flap is reflected, and a perforating defect is seen in the buccal cortex over the periapex of tooth #10. Curettage of the apical lesion is performed, and the root surface can be visualized to reveal a 6 mm vertical root fracture from the mid-root to the apex of the tooth. At this point, the prognosis of the tooth is determined to be guarded and extraction is indicated. Due to treatment planning and esthetic considerations, the extraction will be done at a later date. The area is surgically closed and sutures are placed.

How would you code for this scenario?

D0140 limited oral evaluation – problem focused

D0220 intraoral – periapical first radiographic image

D0364 cone beam CT capture and interpretation with limited field of view – less than one whole jaw

D3501 surgical exposure of root surface without apicoectomy or repair of root resorption – anterior

Note: D3501 describes the procedure of exposing the root surface followed by observation and surgical closure of the exposed area; this procedure is not used for or delivered in conjunction with apicoectomy or repair of root resorption.

Remember, the existence of a code does not mean that this code will be covered by a given patient's dental benefits, despite recommendations by a dental professional.

Clinical Coding Scenario #11:
Pulpal Regeneration

Visit #1: Initial Appointment

A 12-year-old patient presents with a somewhat painful tooth #29. The parent noticed that the child avoids chewing on the tooth.

Clinical examination is performed, and radiographs (one bitewing and one periapical) are taken. There is mild swelling in the vestibule, buccal to tooth #29. It is percussion sensitive, palpation sensitive, slightly mobile (Class I), and there are no probing depths over 3 mm. The tooth is sensitive to biting on the Tooth Slooth® and is non-responsive to pulp vitality testing. The tooth has never been restored and no caries is present, radiographically or clinically. Radiographically, a moderately-sized periapical radiolucency is present. There is a very tall pulp chamber, making the enamel look like a thin shell, rather than a thick band over the occlusal area of the pulp chamber. The apex of the tooth has an immature foramen with no apical constriction, and the apical opening is over 1 mm wide. The tooth appears 3–5 mm shorter than adjacent tooth #28.

A diagnosis of pulpal necrosis and acute apical abscess is made. The etiology is determined to be that a dens evaginatus tubercle had previously fractured and led to ingress of bacteria and eventual pulpal necrosis. A treatment plan for pulpal regeneration is discussed, and with the parent's consent, treatment is initiated.

Local anesthetic is administered, a rubber dam is placed, and an access opening is made. The canal is appropriately instrumented and irrigated according to established protocols. Calcium hydroxide or antibiotic paste is placed as an intracanal medicament and a temporary restoration is placed.

What CDT codes are applicable for the procedures delivered during this visit?

Visit #1

D0140	**limited oral evaluation – problem focused**
D0220	**intraoral – periapical first radiographic image**
D0270	**bitewing – single radiographic image**
D0460	**pulp vitality tests**
D3355	**pulpal regeneration – initial visit**

Continued on next page

Visit #2

The patient is asymptomatic at the second visit, three weeks after initiation of treatment. There is no swelling, and the tooth is not abnormally mobile, but the patient is unable to chew normally upon tooth #29. Local anesthetic is administered, a rubber dam is placed, the tooth is re-instrumented, re-irrigated, and re-medicated, and a temporary restoration is placed.

The CDT code for the second visit is:

D3356 pulpal regeneration – interim medication replacement

#3

Three weeks have passed since the second visit. The tooth is now completely normal; all symptoms have resolved. Local anesthetic is administered, a rubber dam is placed, and the canal space is re-irrigated to remove all intracanal medicament. Apical bleeding is initiated, a bioceramic barrier is placed in the cervical area of the root canal, and a composite restoration is placed in the access opening. A final radiograph is taken for documentation and to be used as a baseline for future follow up. Regular follow-up visits are recommended to monitor the maturation of the root of tooth #29.

The CDT codes for this third visit are:

D3357 pulpal regeneration – completion of treatment

D2391 resin-based composite – one surface, posterior

Clinical Coding Scenario #12:
Decoronation

A 10-year-old patient of record returns to the office for periodic review tooth #8 with a history of dental trauma and avulsion 2 years ago. At that time, the tooth was reimplanted and root canal therapy was completed. Clinical examination reveals that the tooth exhibits 2 mm infra-positioning, and radiographic examination with periapical radiographs and CBCT reveals evidence of advanced replacement root resorption. The tooth was deemed non-savable and treatment planned for decoronation to retain the root and preserve ridge height and width until patient reaches suitable age for implant placement.

The patient returns for the decoronation procedure, and a mucosal flap is reflected and the tooth is decoronated at the level of the osseous crest. The root canal obturation material is removed to facilitate osseous integration, and the flap is re-approximated and sutured. A post-treatment radiograph is taken. The patient returns for suture removal.

What procedure codes would be used to document and report the services provided during each of these visits?

Visit #1

D0120 **periodic oral evaluation – established patient**

D0220 **intraoral – periapical first radiographic image**

D0364 **cone beam CT capture and interpretation with limited field of view – less than one whole jaw**

Visit #2: Decoronation

D3921 **decoronation or submergence of an erupted tooth**

Visit #3: Post-operative Follow Up, Sutures Removed

D0171 **re-evaluation – post-operative office visit**

Note: D3921 describes procedures for Intentional removal of coronal tooth structure for preservation of the root and surrounding bone.

Clinical Coding Scenario #13:
Decompression and Root Canal Therapy

Visit #1: Initial Appointment

A 16-year-old patient presents with facial swelling and pain associated with tooth #8. Prior history of this tooth includes a traumatic injury years previously when the patient was hit in the mouth with a baseball.

Clinical examination is performed, and periapical radiographs (at different angles) are taken. There is significant facial swelling and swelling in the buccal vestibule, buccal to tooth #8. The tooth is painful to percussion and palpation and is the only tooth in the area which is non-responsive to pulp vitality testing. The tooth has never been restored and no caries is present, radiographically or clinically. Radiographically, a large apical lucency is seen to encompass the apices of teeth #7 and #9.

A diagnosis of pulpal necrosis and acute apical abscess is made. A treatment plan for initiation of root canal therapy, with the possible need for further intervention is discussed, and with the parent's consent, treatment is initiated.

Local anesthetic is administered, a rubber dam is placed, and an access opening is made. Significant purulent drainage exudes from the canal. The canal is appropriately instrumented and irrigated according to established protocols. Calcium hydroxide is placed as an intracanal medicament and a temporary restoration is placed.

What CDT codes are applicable for the procedures delivered during this visit?

Visit #1

D0140	**limited oral evaluation – problem focused**
D0220	**intraoral – periapical first radiographic image**
D0270	**bitewing – single radiographic image**
D0364	**cone beam CT capture and interpretation with limited field of view – less than one whole jaw**
D0460	**pulp vitality tests**
D3221	**pulpal debridement, primary and permanent teeth**

Continued on next page

Visit #2

The patient returns three weeks after initiation of treatment. Although the facial swelling has resolved, there is still swelling in the vestibule. Local anesthetic is administered, a rubber dam is placed, the tooth is accessed, and significant purulent exudate can be expressed from the canal with gentle pressure on the vestibular swelling. The tooth is re-instrumented, re-irrigated, and re-medicated with Calcium Hydroxide, and a temporary restoration is placed. Further discussion with the patient's parents about the persistence of the large cyst-like infection includes the recommendation for decompression, as conservative treatment with decompression may allow healing with periapical surgery. With the parents' consent, a vestibular incision is made and a surgical catheter is placed. The patient is given home care instructions to irrigate through the catheter daily.

D7509   marsupialization of odontogenic cyst
Surgical decompression of a large cystic lesion by creating a long-term open pocket or pouch.

Note: D7509 is a code effective January 1, 2023 to report surgical decompression of a large cystic lesion. This code is not used to document surgical excision of a periradicular cyst.

Visits #3, 4, and 5

The patient returns two, six, and ten weeks later for evaluation of healing. He is comfortable and the swelling has not returned. The patency of the surgical catheter is confirmed at each visit and the lesion is irrigated with sterile saline through the catheter.

D0171   re-evaluation – post-operative visit

Visit #6

At this visit, the catheter is removed and root canal therapy is completed. Local anesthetic is administered, a rubber dam is placed, and the tooth is accessed with no signs of purulent drainage. The canal is irrigated, the Calcium Hydroxide is removed, and the canal is obturated. A final restoration with composite is used to close the access opening.

D3310   endodontic therapy, anterior tooth (excluding final restoration)

D2391   resin-based composite – one surface, posterior

Coding Q&A

1. *Are the pretreatment evaluation and preoperative radiographs included in the code for root canal therapy?*

   No, the CDT manual guidelines specifically state that endodontic therapy does not include diagnostic evaluation, testing, and radiographs/diagnostic images. Prior to initiating endodontic therapy, the practitioner can and should use CDT codes to record the services provided to the patient. All intraoperative images, however, are included in the CDT category for endodontic therapy.

2. *I submitted the CDT code **D3911 intraorifice barrier** to my insurance company and they have disallowed the code saying that it is a part of the endodontic treatment, and will not allow me to collect a fee from the patient. Should I just stop using the code?*

   CDT codes are to be used to document the procedures performed. In this case, if an intraorifice barrier is placed, the practitioner is justified to submit the code for the procedure performed. Many times insurers will try to "bundle" procedures that the Code Maintenance Committee determines to be a distinct procedure into a larger procedure code. In addition, third party payers have policies, based upon the agreement with the subscribers, on what they will or will not cover. Nevertheless, as practitioners it is important to record procedures performed through use of the CDT codes. This information will allow for a record of the frequency of use of the codes and may also allow the information to be used for future metrics on prognosis studies. The hope is that this can influence insurers to change their policies and fairly recognize the procedures performed.

3. *I worked really hard on a tooth that had six root canals in it and it seems like I should be able to have a code to express the difficulty of the case.*

   CDT codes for documenting and reporting endodontic therapy procedures by tooth type or location (e.g., anterior, premolar, molar) were established with CDT-1, effective January 1, 1990. This change replaced dental procedure codes based on number of canals per tooth (2, 3, or 4), plus a separate code for "each additional canal" that is used when needed. The rationale was that tooth anatomy or location better reflects the degree of difficulty most often encountered in clinical situations.

4. *I want to use an expensive adjunct irrigant or irrigating device instead of, or in addition to, the traditional sodium hypochlorite that is commonly used. What code can I use to reflect the additional expertise and expense?*

Irrigation as well as other aspects of endodontic therapy are considered part of the procedure itself and are included in the code set for the type of tooth for which the root canal is performed. Separating out what is generally considered part of the procedure is often called "unbundling." From an ethical perspective, intentional unbundling by a dentist to increase reimbursement and intentional bundling by a third-party payer to decrease reimbursement are both considered inappropriate.

5. *How can I use the CDT Code to describe that I have done an endodontic therapy in two visits instead of one visit? It costs the dentist more to do it in two visits, and I think that should be reflected.*

This is a common inquiry made to the American Association of Endodontists that has multiple considerations. One question is about how to document the two visits. The first visit, when the need for RCT is diagnosed and then started, may be recorded with D3999 for record-keeping purposes. In cases when emergency treatment was performed on the first visit, **D3221 pulpal debridement, primary and permanent teeth** is appropriate. Then, at the second appointment, the typical D3330 code is used to reflect the completion of the treatment.

The second, implied question seems to be more about how to charge more for the procedure than the dentist's established full D3330 fee. There is not a simple answer, as every dentist is responsible for determining their fee and when doing so must consider the legal and ethical ramifications of having different full fees for the same procedure. This consideration should include a review of your participating provider contracts in effect and discussion with your legal counsel.

In addition, coding for a root canal that was never actually finished is a recurring issue. If the code for the root canal is submitted, but the procedure has not been completed, corrections must be made with the dental benefits company involved, and explanations must be made to the patient and any other dentist or specialist who becomes involved in the completion of the treatment. Clear communication using the codes as the language and descriptor for treatment performed is helpful for all parties involved.

6. *What is the difference between using the apexification codes and the pulpal regeneration codes?*

The procedures are very different in their intentions.

Apexification is a procedure that had previously been the only option to treat teeth that had necrotic pulp and open apices and immature root formation. Long-term calcium hydroxide treatment was used until a hard tissue bridge formed over the apex. Gutta-percha could then be safely condensed against that bridge, in a manner that prevented the root filling material from extruding into the periapical tissues.

In contrast, pulpal regeneration is a different way to treat these teeth with necrotic pulp and open apices and immature root formation. Pulpal regeneration involves disinfection of the root canal system and using stem cell technology to stimulate ingrowth of pulp-like tissue into the root canal. This process promotes maturation of the root, including closure of the open apex, and increased length and width of the root canal walls.

7. *When is it appropriate to use* **D3331 treatment of root canal obstruction; non-surgical access**?

This code is used to document a procedure that is delivered infrequently and for extremely difficult cases, such as one where the root canal is more than 50% calcified. The code can also be used when a dentist separates an instrument in the root canal and then refers the case to a specialist who is able to remove it using their expertise and specialized equipment.

8. *I planned to do an apicoectomy but, upon initiating the treatment and removing the pathology around the root, I discovered a root fracture that traveled the length of the root, and the tooth is significantly compromised. I did not proceed with the treatment and recommended further treatment planning for extraction and replacement of the tooth. What is the appropriate code to use for this situation?*

The codes **D3501 surgical exposure of root surface without apicoectomy or repair of root resorption – anterior**, **D3502 surgical exposure of root surface without apicoectomy or repair of root resorption – premolar**, and **D3503 surgical exposure of root surface without apicoectomy or repair of root resorption – molar** are the codes specifically designed for use in this situation.

9. *When retreating a root canal that had a post and core, I had to spend a significant amount of time removing the post prior to performing the retreatment. I submitted the codes for post removal and retreatment, and the dental benefits company denied benefits for the post removal. What should I do?*

    Coding for this scenario is straightforward as there are two separate procedures – **D2955 post removal and D3346 retreatment of previous root canal therapy – anterior** (or D3347 or D3348). In cases when the procedure requires more than one visit, D2955 (post removal) is usually completed and posted on the first visit, and the root canal retreatment (e.g., D3346) is posted on the second or final visit when this separate procedure is completed.

    While post removal is clearly a distinct procedure separate from retreatment of previous root canal therapy, some dental benefit companies "bundle" the post removal into the retreatment for adjudication and reimbursement calculation purposes. According to the ADA, bundling, or the "the systematic combining of distinct dental procedures by third-party payers that results in a reduced benefit for the patient/beneficiary" is frowned upon. Dentists who have signed participating provider agreements with third-party payers may be bound to plan provisions that limit or exclude coverage. Submission of a short narrative with the original claim or appeal, explaining the complexity of the post removal along with radiographs and/or photographs, may be helpful in obtaining full available reimbursement for both procedures.

10. *A patient was referred to me after a dentist attempted endodontic treatment and perforated the furcation of tooth #19. I repaired the perforation with bioceramic putty internally and completed the endodontic therapy. How do I code for the placement of the bioceramic putty?*

    D3333 internal root repair of perforation defects is used for the perforation repair procedure. The use of bioceramic putty is not relevant as the CDT code entry does not specify (i.e., limit) the material that the dentist may select to repair the perforation defect.

11. *What do I need to know about a dental dam, its use in endodontic treatment and the applicable CDT code for documentation and reporting?*

    A dental dam is a sheet of latex or rubber-like material with a punched hole to allow placement around a tooth prior to an endodontic procedure. Dental dam isolation minimizes the risk of contaminating the root system by oral bacteria during endodontic treatment. Additional benefits of dam placement include aiding in visualization by providing a clean operating field and preventing ingestion or aspiration of dental materials, irrigants and instruments. Dental dam placement is documented using CDT code **D3910 surgical procedure for isolation of tooth with rubber dam**.

Summary

Endodontic procedure coding can be relatively straightforward given that most of the codes are self-explanatory. CDT codes effective on the date of service are integral to a complete patient record as they describe the endodontic treatment that has been performed. "Code for what you do" is the fundamental rule in all coding situations. The existence of a procedure code does not necessarily mean that it is a covered service of a given dental benefit plan. Unless a code is used appropriately and submitted, dental benefit plans will not have a history of the frequency of use or fees associated with the procedures performed. By consistently coding for endodontic procedures as they are performed, we may influence third-party payers for consideration of coverage in the future.

Contributor Biography

Elizabeth Shin Perry, D.M.D., is a board-certified endodontist and has been in private practice in Westfield, Massachusetts since 1995. She holds a faculty appointment at the Harvard School of Dental Medicine where she is a clinical instructor in the Advanced Graduate Program in Endodontics. Dr. Perry is a graduate of the University of Pennsylvania and the Harvard School of Dental Medicine. She completed her post-doctoral residency in endodontics at the University of Connecticut. Dr. Perry currently serves on the Board of Directors of the American Association of Endodontists. She is past chair of the Practice Affairs Committee and has also served on the Regenerative Endodontics and Nominations Committees of the American Association of Endodontists. She is a Fellow of the International College of Dentists. Dr. Perry has been active in code maintenance nationally since 2016 and also represents the AAE as a voting member of the American Dental Association's Code Maintenance Committee.

By Marie Schweinebraten, D.M.D.

Introduction

Periodontal treatment has seen many changes over time. For example, different types of grafting materials, both autogenous and non-autogenous, are more common. Dental implants are often included in periodontal treatment planning. Bone regeneration has become more predictable with the availability of new products and techniques. Periodontal procedure coding has grown with these changes as has the knowledge base required to code correctly and obtain reimbursement for the treatment completed.

Periodontics has always been a category that includes both non-surgical and surgical procedures. What complicates matters is that some of the coded procedures are site specific while others are tooth or quadrant (four or more teeth; one to three teeth) specific. Adding to the confusion is that procedure codes have become differentiated as to the type of material used as well as whether the procedure is performed on a tooth or implant. Many periodontal procedures overlap with procedures from other categories, resulting in additional considerations for coding correctly.

Thus, for a given outcome, there could be a number of separate procedures involved, each documented with its individual CDT code. Grafts are an example of such "á la carte" coding. Bone graft materials are listed separately from the procedure for achieving access – osseous surgery (D4260 or D4261) or gingival flap (D4240 or D4241). There are separate codes for other procedures that may be required in a graft case, including placement of barriers or biologic materials to aid in regeneration.

It is especially important in the Periodontics category to realize that procedure codes are meant to describe the treatment rendered, not the means that are used to accomplish the treatment. For example, a gingivectomy can be done utilizing several techniques, including a blade, a periodontal knife, or a laser. The code for the procedure, however, is the same.

With attention to detail and a basic understanding of periodontal treatment and the accompanying codes, including required attachments to be submitted, a dental office can prevent confusion for the patient and misunderstanding of plan coverage while at the same time obtaining reimbursement as effectively and efficiently as possible.

Key Definitions and Concepts

Full quadrant: The mouth is divided into four quadrants. A full quadrant is defined for coding purposes as four or more teeth.

> The ADA Glossary definition of **quadrant** is "One of the four equal sections into which the dental arches can be divided; begins at the midline of the arch and extends distally to the last tooth."

Partial quadrant: One to three contiguous teeth or bounded tooth spaces, when present within the same quadrant, is defined for coding purposes as a partial quadrant.

Site: The term site is used to describe a single area or position. "Site" is frequently used to describe an area of recession on a single tooth or an osseous defect adjacent to a single tooth. It can also apply to soft tissue or osseous defects in an edentulous area.

For example:

- If two contiguous teeth have areas of recession, each tooth is considered a single site.

- If two contiguous teeth have adjacent but separate osseous defects, each defect is a single site. If these defects communicate, however, they would be considered a single site.

- Up to two contiguous tooth positions in an edentulous area may be considered a single site.

> The ADA Glossary definition of **site** is "A term used to describe a single area, position, or locus. For periodontal procedures, an area of soft tissue recession on a single tooth or an osseous defect adjacent to a single tooth; also used to indicate soft tissue defects and/or osseous defects in edentulous tooth positions."

Autogenous soft tissue graft: Donor graft material is taken from the patient's mouth resulting in a second surgical site.

> The ADA Glossary definition of **autogenous graft** is "Taken from one part of a patient's body and transferred to another."

Key Definitions and Concepts

Non-autogenous: There is no second surgical site in the patient's mouth. The graft material comes from another source.

> The ADA Glossary definition of **non-autogenous** is "A graft from donor other than patient."

Notes:

> The term "non-autogenous" is commonly understood to be any type of graft material that is not from the patient's body. In other words allogenic, alloplastic, allograft and xenograft materials are considered non-autogenous.
>
> Non-autogenous or synthetic soft or hard tissue graft materials include AlloDerm®, Fibro-Gide®, Oracell®; and "bone out of a bottle" products such as Bio-Oss® or OSSIF-i sem™.
>
> More information about grafts and procedures is in the ADA Guide to Graft Material Collection Procedures that is available on the *CDT Coding Education web page*.

Changes to This Category

The Periodontics category in CDT 2023 includes one addition and six revisions.

The addition is:

D4286   removal of non-resorbable barrier

There were no deletions.

The revisions are:

D4240   gingival flap procedure, including root planing – four or more contiguous teeth or tooth bound spaces per quadrant
A soft tissue flap is reflected or resected to allow debridement of the root surface and the removal of granulation tissue. Osseous recontouring is not accomplished in conjunction with this procedure. May include open flap curettage, reverse bevel flap surgery, modified Kirkland flap procedure, and modified Widman surgery. This procedure is performed in the presence of moderate to deep probing depths, loss of attachment, need to maintain esthetics, need for increased access to the root surface and alveolar bone, or to determine the presence of a cracked tooth, or fractured root ~~or external root resorption~~. Other procedures may be required concurrent to D4240 and should be reported separately using their own unique codes.

D4241   gingival flap procedure, including root planing – one to three contiguous teeth or tooth bound spaces per quadrant
A soft tissue flap is reflected or resected to allow debridement of the root surface and the removal of granulation tissue. Osseous recontouring is not accomplished in conjunction with this procedure. May include open flap curettage, reverse bevel flap surgery, modified Kirkland flap procedure, and modified Widman surgery. This procedure is performed in the presence of moderate to deep probing depths, loss of attachment, need to maintain esthetics, need for increased access to the root surface and alveolar bone, or to determine the presence of a cracked tooth, or fractured root, ~~or external root resorption~~ Other procedures may be required concurrent to D4241 and should be reported separately using their own unique codes.

D4266 **guided tissue regeneration, natural teeth – resorbable barrier, per site**
This procedure does not include flap entry and closure, or, when indicated, wound debridement, osseous contouring, bone replacement grafts, and placement of biologic materials to aid in osseous regeneration. This procedure can be used for periodontal defects around natural teeth and peri-implant defects.

D4267 **guided tissue regeneration, natural teeth – non-resorbable barrier, per site (includes membrane removal)**
This procedure does not include flap entry and closure, or, when indicated, wound debridement, osseous contouring, bone replacement grafts, and placement of biologic materials to aid in osseous regeneration. This procedure can be used for periodontal defects around natural teeth and peri-implant defects.

D4355 **full mouth debridement to enable a comprehensive oral periodontal evaluation and diagnosis on a subsequent visit**
Full mouth debridement involves the preliminary removal of plaque and calculus that interferes with the ability of the dentist to perform a comprehensive oral evaluation. Not to be completed on the same day as D0150, D0160, or D0180.

D4921 **gingival irrigation with a medicinal agent – per quadrant**
Irrigation of gingival pockets with a prescription medicinal agent. Not to be used to report use of over the counter (OTC) mouth rinses or non-invasive chemical debridement.

Clinical Coding Scenario #1:
Periodontal Abscess

A patient presented in pain and complained about swelling around one tooth. The doctor's emergency evaluation included two periapical radiographic images and pocket measurements of the teeth in the area. The swelling was clearly adjacent to tooth #3, and when the sulcus was probed, both bleeding and suppuration were seen.

The doctor treated the patient for a periodontal abscess by debridement and draining of the sulcus and irrigation of the pocket with chlorhexidine. Before leaving the dentist gave the patient a prescription for an antibiotic.

How could this encounter be coded?

Since the evaluation was problem-focused, the appropriate codes for diagnostic procedures would be:

D0140 limited oral evaluation – problem focused

D0220 intraoral – periapical first radiographic image

D0230 intraoral – periapical each additional radiographic image

In this case, there are a number of codes that might be used to document the operative services, alone or in combination. Possible procedure coding options are:

D9110 palliative treatment of dental pain – per visit

Use of this code to document the service provided may require a narrative to describe the exact treatment rendered. It may be the most appropriate code to use in this case.

An alternative code if drainage was achieved through the periodontal sulcus could be:

D7510 incision and drainage of abscess – intraoral soft tissue
        Involves incision through mucosa, including periodontal origins.

Irrigation of the abscess would be coded as:

D4921 gingival irrigation with a medicinal agent – per quadrant

Clinical Coding Scenario #2:
Periodontitis

A 49-year-old male patient presents for periodontal examination with a chief complaint of sore and bleeding gums. His medical history is significant for type II diabetes being treated with Metformin (Glucophage®) and a beta blocker (naldalol) for hypertension. He smokes one pack of cigarettes a day. His last dental appointment was five years ago, and there are heavy accumulations of plaque and calculus, both supragingival and subgingival.

Since the amount of calculus and plaque prevented a periodontal evaluation from being performed adequately, the patient was seen by the hygienist that same day. Without using any anesthesia, she utilized an ultrasonic scaler to debride supragingival calculus and plaque in all four quadrants. After reviewing home care instructions and giving the patient chlorhexidine rinse, provided by the office, the patient was scheduled to return in two weeks for a comprehensive periodontal evaluation and appropriate radiographic images.

How would these visits be coded?

Visit #1: Assessment and Debridement

D0191 **assessment of a patient**

D4355 **full mouth debridement to enable a comprehensive periodontal evaluation and diagnosis on a subsequent visit**

D1330 **oral hygiene instructions**

D9630 **drugs or medicaments dispensed in the office for home use**

Visit #2: Evaluation, Diagnosis, and Treatment Planning

Two weeks later, the patient returned for radiographic images and a complete periodontal evaluation.

The diagnosis is Stage III Grade C periodontitis with pocket depths ranging from 4 to 9 mm, furcation involvement, mobility, and localized recession. The patient also shows signs of xerostomia, with cervical caries present, which may be caused by the beta blocker. Consultation with the patient's internist to evaluate possibility of changing the high blood pressure medication was done by the dentist.

Continued on next page

A complete oral evaluation was done with full mouth periapical radiographic images taken. The diagnostic findings were:

1. Missing teeth #1, #5, #12, #16, #17, #21, #28, and #32. The premolars were extracted for orthodontic reasons when he was a teenager.

2. Bone loss of up to 40 percent around the posterior teeth with pocket depths ranging from 5 to 9 mm in the posterior

3. Heavy accumulations of plaque and calculus supra- and subgingival

4. Furcation involvement on the molars

5. Mobility of teeth

6. Cervical caries: Teeth #3, #4, #13, #22, #27, and #29.

7. Inadequate oral hygiene

The evaluation and diagnosis led to a multiple-appointment treatment plan for this patient – four quadrants of scaling and root planing spread across two appointments and a third appointment four to six weeks after the initial therapy for a post-operative visit to assess the outcome.

Note: Some dental benefit plans will not cover four quadrants of SRP delivered at one appointment.

CDT codes for the services delivered and planned during the second visit follow:

D0180 **comprehensive periodontal evaluation – new or established patient**

D0210 **intraoral – comprehensive series of radiographic images**

D1330 **oral hygiene instructions**

D9311 **consultation with a medical health care professional**

Visit #3: SRP – Two Quadrants

D4341 **periodontal scaling and root planing – four or more teeth per quadrant**

Note: This procedure is reported twice, and the two quadrants treated (e.g., maxillary right and mandibular right) are identified by entering the applicable area of the oral cavity code on the claim.

Continued on next page

Visit #4: SRP – Two Quadrants

D4341   periodontal scaling and root planing – four or more teeth per quadrant

This procedure is reported twice, and the two quadrants treated (e.g., maxillary left and mandibular left) are identified by entering the applicable area of the oral cavity code on the claim.

Visit #5: Four to Six Weeks after SRP Completed

D0171   re-evaluation – post-operative office visit

Re-charting was done at this appointment after healing of the scaling and root planing. Although some improvement was noted, significant pocket depths with bleeding on probing in the posterior quadrants were evident. The dentist felt that the patient would benefit from osseous surgery in the posterior quadrants (D4260) at a later date. The medical consultation from the first appointment was returned, and the physician plans to change the patient's hypertension medication. The necessary restorative procedures to address the cervical caries on teeth #3, #4, #13, #22, #27, and #29 were scheduled for subsequent appointments.

Clinical Coding Scenario #3:
Treatment to Eliminate Periodontal Pocketing

A 60-year-old female has been under care since having scaling and root planing done eight months ago, followed by periodic **D4910 periodontal maintenance** every three months. The patient decided she is ready to proceed with the planned treatment to eliminate periodontal pocketing but is very anxious about the surgery. Before proceeding, the doctor completed a new periodontal chart to assess her current situation. Since the full mouth radiographs were less than a year old, no additional radiographs were necessary.

Note: If additional radiographs are deemed necessary for a better diagnosis, there may not be reimbursement by the dental benefit plan if coverage provisions have diagnostic imaging frequency limitations.

The diagnostic findings are as follows:

1. Missing teeth #1, #2, #16, #17, #18, and #32
2. Bone loss is generalized and ranges from 10–50 percent with periodontal pocket depths up to 5 to 9 mm
3. Furcation involvement in the molar areas
4. Vertical defects on the distal of tooth #19 and the mesial of tooth #21
5. Periodontal bleeding on probing in the periodontal pocket areas
6. Patient apprehension to dental treatment

What CDT code is used to report the periodontal charting completed at this appointment?

Charting is considered to be a part of a D0180 comprehensive periodontal evaluation procedure, which also should include details such as bleeding on probing, furcation involvement, mobility, recession, and clinical attachment loss. These findings may also be part of a D0150 comprehensive oral evaluation. It is recommended that periodontal charting and evaluation be completed annually for patients with a history of periodontitis.

The patient's next appointment was for four quadrants of osseous surgery and bone grafts in conjunction with biologics and barriers to enhance regeneration addressing the defects on teeth #19 and #21. These procedures would be delivered with the patient under conscious sedation due to her anxiety.

Continued on next page

Services delivered during this appointment would be coded as follows:

For four quadrants of osseous surgery:

D4260 **osseous surgery (including elevation of a full thickness flap and closure) – four of more contiguous teeth or tooth bounded spaces per quadrant**

Note: This procedure is reported four times as it is a "per quadrant" service and all four quadrants were involved (maxillary right and left; mandibular right and left) by entering the applicable area of the oral cavity code on the claim on this date of service. A provider should also remember that pre-treatment estimates will help determine plan limitations that may affect reimbursement, such as limiting the number of quadrants allowed at one visit.

For tooth #19 (distal):

D4263 **bone replacement graft – retained natural tooth – first site in quadrant**

D4265 **biologic materials to aid in soft and osseous tissue regeneration, per site**

D4266 **guided tissue regeneration, natural teeth – resorbable barrier, per site**

For tooth #21 (mesial):

D4264 **bone replacement graft – retained natural tooth – each additional site in quadrant**

D4265 **biologic materials to aid in soft and osseous tissue regeneration, per site**

D4266 **guided tissue regeneration, natural teeth – resorbable barrier, per site**

For 2.5 hours of anesthesia:

D9239 **intravenous moderate (conscious) sedation/analgesia – first 15 minutes**

D9243 **intravenous moderate (conscious) sedation – each subsequent 15 minute increment**

Continued on next page

Note: Since the anesthesia procedure took 2.5 hours (150 minutes) and these codes are reported in 15-minute increments, the patient record and claim would document the first 15 minutes of sedation, D9239, once and then document the additional 135 minutes with D9243 and a "Quantity" of nine.

The patient returned for a post-surgery check two weeks later for suture removal, light cleansing of the affected areas, and oral hygiene instructions. At that time, the doctor determined that the patient would benefit from an antimicrobial mouth rinse (chlorhexidine), which the office provided.

CDT codes for this visit are:

D0171   re-evaluation – post-operative office visit

D1330   oral hygiene instructions

D9630   drugs or medicaments dispensed in the office for home use

Clinical Coding Scenario #4:
Scaling in the Presence of Mucositis around an Implant

A patient of record who has been on a D4910 periodontal maintenance treatment plan presents with the complaint of soreness around the implant for tooth #5. Examination revealed bleeding with probing around the implant accompanied by swelling and some suppuration. Resulting pocket depths were 4–5 mm. A periapical radiograph was taken, which indicated bone height comparable to that seen previously after the implant was placed.

The doctor treated this area with debridement and curettage using local anesthesia. The periodontal maintenance procedure was not done at this appointment, but scheduled approximately three to four weeks later when a re-evaluation could be performed on the implant treated.

How would this encounter be coded?

Visit #1: Initial Appointment

D0140 **limited oral evaluation – problem focused**

D0220 **intraoral – periapical first radiographic image**

D6081 **scaling and debridement in the presence of inflammation or mucositis of a single implant, including cleaning of the implant surfaces, without flap entry and closure**

Note: According to this code's descriptor, a D6081 procedure is not performed in conjunction with D1110, D4910, or D4346.

Subsequent Visit

D0171 **re-evaluation – post-operative office visit**

D4910 **periodontal maintenance**

Chapter 5: D4000–D4999 Periodontics

Clinical Coding Scenario #5:
Overdue Patient with Gingivitis

A patient of record in the office has not been seen for over two years. When they arrive for a routine prophylaxis, the evaluation reveals heavy plaque, some supragingival and subgingival calculus, and moderate stain. Bleeding on probing is noted on most teeth, accompanied by edema and swelling. No bone loss is seen on the vertical bitewing radiographs that are taken. From the clinical evaluation, a diagnosis of generalized moderate to severe gingivitis is made. The hygienist proceeds with full mouth scaling, not a prophylaxis, noting that this scaling procedure requires more time than needed for a prophylaxis.

How should this appointment be coded for reimbursement?

Since the patient has not been seen in the office for over two years, a comprehensive periodontal evaluation should be done. This includes both dental and periodontal charting, with pocket depths, bleeding points, and any additional findings such as suppuration and edema.

D0180 **comprehensive periodontal evaluation – new or established patient**

As mentioned, bitewing radiographs were also taken, so you would also use the following code regardless of whether the radiographs were vertical or horizontal:

D0274 **bitewings – four radiographic images**

Note: If the need for a panoramic radiograph is indicated (i.e., it has been five or more years since the patient has had a panoramic or full mouth series of radiographs), that procedure would be reported separately with **D0330 panoramic radiographic image**.

In this case, a comprehensive periodontal evaluation has been done and treatment will be done at the same visit. Since the diagnosis is generalized moderate to severe gingivitis, a routine adult prophylaxis is not appropriate – the applicable procedure is:

D4346 **scaling in the presence of generalized moderate or severe gingival inflammation – full mouth, after oral evaluation**
The removal of plaque, calculus and stains from supra- and subgingival tooth surfaces when there is generalized moderate or severe gingival inflammation in the absence of periodontitis. It is indicated for patients who have swollen, inflamed gingiva, generalized suprabony pockets, and moderate to severe bleeding on probing. Should not be reported in conjunction with prophylaxis, scaling and root planing, or debridement procedures.

Continued on next page

This scenario emphasizes that an evaluation can be done the same day as treatment when scaling is coded as D4346. The D4346 procedure differs from **D4355 full mouth debridement to enable a comprehensive periodontal evaluation and diagnosis on a subsequent visit** as the full mouth debridement procedure addresses removal of accumulations and inflammation present that do not allow a comprehensive periodontal evaluation to be done. For example, pocket depths cannot be recorded due to the amount of calculus present both supragingivally and subgingivally, and inflammation will need to subside before pocket depths can be adequately evaluated to determine further treatment.

Also note that D4346 is a full mouth procedure. It cannot be coded multiple times by quadrant.

Many times, a second procedure of scaling may be necessary to accomplish adequate debridement for patients who have had the D4346 procedure. For example, a re-evaluation (**D0171 re-evaluation – post-operative office visit**) might be appropriate, or a second appointment for a D1110 prophylaxis if inflammation and pocket depths have decreased.

As with all codes, carriers differ as to the benefit allowed for D4346. A clinician should code for what they do, not code for reimbursement. Also remember that unless a code is used appropriately and submitted, carriers will not have a history of the frequency of use or the dentist's full fee for the procedure.

Note: The procedure documented with D4346 is intended to treat patients who have widespread gingival inflammation but no bone or attachment loss. Patients with generally healthy periodontium receive preventive care, and those with periodontal disease involving bone and attachment loss receive therapeutic care. D4346 is not considered treatment for periodontitis and so does not make the patient eligible for periodontal maintenance D4910. Code D4346 documents the procedure that lies between a prophylaxis and a scaling and root planing. The ADA has published a separate document that contains a detailed discussion of the nature, scope, and decision-making process that leads to delivery of the D4346 procedure. This guidance document and its related webinar are found on the "Coding Education" web page linked to the ADA's Code on Dental Procedures and Nomenclature (CDT Code) web page – *ADA.org/CDTEducation.*

Clinical Coding Scenario #6:
Areas of Scaling and Root Planing Involving Three Quadrants

A new patient presents at the office, and during the evaluation that accompanied the prophylaxis, it was determined that areas within three of the oral cavity's four quadrants need scaling and root planing. One quadrant has no periodontal disease, but does require a prophylaxis. All treatment is completed after two appointments.

How could these visits be coded?

Visit #1: Evaluation, Diagnosis, and Treatment Planning

It would be correct to code for an evaluation and the adult prophylaxis.

D0180   comprehensive periodontal evaluation – new or established patient

Note: Periodontal charting including pocket depths and current radiographs will be necessary to support the need for scaling and root planing. A comprehensive periodontal evaluation procedure includes probing and charting as well as clinical evaluation of the patient's overall oral health as described in the D0180 descriptor. If definitive periodontal treatment (SRP) is to be done, full mouth periodontal charting must be completed.

D1110   prophylaxis – adult

Visit #2: SRP – Three Quadrants of Scaling and Root Planing

At a subsequent appointment, the scaling and root planing procedure is delivered, reported by quadrant, and reported with the SRP code applicable to the number of teeth treated in the quadrant.

D4342   periodontal scaling and root planing – one to three teeth per quadrant

or

D4341   periodontal scaling and root planing – four or more teeth per quadrant

D4342 or D4341, or both, are reported depending on the number of teeth treated in the quadrant. The claim service line for each code reported includes the applicable area of the oral cavity code to identify the specific quadrant; specific tooth numbers of the teeth treated may also be reported.

Continued on next page

Notes:

- It is always advisable to request a pre-treatment estimate prior to any periodontal therapy since carriers may have plan limitations that may affect reimbursement. For example, some carriers will only reimburse a maximum of two quadrants of scaling and root planing per appointment.

- In some instances, performing a prophylaxis prior to scaling and root planing can decrease the inflammation and allow a more thorough debridement during scaling and root planing since bleeding will be reduced and access to subgingival calculus and toxins improved.

- In this scenario the dates of service reported for the prophylaxis performed at visit #1, is not the same as the date of service reported for the three quadrants of scaling and root planing delivered during visit #2.

Clinical Coding Scenario #7:
Recession

During a prophylaxis, the patient complains of sensitivity and soreness in the lower anterior area. A comprehensive periodontal evaluation is completed. Findings include 3–4 mm of recession with either no attached gingiva or 1 mm of attached gingiva on teeth #22–#25 and tooth #28, as well as the implant in the area of #29. The threads of the implant are visible on the facial where recession has occurred. Pocketing is 2–3 mm, but the tissue bleeds easily and edema is present. There is no mobility present, but the incisors exhibit slight fremitus with occlusion.

During this initial appointment, there were several other procedures in addition to the routine prophylaxis and oral evaluation. Periapical radiographs were taken of teeth #22–#25 and #28–#29, the teeth with recession. Two intraoral photographs were also taken to visually document the amount of recession, lack of attached gingiva, and the inflammation present. The occlusion was adjusted on the mandibular incisors and homecare (oral hygiene) instructions were provided. This visit concluded with discussion of the treatment plan that addressed the oral evaluation findings.

How could these visits be coded?

Visit #1: Initial Appointment Procedure Coding

D1110 **prophylaxis – adult**

D1330 **oral hygiene instructions**

D0180 **comprehensive periodontal evaluation – new or established patient**

D0220 **intraoral – periapical first radiographic image**

D0230 **intraoral – periapical each additional radiographic image**

(Report the number of additional periapical images in the claim service line's "Quantity" field.)

D0350 **2D oral/facial photographic image obtained intra-orally or extra-orally**

(Report "2" in the "Quantity" field of the claim service line where D0350 is posted.)

D9951 **occlusal adjustment – limited**

Continued on next page

Treatment Plan Notes (Examples)

Evidence of clinical attachment loss with recession and lack of keratinized tissue accompanied by inflammation indicates that soft tissue grafts should be performed on teeth #22–#25 and #28–#29. The patient prefers that all grafts be completed at the same appointment with a local anesthetic.

Non-autogenous connective tissue grafts using AlloDerm™ are to be completed at one appointment. Suture removal is done two weeks after the surgery, and a final check of the surgical areas is completed six weeks later. Homecare is stressed during all subsequent appointments.

Pre-Treatment Estimate

It is important to obtain a pre-treatment estimate in this case so that the patient clearly understands coverage for the soft tissue grafts, which varies between plans. Some plans may request additional attachments, such as radiographs or photographs, for soft tissue grafts. Once the pre-treatment is obtained, the date of surgery only is the additional information required to receive benefits.

Visit #2: Graft Procedures Delivered

Codes for the procedures to be delivered at this scheduled appointment are listed by teeth being treated.

Teeth #22–#25

D4275 **non-autogenous connective tissue graft (including recipient site and donor material) first tooth, implant, or edentulous tooth position in graft**

D4285 **non-autogenous connective tissue graft procedure (including recipient surgical site and donor material) – each additional contiguous tooth, implant or edentulous tooth position in same graft site**

(Repeat D4285 three times.)

Tooth #28 and Implant #29

D4275 **non-autogenous connective tissue graft (including recipient site and donor material) first tooth, implant, or edentulous tooth position in graft**

D4285 **non-autogenous connective tissue graft procedure (including recipient surgical site and donor material) – each additional contiguous tooth, implant or edentulous tooth position in same graft site**

Continued on next page

For soft tissue grafts, each separate tooth or implant is considered a site. When they are contiguous, meaning adjacent, and the graft site is only one surgical area, the coding includes the first tooth, and each additional tooth in that surgical area is listed with a separate code. As a result, in this case, for tooth #22, one D4275 is needed, and for teeth #23–#25, the D4285 is reported three times.

Tooth #28 and the implant for #29 are coded separately since they are not adjacent to the other surgical site. That is, there are several teeth between the areas treated. Therefore the same codes for soft tissue grafts apply for both teeth and implants. As a result, the coding for these teeth is very similar, with tooth #28 coded with D4275 and the #29 implant D4285.

D1330   oral hygiene instructions

Visit #3: Suture Removal

At the suture removal appointment:

D1330   oral hygiene instructions

D0171   re-evaluation – post operative visit

There is no separate CDT code for suture removal. For reimbursement purposes, most third-party payers consider suture removal as a component part of the surgical procedures (grafts) reported with the codes for Visit #2.

Visit #4: Post-surgery Appointment

At the final check appointment six weeks after surgery:

D0171   re-evaluation – post-operative office visit

or

D9430   office visit for observation (during regularly scheduled hours) – no other services performed

D1330   oral hygiene instructions

Visit #4 is considered a post-operative visit after the surgical treatment. At the fourth (final) visit D0171 would be reported if any additional procedures were delivered; D9430 would be reported only if there are no additional treatments delivered. It is important to code for what you do whether or not the procedure is reimbursed. Precise documentation is necessary for both medical and legal reasons.

Clinical Coding Scenario #8:
Treatment and Maintenance of Hybrid Appliance

Visit #1

A new patient was scheduled for a prophylaxis and evaluation. Once in the office, a medical history was taken, and a comprehensive oral evaluation was performed. Previous treatment included periodontal surgery in the mandibular arch five years ago and placement of a hybrid restoration in the maxilla with six implants placed in the arch. The patient did not have any radiographs from his previous dentist, so a panoramic radiograph was taken with vertical bitewings to include the maxillary implants. Some inflammation was noted surrounding the implants.

It was decided that at the next visit a periodontal maintenance procedure was necessary rather than a routine prophylaxis. Another appointment would be indicated if the inflammation surrounding the implants did not resolve after the maintenance appointment. If so, at a subsequent visit it would be necessary to remove the appliance due to the mucositis surrounding the implants.

The second appointment was scheduled.

How would this initial appointment be coded?

D0150 comprehensive oral evaluation – new or established patient

or

D0180 comprehensive periodontal evaluation – new or established patient

D0330 panoramic radiographic image

D0277 vertical bitewings – 7 to 8 radiographic images
> This does not constitute a full mouth intraoral radiographic series.

Visit #2

The patient was delayed returning for his periodontal maintenance and was seen two months later. Treatment included supra- and subgingival plaque and calculus removal. Implants in the maxillary arch were debrided using air abrasion as well as hand instrumentation. The patient received homecare instructions and was scheduled for a re-evaluation in four weeks.

How could visit #2 be coded?

D4910 periodontal maintenance

D0120 periodic oral evaluation – established patient

D1330 oral hygiene instructions
> This may include instructions for home care. Examples include tooth brushing technique, flossing, and use of special oral hygiene aids.

Continued on next page

In this case, a periodic evaluation is necessary to determine if any additional changes had occurred in the two months since the last appointment. If the patient had been seen a week after the evaluation, D4910 would be the only code necessary. In some cases, state law requires an examination at a maintenance appointment, so a D0120 would also be used in this situation. The primary goal of the evaluation is to determine if further treatment is needed in the maxillary arch. In this case, a re-evaluation is scheduled to permit the tissues to heal and then determine if further treatment is necessary.

Visit #3

Periodontal charting is done, and it is determined that the patient will require further therapy, removing the appliance and treating the mucositis present around the implants in the maxillary arch.

How could visit #3 be coded?

D0171   re-evaluation – post-operative office visit

Note: As there is no D0171 descriptor, the dentist's decision to proceed with periodontal charting and document the encounter with this code is appropriate.

Visit #4

The hybrid appliance is removed, resulting in the implants being more accessible to address the mucositis. Using local anesthesia, scaling and debridement is completed. The appliance is replaced after being examined and cleaned. Instructions for post-operative and daily care of the implants are given. The patient is then placed on a three-month maintenance schedule.

How could visit #4 be coded?

D6080   implant maintenance procedure when prostheses are removed and reinserted, including cleansing of prostheses and abutments
This procedure includes active debriding of the implant(s) and examination of all aspects of the implant system(s), including the occlusion and stability of the superstructure. The patient is also instructed in thorough daily cleansing of the implant(s). This is not a per implant code, and is indicated for implant supported fixed prostheses.

D6081   scaling and debridement in the presence of inflammation or mucositis of a single implant, including cleaning of the implant surfaces without flap entry and closure
This procedure is not performed in conjunction with D1110, D4910, or D4346.

Note: D6081 is a code for treatment of a single implant. In this case, six implants are present, so it should be coded six times.

Clinical Coding Scenario #9:
Generalized Periodontitis Treatment

How could the following visits be coded?

Visit #1

A 55-year-old patient presents with a maxillary denture and natural teeth in the mandible. A cursory examination reveals periodontal disease to be her primary problem, so a comprehensive evaluation is performed. A panoramic radiograph and seven periapical radiographs are taken to determine a diagnosis and develop a treatment plan.

The evaluation reveals isolated pocket depths of 5–6 mm generally, with 7 mm between teeth #24 and #25. Bone loss is primarily horizontal in the coronal third of the root except in the central incisor area where it is approximately 50% of the root, with a moderate crater. Mobility is noted on the incisors. Except for the third molars, all teeth are present in the mandible. Oral hygiene is fair, with some supragingival and subgingival calculus. Medical history includes medication for high blood pressure, which is controlled. The patient smokes four to five cigarettes per day. Further questioning reveals that the maxillary teeth were not lost from periodontal disease but rather from extensive caries. Diagnosis: Periodontitis: Stage III, Grade B.

How would this visit be coded?

D0180 **comprehensive periodontal evaluation – new or established patient**

D0330 **panoramic radiographic image**

D0220 **intraoral – periapical first radiographic image**

D0230 **intraoral – periapical each additional radiographic image**

Note: D0230 should be recorded six times as a total of seven periapical images were acquired and interpreted.

Continued on next page

During the second visit, the treatment plan included scaling and root planing, as well as splinting the mandibular anterior teeth. The mandible was anesthetized with local anesthetic and, two quadrants of scaling and root planing were completed. A splint was placed from teeth #22–#27, using orthodontic archwire and composite on the lingual of these anterior teeth to reduce mobility. Oral hygiene instructions were given, particularly for the teeth included in the splinting.

How would visit #2 be coded?

D4341   periodontal scaling and root planing – four or more teeth per quadrant

Note: D4341 is recorded two times, noting the applicable area of the oral cavity code where the procedure was delivered.

D4323   splint – extra-coronal; natural teeth or prosthetic crowns

Note: This is an additional procedure that physically links individual teeth or crowns to provide stabilization and additional strength. Although only one code is submitted, the teeth numbers should be indicated on the claim.

D1330   oral hygiene instructions

Visit #3

Pocket depths were recorded, and home care was again addressed, as well as the patient's smoking habit. It was determined that osseous surgery would be necessary in both quadrants of the mandibular arch. No bone grafts were necessary although the dentist decided that it would be advantageous to place a biologic material in between teeth #24 and #25 when the patient returns for the surgery procedure.

How would visit #3 be coded?

D0171   re-evaluation – post-operative office visit

D1330   oral hygiene Instructions

D1320   tobacco counseling for the control and prevention of oral disease

Continued on next page

Visit #4

The patient was sedated with oral medication and nitrous oxide. Using local anesthetic, flaps were elevated and the mandible was debrided, roots scaled and planed, and some osteoplasty where needed. Before replacing the flaps, Emdogain®, a biologic material, was placed between the central incisors. Sutures and periodontal dressing were placed. Post-surgical instructions were given and the patient was dismissed to a relative.

How would visit #4 be coded?

D9248 non-intravenous conscious sedation

D9230 inhalation of nitrous oxide/analgesia, anxiolysis

D4260 osseous surgery (including elevation of a full thickness flap and closure) – four or more contiguous teeth or tooth bounded spaces per quadrant

Note: D4260 is reported twice, along with the appropriate quadrant code.

D4265 biologic materials to aid in soft and osseous tissue regeneration, per site

A site is defined as a single area, position, or locus. It includes an osseous defect on a single tooth, or defects in edentulous positions. For example, if two contiguous teeth have osseous defects that are separate, then this would be considered two sites. On the other hand, if two adjacent teeth have an interproximal defect that communicates, then this would be considered a single site. In this case, it is only reported one time.

Visit #5

Two weeks later, sutures were removed, healing evaluated, and the patient was given oral hygiene instructions.

How would visit #5 be coded?

At the suture removal appointment:

D1330 oral hygiene instructions

D0171 re-evaluation – post operative visit

There is no separate CDT code for suture removal. For reimbursement purposes, most third-party payers consider suture removal as a component part of the surgical procedures (grafts) reported with the codes for Visit #4.

Clinical Coding Scenario #10:
Flap Surgery for Debridement and Evaluation

How could the following visits be coded?

A patient is evaluated for a problem on tooth #3. Symptoms include pain when biting, a pocket on the distobuccal of 8 mm, and edema with bleeding on probing but no suppuration. A root canal was completed on this first molar five years ago, but the patient did not have a definitive restoration (crown) placed, as recommended at that time.

A radiograph indicates minimal bone loss in the area with no pathology at the apex. The patient has a history of periodontal treatment including osseous surgery six years ago but has had quarterly maintenance appointments alternating between the general dentist and periodontist. It was decided to schedule the patient for osseous surgery to treat the continued deterioration.

D0140 limited oral evaluation – problem focused

D0220 intraoral – periapical first radiographic image

Visit #2

The patient was anesthetized using local anesthesia. A flap was elevated and the area of concern debrided. Once exposed, it was found that a vertical fracture of the distobuccal root had occurred. After conferring with the patient, the best treatment option was determined to be extraction and a bone graft in anticipation of eventual placement of an implant. A resorbable barrier was placed in conjunction with the bone graft as well as a biologic materials to encourage regeneration.

D4241 gingival flap procedure, including root planing – one to three contiguous teeth or tooth bounded spaces per quadrant

D7140 extraction, erupted tooth or exposed root (elevation and/or forceps removal)

D7953 bone replacement graft for ridge preservation – per site

D7956 guided tissue regeneration, edentulous area – resorbable barrier, per site

D4265 biologic materials to aid in soft and osseous tissue regeneration, per site

Continued on next page

A post-operative visit was done, removing sutures and evaluating healing of the surgical site. The patient will be seen for follow-up over the next three months prior to implant placement.

D0171   re-evaluation – post-operative office visit

There is no separate CDT code for suture removal. For reimbursement purposes, most third-party payers consider suture removal as a component part of the surgical procedures (grafts) reported with the codes for Visit #2.

Clinical Coding Scenario #11:
Recession and Frenum Pull

How could the following visits be coded?

Visit #1

A 25-year-old presents with a strong frenum attachment facially between teeth #24 and #25. These central incisors also have 3–4 mm of recession on the facial. A periapical radiograph was taken to determine the prognosis of the teeth involved. A photo of the mandibular anterior was also taken. Orthodontic treatment is planned, and periodontal treatment should be completed prior to starting the orthodontic therapy. The patient is scheduled for a frenectomy and two connective tissue grafts.

D0140 **limited evaluation – problem focused**

D0220 **intraoral – periapical first radiographic image**

D0350 **2D oral/facial photographic image obtained intra-orally or extra-orally**

Visit #2

A frenectomy was done and connective tissue grafts were performed on teeth #24 and #25 using donor tissue from the patient's palate. After sutures were placed, the patient was given post-operative instructions, and an appointment in two weeks for suture removal was scheduled.

D7961 **buccal / labial frenectomy (frenulectomy)**

D4273 **autogenous connective tissue graft procedure (including donor and recipient surgical sites) first tooth, implant or edentulous tooth position in graft**

D4283 **autogenous connective tissue graft procedure (including donor and recipient surgical sites) – each additional contiguous tooth, implant or edentulous tooth position in same graft site**

Both the frenectomy and the soft tissue grafts are reported separately. Some carriers will benefit only the most inclusive procedures done at the same visit. In this case, those are the soft tissue grafts.

Continued on next page

Visit #3

The sutures were removed. The patient was given oral hygiene instructions and appointed for follow-up three weeks later.

Coding for the follow up and suture removal appointment is:

D1330   oral hygiene instructions

D0171   re-evaluation – post operative visit

There is no separate CDT code for suture removal. For reimbursement purposes, most third-party payers consider suture removal as a component part of the surgical procedures (grafts) reported with the codes for Visit #2.

Clinical Coding Scenario #12:
Periodontal Pocketing and Subgingival Decay

Visit #1

A patient is seen with a chief complaint of pain in the mandibular left. An examination revealed decay on tooth #19 with periodontal disease present on multiple posterior teeth. A comprehensive periodontal evaluation is completed with full mouth radiographs. The diagnosis includes subgingival decay tooth #19 distal with localized moderate periodontitis on teeth #18, #19, and #20. Pocket depths are 7 mm on tooth #18 distal and 5–6 mm on teeth #19 distal and mesial and #20 distal. The final treatment plan includes osseous surgery to address the pocketing present and crown lengthening for tooth #19.

> **D0180** **comprehensive periodontal evaluation – new or established patient**
>
> **D0210** **intraoral – comprehensive series of radiographic images**

Visit #2

A full thickness flap is elevated from teeth #18–#21, including a distal wedge on tooth #18. After debridement, osseous contouring is performed, flattening the shallow crater on the distal of the second molar. The interproximal bone between teeth #18 and #19 is reduced to eliminate pocketing and allow access for restorative in the area of decay. Some bone contouring is also completed on the mesial of tooth #19 and distal of tooth #20 to eliminate pocketing. The flap is repositioned apically with sutures, and periodontal dressing is placed. Post-operative instructions are given.

> **D4261** **osseous surgery (including elevation of a full thickness flap and closure) – one to three contiguous teeth or tooth bounded spaces per quadrant**
>
> **D4249** **clinical crown lengthening – hard tissue**

As with other procedures, such as soft tissue grafts, carriers may reimburse based on the most inclusive procedure, in this case osseous surgery. Providers should always code for what is done, so both the osseous surgery and the clinical crown lengthening are documented in the patient record and reported on the claim.

Continued on next page

Visit #3

The patient is evaluated, and the sutures removed. Oral hygiene instructions are given, and the patient is appointed for a check in three weeks.

Coding for the follow up and suture removal appointment is:

D1330   oral hygiene instructions

D0171   re-evaluation – post operative visit

There is no separate CDT code for suture removal. For reimbursement purposes, most third-party payers consider suture removal as a component part of the surgical procedures (grafts) reported with the codes for Visit #2.

Clinical Coding Scenario #13
Post-Orthodontic Crown Lengthening

A 16-year-old patient is seen after completion of orthodontic therapy over the past few years. Her home care is good and after a prophylaxis removing residual cement and calculus, the periodontal tissues appear healthy with no bone or attachment loss. The patient and her mother both are concerned about esthetics of the maxillary anterior teeth, which appear short, and the tissue appears thick. They also feel she has a "gummy" smile.

After discussing this concern with both, it is decided that some gingival reshaping extending from fist bicuspid to first bicuspid would help resolve the problem and improve esthetics. The patient is scheduled for the procedure at a subsequent visit. Extraoral photographs are taken.

Visit #1:

D0150 comprehensive oral evaluation – new or established patient

D1110 prophylaxis – adult

D0350 2D oral/facial photographic image obtained intra-orally or extra-orally

As with most periodontal surgical procedures, a pre-treatment estimate is strongly recommended. In this case it is particularly true since many plans will not reimburse for cosmetic therapy, which this would fall under.

Visit #2:

D4230 anatomical crown exposure – four or more contiguous teeth or bounded tooth spaces per quadrant

This would be submitted two times for the maxillary left and right. Also note that this procedure is done only when the gingiva is healthy, without any bone loss, and involves removal of excess tissue as well as supporting bone to result in an anatomically correct gingival relationship. Many times it is performed without sutures so follow-up would involve only evaluation of healing and tissue position.

Visit #3:

D0171 re-evaluation – post-operative office visit

Clinical Coding Scenario #14:
Previous Third Molar Extraction Site

A patient presents with discomfort and swelling distal to tooth #18. Tooth #17 had been extracted several years previously, and the area had never been a problem before. After obtaining a periapical radiograph, utilizing a local anesthesia, the distal of this second molar was debrided, with some suppuration noted. After irrigation, the patient was placed on an antibiotic and told to return in ten days to evaluate the area.

At the second appointment, the patient stated the tooth was feeling much better but it was difficult to clean. Re-evaluation revealed that the tissue, although not inflamed, was fibrotic extending to the occlusal height of the second molar. Pocket depths were in the 6–7 mm range. Although no bone loss was evident radiographically, it was decided to remove the excess tissue distal to tooth #18 to provide better access for home care and prevent the problem from returning.

Visit #1:

D0140 **limited oral evaluation – problem focused**

D0220 **intraoral – periapical first radiographic image**

D9110 **palliative treatment of dental pain – per visit**

D4921 **gingival irrigation with a medicinal agent – per quadrant**

Visit #2:

D0171 **re-evaluation – post-operative office visit**

D4274 **mesial/distal wedge procedure, single tooth (when not performed in conjunction with surgical procedures in the same anatomical area)**

If there is bone loss in the area, and osseous contouring is necessary, even if the area treated is still only the distal of the molar, then the code would change to **D4261 osseous surgery (including elevation of a full thickness flap and closure) – one to three contiguous teeth or tooth bounded spaces per quadrant**.

Clinical Coding Scenario #15
Six mm Pocketing – a Periodontics Problem or Something Else (Root Resorption?)

A patient is seen for a routine prophylaxis. During the evaluation, a 6mm pocket is noted on the distolingual of tooth #8. This tooth has never had more than 2–3 mm pocketing previously. Mild inflammation is present, although the patient denies any sensitivity or bleeding. A periapical radiograph reveals a suspicious area subgingivally. It is decided to elevate a flap and evaluate the lesion, eliminating the pocket if possible without compromising esthetics.

At the next appointment, a flap is elevated conservatively with the papilla, and the tooth debrided. Root resorption is found on tooth #8DL. Since access is present, a restoration is placed, and the tissue positioned to retain the interproximal area. The tooth will be monitored in the future to determine if endodontic therapy is needed.

Visit #1:

D1110 **prophylaxis – adult**

D0220 **intraoral – periapical first radiographic image**

D0120 **periodic evaluation – established patient**

Visit #2:

D3471 **surgical repair of root resorption – anterior**

D2330 **resin – based composite – one surface, anterior**

Visit #3:

D0171 **re-evaluation – post-operative office visit**

In this case, what began as a periodontal problem ended up as a problem requiring endodontic treatment. If root resorption had not been present, but rather periodontal bone loss or a fracture existed, then the procedure would be coded as **D4241 gingival flap procedure, including root planing – one to three contiguous teeth or tooth bounded spaces per quadrant**.

Clinical Coding Scenario #16
Periodontitis and Peri-implantitis

During a comprehensive oral evaluation and prophylaxis, a patient is found to have generalized periodontitis diagnosed as Stage III, Grade B. Overall, 6–8 mm pocketing was found, with inflammation and bleeding on probing. A comprehensive series of radiographs revealed 30–50 percent bone loss on posterior teeth, and furcation involvement on the molars. Adding to the diagnosis was peri-implantitis around implants replacing teeth #19 and #29.

After two appointments of scaling and root planing to control inflammation, four quadrants of osseous surgery were treatment planned over two appointments. These appointments also included a bone graft for tooth #3 using a resorbable barrier and a biologic and bone grafts for both implants with non-resorbable barriers. The left quadrants were completed first with the right posterior areas treated at a subsequent appointment. Coding for the appointments would be as follows:

Visit #1:

D1110   **prophylaxis – adult**

D0210   **intraoral – comprehensive series of radiographic images**

D0180   **comprehensive periodontal evaluation – new or established patient**

Visit #2:

D4341   **periodontal scaling and root planing – four or more teeth per quadrant**

This would be submitted twice with the correct area of the oral cavity indicated.

Visit #3:

D4341   **periodontal scaling and root planing – four or more teeth per quadrant**

This would be submitted twice with the correct are of the oral cavity indicated.

Visit #4:

D0171   **re-evaluation – post-operative office visit**

Continued on next page

D4260 osseous surgery (including elevation of a full thickness flap and closure) – four or more contiguous teeth or tooth bounded spaces per quadrant

This would be submitted twice indicating the maxillary left and mandibular left quadrants.

D6102 debridement and osseous contouring of a peri-implant defect or defects surrounding a single implant and includes surface cleaning of the exposed implant surfaces, including flap entry and closure

D6103 bone graft for repair of peri-implant defect – does not include flap entry and closure

D6107 guided tissue regeneration – non-resorbable barrier, per implant

Visit #5 (and #6) involves treatment of a natural tooth (D4260) in the quadrant and an implant. Treatment of the implant is documented with the D6102, D6103, and D6107 codes.

D4260 osseous surgery (including elevation of a full thickness flap and closure) – four or more contiguous teeth or tooth bounded spaces per quadrant

This would be submitted twice indicating the maxillary right and mandibular right quadrants. For the bone graft on tooth #3:

D4263 bone replacement graft – retained natural tooth – first site in quadrant

D4266 guided tissue regeneration, natural teeth – resorbable barrier, per site

For treatment of the implant #29:

D6102 debridement and osseous contouring of a peri-implant defect or defects surrounding a single implant and includes surface cleaning of the exposed implant surfaces, including flap entry and closure

Continued on next page

D6103 **bone graft for repair of peri-implant defect – does not include flap entry and closure**

D6107 **guided tissue regeneration – non-resorbable barrier, per implant**

Visit #7:

D0171 **re-evaluation – post-operative office visit**

This code can be used to monitor and evaluate healing. At some point, the non-resorbable barrier used for regeneration surrounding the implants must be removed. This would involve a surgical procedure and would be coded as follows:

D4286 **removal of non-resorbable barrier**

Coding Q&A

1. *Our patient has pocketing and an osseous defect on the distal of the last tooth in a quadrant. All other teeth in the quadrant have pockets that are three millimeters or less. We are not sure whether the treatment procedure to report is* **D4261 osseous surgery (including elevation of a full thickness flap and closure) – one to three contiguous teeth or tooth bounded spaces per quadrant** *or* **D4274 mesial/distal wedge procedure, single tooth (when not performed in conjunction with surgical procedures in the same anatomical area).** *Which is appropriate?*

   If there is an osseous defect evident radiographically on the distal of the last tooth in a quadrant, and treatment of the defect includes osseous contouring and possibly a bone graft, then the treatment should be coded as osseous surgery one to three teeth, D4261. If a bone graft is performed, use **D4263 bone replacement graft – retained natural tooth – first site in quadrant** along with appropriate codes for membranes or biologics if they, too, apply.

   If the procedure involves only removal of soft tissue and debridement of the tooth surface, then the mesial/distal wedge procedure would apply. The D4274 descriptor states, "This procedure is performed in an edentulous area adjacent to a tooth, allowing removal of a tissue wedge to gain access for debridement, permit close flap adaptation, and reduce pocket depths." No osseous contouring or regeneration is done, but a flap is elevated and the area debrided including scaling and root planing.

2. *What is the code for reporting platelet rich plasma (PRP)?*

   Platelet rich plasma (PRP) is a concentrated suspension of the growth factors found in platelets. It is a procedure where a patient's blood is drawn and then centrifuged to obtain the PRP. This procedure should be coded using **D7921 collection and application of autologous blood concentrate product**.

3. *We use the bone replacement graft codes D4263 and D4264 for periodontal defects around and adjacent to natural teeth. Do we use the same codes in periodontal defects around existing implants?*

   There are separate codes for bone grafts around natural teeth and for bone grafts around implants. If natural teeth are being treated, then **D4263 bone replacement graft – retained natural tooth – first site in quadrant** and **D4264 bone replacement graft – retained natural tooth – each additional site in quadrant** should be submitted. These codes apply "per site."

   If a bone graft is placed around an existing implant, then **D6103 bone graft for repair of peri-implant defect – does not include flap entry and closure** would be correct. D6103 is applied per implant.

4. *We use the bone replacement graft code D7953 when placing graft material in an extraction socket when removing a natural tooth. But if we place an immediate implant in the extraction site and place a bone graft around the implant, do we still use D7953, or do we use one of the periodontal bone graft codes D4263 or D4264?*

    D7953 bone replacement graft for ridge preservation – per site indicates that this procedure is appropriate to report when the service is for ridge preservation. The code's descriptor also makes reference to "preservation of ridge integrity…clinically indicated in preparation for implant reconstruction." D4263 and D4264 specifically state that they apply to "natural" teeth.

    The only appropriate code to use when placing an immediate implant and simultaneously placing bone graft material around the implant would be **D6104 bone graft** at time of implant placement. Note that the D6104 descriptor states, "Placement of a barrier membrane, or biologic materials to aid in osseous regeneration are reported separately." In the case of placing an implant and using a barrier, **D6106 guided tissue regeneration – resorbable barrier, per implant or D6107 guided tissue regeneration – non-resorbable barrier, per implant** would be used.

5. *If we remove an existing implant and place a bone graft in the site, can we use the D7953 code?*

    Yes. You should be using two codes to describe what you are doing. The first would be **D6100 surgical removal of implant body**, and the second should be **D7953 bone replacement graft for ridge preservation – per site**, for which the descriptor states that the "graft is placed in an extraction or implant removal site at the time of extraction or removal…" This means D7953 is appropriate in this situation.

    If a barrier is also used, then **D7956 guided tissue regeneration, edentulous area – resorbable barrier, per site** or **D7957 guided tissue regeneration, edentulous area** – non-resorbable barrier should be reported depending on the type of barrier material.

6. *What code should I use to report periodontal charting?*

    There is no separate code for periodontal charting. It is considered to be part of a **D0180 comprehensive periodontal evaluation** or may be part of a **D0150 comprehensive oral evaluation**). It could also be considered part of a **D0171 re-evaluation – post-operative office visit**, such as that done after initial therapy.

7. *A patient needs multiple connective tissue grafts in the mandible. There are 3-6 mm of recession on the facial of teeth #23, #24, #25, #26, #27, and #28, with no attached gingiva. There is also no attached gingiva around the implant in the area of #29. The dentist plans on using Alloderm when performing connective tissue grafts on all involved teeth and the implant during one appointment.*

Should I just submit a code for the first tooth and then one code for the remaining teeth since they are contiguous? How do we submit for a soft tissue graft around an implant? And which connective graft code would apply, D4273 or D4275?

In this case, the appropriate code would be **D4275 non-autogenous connective tissue graft (including recipient site and donor material) first tooth, implant, or edentulous tooth position in graft** for the first tooth involved. You would then use **D4285 non-autogenous connective tissue graft procedure (including recipient surgical site and donor material) – each additional contiguous tooth, implant or edentulous tooth position in same graft site** for grafts to each of the additional teeth or implants involved.

In this specific case, D4275 would be submitted one time, and D4285 would be submitted six times, regardless of the fact that the teeth are in two quadrants.

8. *I have many orthodontic patients who come in for a prophylaxis. Sometimes we find the tissue around brackets and wires is hyperplastic and bleeding with generalized pseudo-pocketing. There is no bone loss evident and home care is poor. Although the hygienist spends more time on these patients than she would with a routine prophylaxis patient, is D1110 the only option for coding that we have?*

The code for scaling in the presence of moderate to severe inflammation (D4346) would be appropriate in this case.

D4346 **scaling in the presence of generalized moderate or severe gingival inflammation – full mouth, after oral evaluation**
The removal of plaque, calculus and stains from supra- and subgingival tooth surfaces when there is generalized moderate or severe gingival inflammation in the absence of periodontitis. It is indicated for patients who have swollen, inflamed gingiva, generalized suprabony pockets, and moderate to severe bleeding on probing. Should not be reported in conjunction with prophylaxis, scaling and root planing, or debridement procedures.

The D4346 is a full mouth procedure that is more involved than a routine prophylaxis. Remember that carriers may vary on the documentation required when submitting for reimbursement and limitations on the number of times this procedure is covered.

9. *My patient has had periodontal treatment in the past and is on periodic D4910 periodontal maintenance. The patient changed dental benefit plans and when we filed for our visit, the coverage was denied due to no history of periodontal treatment. What actions would best resolve this issue?*

You should send in the current periodontal charting, radiographs, and the patient's history of prior periodontal treatment. Ask for a review of the claim. Some insurers require periodontal treatment in the prior 24 months to be eligible.

10. *A periodontal maintenance patient presents with a localized area of pocketing with 6 mm probing depths. If I treat this area today, is this included in the* **D4910 periodontal maintenance**, *whose descriptor indicates site specific scaling and root planing? Or can it be coded as* **D4342 periodontal scaling and root planing – one to three teeth per quadrant**?

The descriptor of D4910 includes site specific scaling and root planing. It is considered part of the periodontal maintenance appointment on the same day. If the change is significant, you may want to obtain a current periodontal chart and a radiographic image for the patient and then consider scaling and root planing (D4342) as a separate procedure, which would be performed at a separate visit. It is advantageous to have periodontal charting that demonstrates an increase in pocket depths that support the need for scaling and root planing.

11. *I have a patient who has had periodontal surgery six years ago. Although we have encouraged him to alternate his maintenance appointments with the periodontist, he insists on remaining in our office for recall. How often should I schedule his appointments, and how should I code these maintenance visits since he is not seeing a periodontist? His home care is good and only minimal pocket depths are present in localized areas.*

Since the patient has had periodontal therapy in the past, the **D4910 periodontal maintenance** procedure, as described in the code's nomenclature and descriptor, may be delivered, regardless of whether he is treated in a general dentist's office or a periodontist's office. D4910 includes site-specific scaling and root planing, if needed.

An evaluation procedure should accompany the D4910 procedure. It can be any of the following as determined by the dentist:

D0120 **periodic oral evaluation – established patient**

D0150 **comprehensive oral evaluation – new or established patient**

D0180 **comprehensive periodontal evaluation – new or established patient**

It is recommended that a comprehensive periodontal evaluation, D0180, be completed annually since patients who have had periodontal therapy in the past are at a higher risk for recurrence. The number of maintenance visits annually should be determined by the treating dentist, based on the patient's home care, stability, and risk factors such as smoking or diabetes. Most periodontal maintenance patients require a three-to four-month schedule.

Note: A prophylaxis procedure (e.g., D1110) may also be delivered when the dentist determines that the patient's oral health will benefit from this procedure. However, it is not appropriate to deliver and report a prophylaxis procedure solely for reimbursement purposes (e.g., benefit plan limits on reimbursement for D4910).

12. *What is the difference between anatomical crown exposure and a gingivectomy?*

Anatomical crown exposure (D4230 and D4231) is performed on healthy gingival tissues in order to obtain the correct gingival relationship or contour. Both hard and soft tissues are normally removed. This is a procedure that sometimes is done after orthodontic treatment to provide improved esthetics, for example.

A gingivectomy (D4210, D4211, or D4212) is performed when supragingival pocketing, many times due to fibrotic pseudo pocketing, is present with or without inflammation. No bone is removed, only soft tissue.

Remember: Anatomical crown exposure: No periodontal disease present – healthy soft and hard tissue

Gingivectomy: Periodontal disease may be present – unhealthy soft tissue

13. *When is it necessary to take an intraoral photograph of a periodontal patient?*

When recession is present, a photograph of the area prior to treatment is recommended. A photograph is also helpful in cases where a fracture or subgingival decay is present and visible after a flap has been elevated. In cases where there is an unusual condition that can be seen more visually, photographs can be appropriate for multiple reasons.

Not only will a photograph be helpful if an appeal is necessary when requesting benefits from a third-party carrier, but they are also a means to communicate with the patient the need for treatment. Last but by no means least, photographs are part of your legal documentation.

14. *Can I submit both a frenectomy and a free gingival graft in the same area?*

Yes, but reimbursement for these discrete procedures depends on when they were performed.

In many cases, the frenectomy is completed at the same time as the soft tissue graft, especially when doing a free gingival graft. In this case, both procedures are documented, but in all likelihood a third-party carrier will consider the frenectomy to be part on the soft tissue graft when determining reimbursement. This payer adjudication policy may also be applicable when a connective tissue graft is done the same day as a frenectomy.

There are other instances when the frenectomy is performed separately, with the soft tissue graft done after healing of the frenectomy is complete. This allows for better placement and integration of the graft. In these cases, the two codes may be benefitted separately. It is always best to submit a pre-treatment estimate to avoid misunderstanding among all three parties: the dentist, the patient, and the carrier.

15. *When I expose an implant using a flap, should I code it as D6011 or D4245?*

When coding exposure of an implant as **D6011 surgical access to an implant body (second stage implant surgery),** the primary purpose is to gain access to the implant regardless of the way it is done. For example, it may be a "punch" type procedure, removing tissue with a blade or laser, or a flap that is only partially elevated.

D4245 apically positioned flap would indicate that the tissue elevated is being placed below the original position to primarily preserve the attached gingiva in order to maintain a healthy periodontium around the implant.

Reporting both codes is appropriate when both procedures are performed. However, most carriers would only benefit the most inclusive procedure.

16. *When would it be appropriate to code a procedure as a distal wedge?*

In most instances, a distal wedge will be performed on a tooth that has an edentulous area distal to it. We naturally think of a second molar that has had the third molar removed. The goal is to remove only excess soft tissue that has resulted in pocketing. The distal wedge is done so that the tissue will be repositioned to expose the distal of the tooth, resulting in better access for debridement, placement of a restoration, and/or home care. The tissue after healing will be closely adapted to the tooth without pocketing. In most instances, no bone contouring is performed.

17. *If a quadrant of osseous surgery is performed, and several teeth in the quadrant are having bone grafts that include placing a biologic material, do I only report the procedure code one time for all teeth or do I use the same code several times for each tooth treated?*

The codes for bone grafts, D4263 and D4264, as well as the code for biologic materials, D4265, are specifically per site. Remember that site is defined as a single area, position, or locus. It includes an osseous defect on a single tooth or defects in edentulous positions.

For example, if two contiguous teeth have osseous defects that are separate, this would be considered two sites. On the other hand, if two adjacent teeth have an interproximal defect that communicates, this would be considered a single site.

The term "site" is defined at the beginning of the D4000–D4999 Periodontal category. Bone grafts, biologic materials, and guided tissue regeneration barriers are coded per site.

In this case, the number of individual teeth involved is not pertinent, the number of sites is. Therefore, each site would be separately coded for the bone graft procedure and the biologic material.

18. *When I use local delivery antimicrobial agents, many times it is when a patient is seen for maintenance and has several areas of inflammation and increased pocket depths. Is it appropriate to code each tooth where the agent is placed?*

Yes, it would be appropriate to code D4381 for every tooth that is treated as this procedure is described as "local delivery of antimicrobial agents via a controlled release vehicle into diseased crevicular tissue, per tooth."

However, if this procedure is covered the benefit plan may have limitations on the number of teeth involved. Some limit the number of teeth per quadrant, others have a maximum number of teeth in the mouth. It is best to get a pre-treatment estimate since coverage of local delivery antimicrobials varies greatly among plans.

19. *When a splint is placed for stabilization of periodontally involved teeth, should I code for each tooth involved?*

D4322 splint – intra-coronal; natural teeth or prosthetic crowns and **D4323 splint – extra- coronal; natural teeth or prosthetic crowns** are submitted as one code regardless of the number of teeth or crowns involved. On the claim form, however, it should be noted which teeth are included in the splint.

For example, if a lingual extra-coronal splint is placed from tooth #22 to tooth #27, D4322 would be submitted one time with the tooth numbers for #22, #23, #24, #25, #26, and #27 in the claim's space for reporting tooth number.

20. *When I place a bone graft and use a membrane, should I always use the membrane code in the periodontal category even if I am placing it around an implant?*

This has always been an issue when using barriers in treatment outside that of periodontitis on natural teeth. Previously, yes, you would have to use the **D4266 guided tissue regeneration – resorbable barrier, per site** or **D4267 guided tissue regeneration – non-resorbable barrier, per site**. As of January 1, 2023, coding for GTR procedures has changed to enable more granular documentation and reporting of barrier placement.

- The periodontal guided tissue regeneration codes, D4266 and D4267 are now applicable only when the procedure is delivered to natural teeth.

- When a barrier is used in conjunction with periradicular surgery, the appropriate code is **D3432 guided tissue regeneration, resorbable barrier, per site, in conjunction with periradicular surgery**.

- When placing a barrier in an implant case, the available codes are **D6106 guided tissue regeneration – resorbable barrier, per implant** and **D6107 guided tissue regeneration – non-resorbable barrier, per implant**.

- During oral surgery procedures, if a barrier is used in an edentulous area either after an extraction or for ridge augmentation, the applicable codes are either **D7956 guided tissue regeneration, edentulous area – resorbable barrier, per site** or **D7957 guided tissue regeneration, edentulous area – non-resorbable barrier, per site**.

Chapter 5: D4000–D4999 Periodontics

Summary

Filing for benefits related to periodontal procedures can be frustrating. In order to reduce issues with carriers and patients, some things can be routinely done to avoid problems. Use this checklist as a reminder:

- Obtain proper documentation when evaluating a patient who requires periodontal treatment. Full periodontal charting should be present, which includes not only pocket depths, but also recession, the amount of attached gingiva, furcation involvement, mobility, bleeding on probing, clinical attachment loss, and any other periodontal condition found. The charting should be recent, usually less than six months old. Radiographic images should typically be less than one year old. Periapical images are preferred over bitewing or panoramic images. At times, especially for soft tissue grafts, photographic images may be helpful, but these are not normally submitted with the initial claim.

- A pre-treatment estimate is the best way to avoid problems with reimbursement. Although not a guarantee of benefits, it establishes guidelines for the patient related to payments. With some plans, pre-treatment estimates may be valid for a limited time and this should be taken into consideration. Other times, pre-treatment estimates are required.

- When submitting for periodontal reimbursement, attachments are essential. For periodontal scaling and root planing, as well as osseous surgery, periapical radiographs and charting are necessary. For soft tissue grafting, recession and the amount of attached gingiva must be evident on the charting. If initial therapy has been performed prior to any necessary osseous surgery, many carriers will require periodontal charting after the scaling and root planing has healed and prior to the osseous surgery for comparison pocket depths. This holds true for periodontal maintenance patients also. If it is determined that treatment such as scaling and root planing or osseous surgery is needed and a patient has been on a periodontal maintenance schedule, then previous, as well as recent charting, should be available to demonstrate changes, normally seen as increased pocket depths between appointments.

Contributor Biography

Marie Schweinebraten, D.M.D., is a practicing periodontist in Duluth, GA. She has been active in the dental tripartite, including serving on the ADA Council on Dental Benefit Programs and as Fifth District Trustee. While appointed to the Council on Dental Benefit Programs, she represented the ADA on the Code Maintenance Committees. Presently she serves as Insurance Consultant for the American Academy of Periodontology, representing the AAP on the Code Maintenance Committee the past five years. Dr. Schweinebraten has given code workshops and is a certified insurance consultant.

Betsy K. Davis, D.M.D., M.S.

Introduction

This Prosthodontic category of service describes procedures that replace missing dentition in partially or completely edentulous patients. Stability and retention of a removable prosthesis reported with a code in this category of service is dependent on both hard and soft tissue support. Materials used in prosthesis fabrication have particular characteristics that are reflected in the nomenclatures of several codes used to document prosthesis fabrication and placement.

Because most of the materials used for a well-fitting prosthesis can be modified or repaired, there are a significant number of codes in this category to describe various repair, reline, and adjustment procedures. Such procedures are delivered to maintain or modify a prosthesis when changes occur to the supporting structures. It is important to note that all procedure codes in this category are inherently based on either a partial or complete denture. Moreover, nomenclatures of most codes specifically designate the involved arch – maxillary or mandibular.

Key Definitions and Concepts

The ADA's "Glossary of Dental Clinical Terms" defines the following prosthodontic procedure terms.

Denture: An artificial substitute for some or all of the natural teeth and adjacent tissues.

Complete denture: A prosthetic for the edentulous maxillary or mandibular arch, replacing the full dentition. Usually includes six anterior teeth and eight posterior teeth.

Partial denture: Usually refers to a prosthetic device that replaces missing teeth. See fixed partial denture or removable partial denture.

Fixed partial denture: A prosthetic replacement of one or more missing teeth cemented or otherwise attached to the abutment natural teeth or their implant replacements.

Removable partial denture: A removable partial denture is a prosthetic replacement of one or more missing teeth that can be removed by the patient.

Immediate denture: Prosthesis constructed for placement immediately after removal of remaining natural teeth.

> **Note**: An immediate denture procedure code only applies to the initial insertion appointment. Post-insertion visits for purposes of adjustments, repairs, or relines are documented with the code applicable to the type of denture subject to the procedure.

Overdenture: A removable prosthetic device that overlies and may be supported by retained tooth roots or implants.

Prosthesis: Artificial replacement of any part of the body.

Changes to This Category

There are no additions, revisions, deletions, or editorial changes in CDT 2023.

Clinical Coding Scenario #1:
Flexible Base Immediate Removable Partial Denture

A patient presents with teeth #2–#11 and #15 present on the maxillary arch. The clinical and radiographic examination reveals non-restorable teeth #3, #4, and #5. After presenting the patient the restorative options, the patient elects for extraction for #3, #4, and #5 and an immediate removable partial denture. The patient is adamant about not having metal clasps. Rather than making an impression, the dentist scans the maxillary and mandibular arches and sends it electronically to the laboratory for prosthetic fabrication. The laboratory 3D prints the model to fabricate the flexible base immediate removable partial denture.

How would you code this scenario?

D5227   immediate maxillary partial denture – flexible base (including any clasps, rests and teeth)

D0801   3D dental surface scan – direct

Clinical Coding Scenario #2:
Implant Fixture

A patient presents with implants in #22 and #27 sites. The original plan was to pick up two locator attachments in the patient's existing mandibular complete denture. Upon removing the healing abutment, the implant fixture (body) came out with the healing abutments for both implants.

How would you code this scenario?

D6105   removal of implant body not requiring bone removal or flap elevation

Clinical Coding Scenario #3:
Fabrication of Removable Partial Dentures

A patient presents for fabrication of maxillary and mandibular removable partial dentures. At the first visit, the dentist scans the maxillary and mandibular arches with a TRIOS® intraoral scanner. The purpose of the scan was diagnostic, to determine the location of the rests, guide planes, and clasps.

What CDT code would be selected to document the intra-oral scanning procedure?

The applicable code is **D0801 3D dental surface scan – direct** as the procedure is delivered while the patient is present in the operatory.

Clinical Coding Scenario #4:
Modification of Mandibular Complete Denture to Enable Placement on Implants

A patient presents with an existing mandibular complete denture that needs to be modified prior to placement on two implant fixtures recently integrated into the anterior mandible. Following the implant placement surgery, the denture is relieved in the areas of implant support and retention, and a soft liner or tissue conditioner is placed to re-adapt the denture base.

How would you code these procedures related to changes made to the denture base?

D5875 **modification of removable prosthesis following implant surgery**
Attachment assemblies are reported using separate codes.

D5851 **tissue conditioning, mandibular**
Treatment reline using materials designed to heal unhealthy ridges prior to more definitive final restoration.

Note: D5875 is used to describe the procedure that modifies an existing removable prosthesis following implant surgery.

But, in the event that a completely new implant supported mandibular overdenture will be fabricated with an implant attachment such as a locator, then the following codes in the Implant Services category would apply:

D6111 **implant/abutment supported removable denture for edentulous arch – mandible**

D6192 **semi-precision attachment – placement**

(Report each attachment assembly separately.)

Clinical Coding Scenario #5:
Removable Denture and Bone Loss

A patient presents with an existing mandibular removable partial denture which is supported by remaining anterior dentition, teeth #22 through #27. On examination, multiple teeth exhibit greater than 50 percent bone loss as demonstrated radiographically. Both #22 and #27 have existing PFM crowns, which have defective margins and recurrent decay.

The treatment plan involves removal of the remaining dentition, #22 through #27, with placement of new denture on the now completely edentulous mandible. An immediate mandibular complete denture will be fabricated in advance of the scheduled surgery and inserted with a soft reline on the day of surgery.

How would you code the removable prosthodontic procedures completed in advance of the scheduled surgery?

The correct coding for the removable prosthesis is:

D5140   immediate denture – mandibular

How would you code future reline procedures for the removable denture placed on the day of scheduled surgery?

In this case, a chairside reline at a future visit would be coded as:

D5731   reline complete mandibular denture (direct)

As the immediate denture placed at the time of surgery has not been replaced with another prosthesis (e.g., implant/abutment supported removable denture) it is considered, for maintenance purposes such as relines and rebases, to be the same as a permanent complete denture. There are no codes for reline (and rebase) procedures applicable to any interim prosthesis.

Clinical Coding Scenario #6:
Complete Denture Repair

A patient presents relating that they dropped their maxillary complete denture, resulting in fracture of the buccal flange along the right side including the area comprising the tuberosity. The denture is otherwise in good condition, and the flange is able to be accurately re-assembled and repaired with acrylic resin.

How would you code this procedure?

D5512   repair broken complete denture base, maxillary

Clinical Coding Scenario #7:
Reinforcement of the Denture Base for a Complete Denture

A patient with a history of fracture and repair of the denture base due to an opposing arch of natural dentition and a Class III jaw relationship presents for a new maxillary complete denture. In order to strengthen the denture base, a metal substructure is added to the palatal aspect of the new denture to enhance resistance to fracture during function.

How would code this procedure?

D5876   add metal substructure to acrylic complete denture (per arch)

Clinical Coding Scenario #8:
Fractured Tooth and an Interim Prosthesis

A patient comes in with a fractured #3. The tooth is extracted by the oral surgeon with bone grafting/socket preservation. The oral surgeon requests an interim prosthesis to replace #3 during the healing process until an implant can be placed and an implant crown can be fabricated. The dentist fabricates a unilateral removable partial denture of a resin base to replace tooth #3.

How would you code for this prosthesis?

D5286   removable unilateral partial denture – one piece resin (including retentive/clasping materials, rests, and teeth) – per quadrant

Clinical Coding Scenario #9:
Fractured Teeth and a Removable Partial Denture

An 87-year-old patient presents to the office upon referral from the oral surgeon. The patient fractured teeth #7, #8, #9, and #10 as a result of a fall. The surgeon extracted teeth #7 through #10. A removable partial denture replacing teeth #7–#10 was fabricated by the restorative dentist and inserted immediately at the time of the extractions. After several months of healing the patient is in need of a new prosthesis to be used as an interim measure until the remaining dental work can be completed.

How would you code the prosthesis inserted at the time of extraction?

> **D5221 immediate maxillary partial denture – resin base (including retentive/clasping materials, rests and teeth)**
> Includes limited follow-up care only; does not include future rebasing/relining procedure(s).

What code would be applicable to report the procedure for fabrication and placement of the prosthesis placed after several months of healing?

This interim prosthesis would be reported with **D5820 interim partial denture (including retentive/clasping materials, rests, and teeth), maxillary**.

Clinical Coding Scenario #10:
Second Stage Implant Surgery (Stage II Surgery) and Placement of the Modified Prosthesis

A patient, who has a removable complete denture modified to enable placement on implant bodies, presents for surgery to exposure the previously placed implants. During this visit the dentist will complete the denture modification with placement of locators followed by prosthesis insertion.

What CDT codes are used to document the several procedures involved in this implant case?

D5875 **modification of removable prosthesis following implant surgery**
Attachment assemblies are reported using separate codes.

D6011 **surgical access to an implant body (second stage implant surgery)**
This procedure, also known as second stage implant surgery, involves removal of tissue that covers the implant body so that a fixture of any type can be placed, or an existing fixture be replaced with another. Examples of fixtures include but are not limited to healing caps, abutments shaped to help contour the gingival margins or the final restorative prosthesis.

D6191 **semi-precision abutment – placement**
This procedure is the initial placement, or replacement, of a semi-precision abutment on the implant body.

D6192 **semi-precision attachment – placement**
This procedure involves the luting of the initial, or replacement, semi-precision attachment to the removable prosthesis.

Clinical Coding Scenario #11:
Locator Attachment Repair

A patient presents to the office and is upset that her maxillary denture is loose. She demands that all six locator attachments receive new plastic housings and the dentist evaluates the situation. Upon closer examination the dentist determines that three of the attachments can be repaired, but three of the locator abutments on the implants are worn due to bruxism and cannot be repaired. Hence, three new locator abutments were placed.

How would you code the procedures delivered during this encounter?

D0140 limited oral evaluation – problem focused

D6091 replacement of replaceable part of semi-precision or precision attachment of implant/abutment supported prosthesis, per attachment

Note: This service is reported three times as the nomenclature states it is a "per attachment" procedure.

D6191 semi-precision abutment – placement
This procedure is the initial placement, or replacement, of a semi-precision abutment on the implant body.

Note: This service is reported three times as the nomenclature and descriptor use the singular form to describe the appliance ("abutment") and procedure's nature and scope.

Clinical Coding Scenario #12:
Soft Liner

A patient presents with an existing mandibular complete denture with a chief complaint of looseness of the mandibular denture. Due to a complex medical history, implant placement is not an option for the patient. The dentist recommends a soft liner for her existing denture.

How would you code the soft liner?

D5765 soft liner for complete or partial removable denture – indirect

What if a new complete mandibular denture was first fabricated followed by a soft liner? How would you code the procedures?

D5120 complete denture – mandibular

D5765 soft liner for complete or partial removable denture – indirect

Clinical Coding Scenario #13:
Replacement of Denture Acrylic Material and Teeth

A patient presents with a hybrid prosthesis, and the teeth and the denture acrylic material are worn out and need replacing. The framework, however, is acceptable.

How would you code the replacement of the denture acrylic material and the teeth?

D5725   rebase hybrid prosthesis

D5650   add tooth to existing partial denture

The D5650 nomenclature uses the singular form – tooth. Therefore, if one tooth was added, the code would be reported once; if more than one tooth was added, the patient's record and claim submission would indicate the number or times this procedure was delivered (e.g., five teeth added means D5650 is reported with a Quantity of "5" with the appropriate full fee for the total number of teeth).

Clinical Coding Scenario #14:
Overdenture

A patient has existing teeth #22 and #27 in the mandibular arch. Since #22 and #27 have already had root canals and the coronal tooth structure is mostly composite restorations, it was decided to make #22 and #27 overdenture abutments with attachments and to make a mandibular overdenture.

How would you code this clinical scenario?

D5865   overdenture – complete mandibular

D5862   precision attachment, by report

D5862 would be reported twice – once for the precision attachment involving tooth #22 and the second time for tooth #27.

Coding Q&A

1. *For a patient whose maxillary arch is fully edentulous, when would I report a* **D5130 immediate denture** *procedure, and when would I report a* **D5110 complete denture** *procedure?*

   An immediate denture is a prosthesis that may be placed for aesthetic or clinical reasons and is inserted immediately following extraction of teeth when the definitive prosthesis is not available. A complete denture is the definitive prosthesis. The dentist determines the longevity of an immediate denture.

   Note: The above also applies to immediate partial dentures.

2. *How do I properly code refitting the denture base of an existing removable partial denture when additional teeth are added to this prosthesis?*

   If the entire denture base needs to be updated in an existing removable partial denture, meaning the borders of the edentulous area are developed to re-establish proper extension and contour, then the correct code for this procedure would be either **D5720 rebase maxillary partial denture** or **D5721 rebase mandibular partial denture**.

   The code for adding each additional tooth to this existing partial denture is **D5650 add tooth to existing partial denture**.

3. *How do I code for a partial denture that needs an adjustment and a repair?*

   A maxillary partial denture that has a broken clasp assembly typically requires both a repair and an adjustment once the new clasp assembly is joined to the framework. This should be coded as **D5630 repair or replace broken retentive/clasping materials – per tooth** and **D5421 adjust partial denture – maxillary**.

4. *Is the procedure documented with code* **D5876 add metal substructure to acrylic full denture (per arch)** *applicable to fabrication of a new denture, or to the repair of an existing denture?*

   This procedure may be reported in either situation. Patients who present with a broken denture or who have a history of heavy bruxism may be candidates for a substructure to be added to their denture. Additionally, patients with certain disabilities including the lack of fine motor skills or manual dexterity may need a substructure to prevent breakage of a new denture.

5. *How do I properly code the placement of a locator abutment on an implant?*

   D6191 semi-precision abutment – placement is the proper code for documenting placement of a semi-precision attachment as described on an implant body. This code is recorded for each individual abutment. Code D6191 may be reported for both initial placement and any necessary replacement of the entire abutment.

   Note: When a replaceable part of the abutment is no longer functional, the procedure for replacing the replaceable part only is documented with code **D6091 replacement of replaceable part of semi-precision or precision attachment of implant/abutment supported prosthesis, per attachment**.

6. *A patient has lost tooth #5 and grinds their teeth. The dentist decides to fabricate a unilateral partial denture with a metal base to address these conditions. How would you code this denture procedure?*

   D5282   removable unilateral partial denture – one piece cast metal (including retentive/clasping materials, rests, and teeth), maxillary

7. *A patient recently had insertion of immediate maxillary and mandibular complete dentures. Due to shrinkage, change of anatomical contour, the dentures are worn out and lack retention, stability, and support. However, the patient is not ready for her definitive implant prostheses. She is in need of a new maxillary and mandibular dentures until she can have her definitive implant supported prosthesis. How would you code the dentures?*

   D5810   interim complete denture (maxillary)

   D5811   interim complete denture (mandibular)

   An interim prosthesis (also called "provisional prosthesis") is intended to be used for a limited period of time until the definitive restoration is fabricated and ready for placement.

8. *What is the difference between a rebase and a reline procedure?*

   A rebase procedure is the process of refitting a denture by replacing the base material (see codes D5710—D5725 in the Denture Rebase Procedures subcategory).

   A reline procedure is the process of resurfacing the tissue side of a denture with new base material (see codes D5730–D5761 in the Denture Reline Procedures subcategory).

Note: There is another "reline" code in the Other Removable Prosthetic Services subcategory:

D5765   soft liner for complete or partial removable denture – indirect
A discrete procedure provided when the dentist determines placement of the soft liner is clinically indicated.

D5765 is a code specifically for reporting a soft reline procedure when a patient presents with a complaint that the denture does not fit well or is uncomfortable, and the dentist determines that better retention or comfort is possible with a soft liner.

A silicone material would be used for this procedure. The traditional method of relining dentures is to use acrylic, which is "hard" reline. Appliance retention or comfort, as well as form and function, can be improved by placement of the soft liner on the denture's base, which is why this code is in the Other Removable Prosthetic Services subcategory.

9. *What is the difference between code* **D5765 soft liner for complete or partial removable denture – indirect** *and code* **D5850 tissue conditioning, maxillary** *and* **D5851 tissue conditioning mandibular***?*

Code D5765 is when a soft liner is used as a definitive liner for a removable prosthesis that is placed in the laboratory. Code D5850 and D5851 are used during the healing phase and used chairside.

10. *What is the difference in the codes for complete dentures when they are fabricated digitally or in a conventional manner (impression, etc)?*

There is not any difference in the codes. Codes **D5110 complete denture – maxillary** and **D5120 complete denture – mandibular** are used for digital dentures or conventional dentures. Codes are determined by procedure, not fabrication process.

Summary

The procedure codes listed in this category describe services related to either a partial or complete denture that is natural tooth borne. These removable denture procedures are not the same as those that are implant borne and listed in the CDT Code's Implant Services category. Keeping this concept in mind when coding for a procedure will simplify the correct code decision-making process.

Note: The inclusion of select procedure codes from the Implant Services category illustrates the differences in appropriate code selection.

Contributor Biography

Betsy K. Davis, D.M.D., M.S., is the National Group Director for Maxillofacial Prosthodontics and Dental Oncology for the Sarah Cannon Cancer Institute of HCA Healthcare. She is also the Past-President for the American Academy of Maxillofacial Prosthetics, past Treasurer for the International Society for Maxillofacial Rehabilitation, and a representative for the American College of Prosthodontists and American Academy of Maxillofacial Prosthetics to CMS (Centers for Medicare and Medicaid Services).

Chapter 7: D5900–D5999 Maxillofacial Prosthetics

Betsy K. Davis, D.M.D., M.S.

Introduction

The CDT Code's Maxillofacial Prosthetics category of service is unique as the majority of codes address procedures for devices often used for patients with acquired defects or congenital/craniofacial patients. Due to the various medical conditions of these patients, the majority of the codes and services in this category would be submitted to medical carriers. However, codes for procedures such as medicament carrier fabrication or splints would be covered by dental carriers, not necessarily by medical carriers.

Key Definitions and Concepts

The ADA glossary is the accepted glossary for a description of the various prostheses.

> The ADA Glossary definition of **splint** is "A device used to support, protect, or immobilize oral structures that have been loosened, replanted, fractured or traumatized. Also refers to devices used in the treatment of temporomandibular joint disorders."

> The ADA Glossary does not define stent; however, the Glossary of Prosthodontic Terms defines **stent** as "A prosthetic device which is used to apply pressure to soft tissue to aid in healing and to prevent scarring during healing. It can be used after surgery to aid in tissue closure and healing. Stents are often utilized for procedures post periodontal surgery, such as skin grafting."

The ADA Glossary definition of **obturator** is "A disc or plate which closes an opening; a prosthesis that closes an opening in the palate." Obturators can be classified as interim, surgical, and definitive.

Changes to This Category

There are no additions, revisions, deletions, or editorial changes in this category of service in CDT 2023.

Coding Scenario #1:
Maxillary and Mandibular Arches Scan

A patient presents with a new diagnosis of oral cancer. The head and neck surgeon requests models of the maxillary and mandibular arches to review prior to surgery.

If the maxillary and mandibular arches are scanned, how would you code it?

D0801   3D dental surface scan – direct

If impressions had to be made of the maxillary and mandibular arches with impression material, how would you code it?

D0470   diagnostic casts

Coding Scenario #2:
Scan with 3D Model

A patient presents with nasal cancer. It was decided at Tumor Board that the patient would undergo surgical resection of nasal cancer along with surgical reconstruction. The reconstructive surgeon requests a model of the nose. The nose is scanned and 3D printed for the surgeon.

How would you code it?

D0803   3D facial surface scan – direct

Coding Scenario #3:
Complete Denture and Prosthesis for Edentulous Patient

A patient who is edentulous on both the maxillary and mandibular arches has mandibular cancer. The patient underwent surgical resection/reconstruction with a fibular free flap. At the time of reconstruction, four dental implants were placed in the fibula. The patient did not require postoperative radiation therapy. The restorative plan is to make a maxillary complete denture, a mandibular prosthesis with ramps, and four locator attachments.

How would you code it?

D5110   complete denture – maxillary

D5934   mandibular resection prosthesis with guide flange

D6191   semi-precision abutment – placement

Report four times.

D6192   semi-precision attachment – placement

Report four times.

Coding Scenario #4:
Removable Partial Denture for Hard Palate Cancer

A patient who has teeth #2–#15 present finds out that she is going to lose teeth #10–#15 due to hard palate cancer. The plan is to do a surgical resection/reconstruction with a fibula free flap. At the time of surgery, three implants will be placed in the fibula to retain a removable partial denture. The plan is to place 3 locator abutments on the implants and fabricate a removable partial denture.

How would you code it?

D5213   maxillary partial denture – cast metal framework with resin denture bases (including retentive/clasping materials, rests and teeth)

D6191   semi-precision abutment – placement

Report three times.

D6192   semi-precision attachment – placement

Report three times.

Clinical Coding Scenario #5:
Implant Placement Guide

Four months after an extraction and socket preservation, a patient returns for endosteal implant placement at site #30. You fabricate a guide for the implant placement surgery. In the past, you have used **D5982 surgical stent** and you were recently told this is wrong.

How would you code this encounter?

The correct code to report for this scenario is **D6190 radiographic/ surgical implant index, by report**, which is in another CDT Code category of service (Implant Services). Code D5982 in Maxillofacial Prosthetics is not the appropriate code to report in this case as it is applicable when reporting a surgical stent to apply pressure to soft tissues to facilitate healing and prevent cicatrization or collapse.

Clinical Coding Scenario #6:
Obturator for Cancer Patient

A patient was referred to you for fabrication of an obturator. The patient was recently diagnosed with mucoepidermoid carcinoma of the maxilla. He currently has a surgical obturator that was fabricated for him pre-operatively but no longer fits well. You plan on fabricating another obturator for him instead of modifying the ill-fitting prosthesis.

What other obturator(s) might you fabricate for your patient, and how would you code for this prosthesis?

The provider can provide the patient with either an interim (D5936) or a definitive (D5932) obturator depending on the clinical condition. If the patient requires an interim obturator they will likely require the fabrication of a definitive prosthesis once healing is complete.

Clinical Coding Scenario #7:
Obturator for Palatal Perforation Due to Cocaine Use

A patient with a history of cocaine abuse presents with palatal perforation and nasal communication due to snorting cocaine. The patient states that they are having a hard time eating and drinking. You decide to make an obturator for your patient. The patient is not pursuing surgical treatment at this time.

How would you code for fabricating the appliance used in this treatment?

> **D5932** obturator prosthesis, definitive

What other obturator(s) might you fabricate for your patient, and how would you code for this?

If the patient decides to pursue surgical treatment you can code **D5931 obturator prosthesis, surgical**. Any obturator adjustments (to the surgical or definitive obturator) can be coded with **D5933 obturator prosthesis, modification**.

Clinical Coding Scenario #8:
Appliance for Patient Undergoing Radiation Therapy

Your patient is diagnosed with squamous cell carcinoma and is scheduled to undergo radiation therapy. In order to best protect the unaffected tongue and oral mucosa, you decide to fabricate an oral appliance.

How would you code this appliance fabrication procedure?

You would use **D5984 radiation shield**.

Clinical Coding Scenario #9:
Protecting Dentition During Cancer Treatment

A patient was recently diagnosed with cancer of the tongue and will be undergoing radiation therapy in the very near future. The patient's oncologist suggested the patient see you to discuss ways to protect the dentition during cancer therapy. The doctor recommends fluoride trays for the patient.

How would you code for the fluoride tray fabrication?

D5986 fluoride gel carrier

Synonymous terminology: fluoride applicator.

A prosthesis, which covers the teeth in either dental arch and is used daily to apply topical fluoride in close proximity to tooth enamel and dentin for several minutes daily.

Clinical Coding Scenario #10:
Snoring and Treatment Appliances

A patient comes in stating that his wife complained his snoring is so loud at night that some nights she sleeps in the other room. He has seen his medical doctor and has been told that he does not have obstructive sleep apnea; he is just a loud snorer and his snoring seems to be worse after a high stress day.

The doctor fabricates a snore guard for the patient.

How would you code for this appliance fabrication?

Many people are unaware that the Maxillofacial Prosthetics category includes a number of non-orthodontic treatment appliances. However, there is not a specific code for the snore guard. Since such an appliance is similar to other appliances in the Maxillofacial Prosthetics category, it would be appropriate to use this code:

D5999 unspecified maxillofacial prosthesis, by report

Note: If the patient was diagnosed with obstructive sleep apnea (OSA) and the dentist received a prescription to fabricate and place an OSA appliance, the appropriate code for this procedure is in the CDT Code's Adjunctive General Services category – **D9947 custom sleep apnea appliance fabrication and placement.**

Clinical Coding Scenario #11:
Mouth Lesions

A 50-year-old woman comes to the office stating that she has painful lesions in her mouth. Upon clinical inspection it is noted that the tissue is erythematous and the lesions look erosive in nature, and there are some bullae present. You suspect that the patient has pemphigus vulgaris. The patient states that the lesions have been there for four days and that she has been self-treating with salt water rinses. You prescribe a topical steroid for the lesions and arrange for the lab to create a medicament carrier that will cover the affected areas.

How would you code for fabricating this type of medicament carrier?

D5991   vesiculobullous disease medicament carrier
A custom fabricated carrier that covers the teeth and alveolar mucosa, or alveolar mucosa alone, and is used to deliver prescription medicaments for treatment of immunologically mediated vesiculobullous diseases.

Clinical Coding Scenario #12:
Post-radiation Trismus

A 67-year-old female patient has recently completed her radiation treatment for pT4N2M0 squamous cell carcinoma. The patient reports that since completing radiation she has had a difficult time opening her mouth more than 15 mm. The patient's TMJs are asymptomatic bilaterally. She is worried that lack of mouth opening will harm her oral health and lead to increased weight loss. Her lip opening is within normal limits.

The doctor fabricates a trismus appliance.

How would you code for this fabrication procedure?

D5937   trismus appliance (not for TMD treatment)

This prosthesis can be used to aid in opening the bite of a patient with trismus for causes other than TMJ dysfunction (i.e., radiation treatment).

Clinical Coding Scenario #13:
Malignant Neoplasm of the Hard Palate

Your patient has been diagnosed with a malignant neoplasm of the hard palate, and the planned treatment includes surgical removal of the neoplasm and radiation therapy. Prior to delivery of these treatments you fabricate a surgical obturator to be placed after the removal of the neoplasm, and a radiation shield. After the surgery, the plan is to fabricate both interim and definitive obturator prostheses.

After the surgery however, due to the fit of the surgical obturator, an interim prosthesis is not needed by the patient and only the definitive prosthesis is created.

How would you code these appliance procedures?

    D5984 **radiation shield**

    D5931 **obturator prosthesis, surgical**

Note: If the surgical obturator is to be modified prior to placement of a definitive obturator, the modification procedure would be reported with **D5992 adjust maxillofacial prosthetic appliance, by report**.

    D5932 **obturator prosthesis, definitive**

Maintenance of the definitive obturator would be coded as:

    D5993 **maintenance and cleaning of a maxillofacial prosthesis (extra- or intra-oral) other than required by adjustments, by report**

Clinical Coding Scenario #14:
Gunshot Wound and Ocular Prosthesis

A 30-year-old male was involved in an altercation and sustained a gunshot wound to the left side of his head. Evaluation and imaging obtained in the emergency department revealed left side orbital blow out fracture and left side globe rupture. The patient was taken emergently to the operating room for enucleation of the left globe and repair of facial fractures. His left eye was removed during surgery. The patient is seen in your clinic post-operatively to be evaluated for prosthesis for his left eye to replace the eye that was removed.

How would you code for the post-operative encounter services?

D0999 unspecified diagnostic procedure, by report

This "999" code is applicable to the in-clinic evaluation that led to fabrication of the prosthesis for the patient's left eye.

D5916 ocular prosthesis

Synonymous terminology: artificial eye, glass eye.

A prosthesis, which artificially replaces an eye missing as a result of trauma, surgery or congenital absence. The prosthesis does not replace missing eyelids or adjacent skin, mucosa or muscle.

Ocular prostheses require semiannual or annual cleaning and polishing. Occasional revisions to re-adapt the prosthesis to the tissue bed may be necessary. Glass eyes are rarely made and cannot be re-adapted.

Clinical Coding Scenario #15:
Patient with Maxillary Hypoplasia

An 18-year-old female patient presents with maxillary hypoplasia. The treatment plan for her is a LeFort 1 (three pieces) for which a surgical splint needs to be fabricated.

How do you code for the surgical splint?

D5988 surgical splint

Synonymous terminology: Gunning splint, modified Gunning splint, labiolingual splint, fenestrated splint, Kingsley splint, cast metal splint.

Splints are designed to utilize existing teeth and/or alveolar processes as points of anchorage to assist in stabilization and immobilization of broken bones during healing. They are used to re-establish, as much as possible, normal occlusal relationships during the process of immobilization. Frequently, existing prostheses (e.g., a patient's complete dentures) can be modified to serve as surgical splints. Frequently, surgical splints have arch bars added to facilitate intermaxillary fixation. Rubber elastics may be used to assist in this process. Circummandibular eyelet hooks can be utilized for enhanced stabilization with wiring to adjacent bone.

Clinical Coding Scenario #16:
Patient with Nasal Defect

A patient who lost her nose due to cancer presents after surgery and is in need of a nasal prosthesis. After consultation with her surgeon, it was decided to place two craniofacial implants to retain the nasal prosthesis along with magnet attachments on the craniofacial implants.

How do I code for all the procedures delivered in this case?

Proper documentation requires codes from four of the CDT Code's categories of service – Maxillofacial Prosthetics; Implant Services; Prosthodontics, fixed; Oral & Maxillofacial Surgery.

> **D5913** nasal prosthesis
>
> **D6011** surgical access to an implant body (second stage implant surgery)
>
> **D6950** precision attachment
>
> **D7993** surgical placement of craniofacial implant – extra-oral

Notes: D5913 is reported once as only one prosthesis is required. D6011, D6950, and D7993 are all reported twice as there are two implants included in the patient's treatment plan. D6950 is the procedure appropriate to report delivery of the two magnetic attachments.

Coding Q&A

1. *What is the difference between a surgical, interim, and definitive obturator? The terms are so confusing!*

   A surgical obturator is created and used during surgery and immediately post-operatively. The interim prosthesis is used for the duration of the healing, which can be anywhere from two to six months. After about six months, the definitive prosthesis is given to the patient, and it may last for many years.

2. *A patient has an obturator fabricated pre-operatively for placement immediately after a tumor removal surgery. Due to the excellent fit and comfort of this obturator, the patient decides they do not want another until the final prosthesis is fabricated. Sometime later, that patient returns and states that the obturator does not fit as well as it had before. What code would you use to document the necessary adjustment?*

   You would use **D5933 obturator prosthesis, modification**.

3. *Are obturators used only for cancer patients?*

   No, obturators can be used for patients with a various medical conditions. Patients with palatal perforations due to infection, disease, recreational drug use, or cleft palate may require an obturator as part of their treatment. Not all patients will require a definitive obturator. Some may need a surgical or interim obturator while receiving treatment or in between reconstructive surgeries.

4. *I'm still a little confused about the different types of obturators and when they're used. Can you go into more detail?*

   Surgical obturators (D5931) are delivered to the patient on the date of surgery in the operating room. It may not fit exactly and will likely require some adjustment. The surgical obturator is either wired or screwed in place for 7 to 14 days. The patient then undergoes an unpacking procedure. At that time, a modification of the surgical obturator is made or an interim obturator is delivered. An interim obturator (D5936) is intended to be used prior to the fabrication of a definitive obturator during the healing period. The patient will likely have this for a number of months. A definitive obturator (D5932) is fabricated after healing has occurred. It is designed to be the patient's "final" obturator, though if the patient has it for a number of years it will likely need to be replaced.

5. *I noticed there's a code for a feeding aid (D5951). When would I use this?*

   A feeding aid is used in infants with cleft palates prior to surgery. The prosthesis is placed in the infant's mouth during feeding to help aid in suckling and swallowing. After surgery, the device is not needed. Its use is meant to be intermittent and interim in nature.

6. *What is the difference between* **D5986 fluoride gel carrier** *and* **D5995 periodontal medicament carrier with peripheral seal – laboratory processed – maxillary***?*

   A fluoride gel carrier is used for application of topical fluoride only and it only covers the teeth. The periodontal medicament carrier, however, covers both the teeth and the alveolar mucosa. It is used to deliver medications to tissues (gingiva), membranes (alveolar mucosa), and into periodontal pockets. Report D5995 for a maxillary medicament carrier and D5996 for a mandibular medicament carrier.

7. *In dental coding, is there a separate code for a snoring appliance versus an appliance for patients with sleep apnea?*

   There is not a specific CDT code for a snoring appliance. The best choice of code is to use **D5999 unspecified maxillofacial prosthesis, by report**. However, there is a separate code (D9947) for a sleep apnea appliance.

   For medical coding, it is important to remember that while many patients with sleep apnea do snore, not all patients who snore have sleep apnea and the medical codes for the various appliances are very different. Diagnosis of obstructive sleep apnea from a physician is required to bill for an oral sleep apnea (OSA) appliance to a medical benefit plan.

8. *Is a sleep study required before I can code for a sleep apnea appliance?*

   The patient will need to have a formal diagnosis of obstructive sleep apnea from a physician. This usually includes a sleep study.

   If you file a claim with the patient's medical benefit plan the following codes are applicable:

   - HCPCS procedure – E0486 oral device/appliance used to reduce upper airway collapsibility, adjustable or non-adjustable, custom fabricated, includes fitting and adjustment
   - ICD-10-CM diagnosis – G47.33 Obstructive Sleep Apnea

9. *What is the difference between a trismus appliance and a commissure splint?*

    Both a trismus appliance (D5937) and a commissure splint (D5987) aim to accomplish the same goal: increasing the mouth opening of the patient. Commissure splints are used to increase the opening of the lips specifically. Trismus appliances are used to increase the opening of the oral aperture, not the lips themselves.

10. *What are some examples of vesiculobullous diseases?*

    Examples of vesiculobullous diseases include:

    - Paraneoplastic pemphigus
    - Pemphigus vulgaris
    - Bullous pemphigoid
    - Erythema multiforme
    - Herpes Simplex

11. *A patient requires medication to be delivered to soft tissue areas in the oral cavity due to painful ulcerated lesions. Which type of carrier would be fabricated and how would it be coded?*

    The patient would require a disease medicament carrier, not a periodontal medicament carrier, as a seal is not required. The applicable procedure is documented with CDT code **D5991 vesiculobullous disease medicament carrier**.

12. *Can I use the "periodontal medicament carrier" and "vesiculobullous disease medicament carrier" codes on the same patient? Are these codes somewhat interchangeable?*

    These two codes are not interchangeable. While both are used to describe medicament carriers, the need for these two appliances are quite different. **D5991 vesiculobullous disease medicament carrier** can only be used for patients who have a vesiculobullous disease. The periodontal medicament carrier (D5995 or D5996 depending on the involved arch) is used primarily to treat periodontal disease and deliver medications targeted at the pathogens that cause various periodontal diseases. These appliances are treating two different disease processes. D5995 or D5996 is used to treat diseases that are periodontal in nature, while D5991 is used to treat mucocutaneous diseases involving mucous membranes and skin.

13. *I have a patient who is eight years old and who has a speech impediment due to a palatal defect. The patient is not yet ready for surgery and is having a difficult time with socialization. How can I code for the prosthesis I made?*

The correct code for this scenario would be **D5952 speech aid prosthesis, pediatric**. This prosthesis is used temporarily, or as an interim prosthesis to close a palatal defect. The defect may be developmental or surgical in nature.

It is not intended to be used as a permanent prosthetic device.

14. *I have a patient that has a nasal prosthesis and now needs a new one fabricated. She has been wearing the prosthesis for several years after having extensive surgery on her nose to treat her diagnosis of skin cancer. We still have her original mold. How do I code for the new nasal prosthesis?*

The correct code to report would be **D5926 nasal prosthesis, replacement** as the patient's new artificial nose is produced from the previously made mold. A replacement prosthesis does not require fabrication of a new mold.

15. *A patient well known to your practice presents with an obturator that they have had for eight years stating that one of the clasps broke off last night. You offer to send the prosthesis to the lab for replacement of the clasp. How do I code for this repair procedure?*

In this case, the correct code is **D5993 maintenance and cleaning of a maxillofacial prosthesis (extra- or intra-oral) other than required adjustments, by report**.

16. *I am a maxillofacial prosthodontist working in a large academic setting. The patients I am treating have some pretty significant medical conditions. What are the codes I would use to bill to a dental carrier and a medical carrier for the surgical, interim, and definitive obturator prosthesis?*

CDT codes are used on claims filed with dental benefit plans; CPT codes are used on claims filed with medical benefit plans.

Surgical obturator: CDT code is D5931; CPT code is 21076.

Interim obturator prosthesis: CDT code is D5936; CPT code is 21079.

Definitive obturator prosthesis: CDT code is D5932; CPT code is 21080.

If the claim is being filed with the patient's medical benefit plan using the medical claim format (1500 Health Care Claim; 837P HIPAA electronic professional claim transaction), an ICD-10-CM diagnosis code is required. One example of an ICD-10-CM diagnosis code applicable in this scenario is: **C05.0 Malignant neoplasm of the hard palate**. Keep in mind the diagnosis code reported on the claim must be supported by the documentation in the patient's healthcare record.

17. *A patient presents with cancer of the hard palate and is in need of a surgical obturator initially, an interim obturator to be used during postoperative radiation therapy, and then a definitive obturator. She has both medical and dental insurances. Can I bill both insurances for each of the respective type of obturators?*

It is advisable to bill the medical insurance first on a medical insurance claim form ("1500" paper; 837P electronic) and have them pay first. The medical code is then converted into the respective dental code and submitted with the ADA dental claim form along with the EOB (explanation of benefits) from the medical insurance.

18. *What other medical codes can be used for maxillofacial prostheses?*

The medical procedure codes (CPT) with the corresponding dental procedure codes (CDT) are listed in the following table:

CPT Code	Corresponding CDT Code
21076 immediate surgical obturator	**D5931 obturator prosthesis, surgical**
21077 orbital prosthesis	**D5915 orbital prosthesis**
21079 interim obturator	**D5936 obturator prosthesis, interim**
21080 definitive obturator	**D5932 obturator prosthesis, definitive**
21081 resection appliance mandible	**D5934 mandibular resection prosthesis with guide flange**
	D5935 mandibular resection prosthesis without guide flange
21082 palatal augmentation prosthesis	**D5954 palatal augmentation prosthesis**
21083 palatal lift prosthesis	**D5955 palatal lift prosthesis, definitive**
21084 speech aid prosthesis	**D5953 speech aid prosthesis, adult**
	D5952 speech aid prosthesis, pediatric
21085 oral surgical splint	**D5988 surgical splint**
21086 auricular prosthesis	**D5914 auricular prosthesis**
21087 nasal prosthesis	**D5913 nasal prosthesis**

19. *When do I use a speech aid prosthesis versus a palatal lift prosthesis?*

    A palatal lift is used when the soft palate is velopharyngeal incompetent. A palatal lift is usually used for stroke patients in which the complete soft palate is present but there is no movement of the soft palate. A speech aid prosthesis is used when the soft palate is velopharyngeal insufficient. A speech aid prosthesis is usually used for cleft palate patients or patients with acquired defect. It is used when the soft palate is insufficient to make contact with the lateral and posterior walls of the pharynx.

20. *What are the differences between codes* **D5912 facial moulage (complete), D5911 facial moulage (sectional) and codes D0803 3D facial surface scan – direct** *and* **D0804 3D facial surface scan – indirect***?*

    Codes **D5912 facial moulage (complete)** and **D5911 facial moulage (sectional)** are used when an impression is made of the whole or partial face. Code **D0804 3D facial surface scan – indirect** is used when the model is scanned into the virtual environment. Code **D0803 3D facial surface scan – direct** is used when the face is scanned into the virtual environment.

21. *What are the differences between* **D5934 mandibular resection prosthesis with guide flange** *and* **D5935 mandibular resection prosthesis without guide flange***?*

    Code D5934 is applicable when the prosthesis has ramps or a flange to guide the mandible; code D5935 is applicable when the prosthesis does not have a ramp or flange.

Summary

Due to the severity of the medical condition of so many of the patients seen by maxillofacial prosthodontists (i.e., cancer, gunshot wound, cleft, ameloblastoma, etc.), the majority of the procedures will be billed to medical carriers. Thus, it is important to ensure that you are using the proper CPT code if there is one (there are not always individual CPT codes for all CDT codes) when coding. If there is no specific CPT code, you may bill the medical carrier using the CDT code.

The other pitfall to coding for these procedures for the coder (not necessarily the provider) is a clear understanding of what is actually happening and why is the prosthesis being fabricated in the first place. The definitions are very specific and it is necessary to understand the nuances and differences between them.

Contributor Biography

Betsy K. Davis, D.M.D., M.S., is the National Group Director for Maxillofacial Prosthodontics and Dental Oncology for the Sarah Cannon Cancer Institute of HCA Healthcare. She is also the Past-President for the American Academy of Maxillofacial Prosthetics, past Treasurer for the International Society for Maxillofacial Rehabilitation, and a representative for the American College of Prosthodontists and American Academy of Maxillofacial Prosthetics to CMS (Centers for Medicare and Medicaid Services).

Implant Services

By Linda Vidone, D.M.D.

Introduction

The CDT Code's Implant Services category is somewhat unique and challenging compared to other categories of service because it includes separate entries for procedures that address:

- Surgical placement of the implant post (or body or fixture)

- Placement of connecting components when needed

- The final prosthetic restoration (single crowns, bridges, or dentures)

Once these three basic concepts of implant procedures (addressed in greater detail later in this chapter) are understood, it will become less challenging and even easy to select the appropriate CDT code to document the procedures performed.

Note: When performing implant procedures, it's important to remember that not all codes are in the Implant Services category. For example, the code for removal of non-resorbable barrier (D4286) is in the Periodontics category (D4000–D4999) and codes for sinus augmentation (D7951 and D7952) are in the Oral & Maxillofacial Surgery category (D7000–D7999).

Key Definitions and Concepts

Basic Implant

This image illustrates all components of a single implant. Please note that the connecting element (abutment) may not be present in all cases. The dentist's clinical decision-making determines whether the implant crown will be supported and retained by an intermediary abutment, or if it may be placed directly on the implant body.

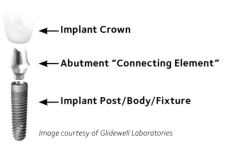

←— **Implant Crown**

←— **Abutment "Connecting Element"**

←— **Implant Post/Body/Fixture**

Image courtesy of Glidewell Laboratories

Implant Post/Body/Fixture

The two most common types of implant posts are endosteal and mini implants. The size and type of implant fixture determines the proper code to document the surgical implant placement procedure.

Surgical Placement of an Implant Body: Endosteal Implant (D6010): Placement of full-sized implant fixture into the jawbone.

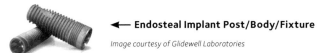

←— **Endosteal Implant Post/Body/Fixture**

Image courtesy of Glidewell Laboratories

Surgical Placement of Mini-Implant (D6013): Placement of mini implant fixture into the jawbone. These are smaller in diameter than full sized implants, yet are still considered permanent. They are typically used to support removable prostheses, but Implant-supported crowns can be placed on the mini-implants as well.

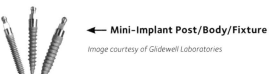

←— **Mini-Implant Post/Body/Fixture**

Image courtesy of Glidewell Laboratories

Connecting Elements for Implant Crowns, Implant Retainer Crowns, and Implant Prostheses

Abutments, both prefabricated (D6056) and custom (D6057), are the "connecting elements" that are placed, when needed, between the implant post and the restorative crown (definitive prosthesis), retainer crown (for a fixed partial denture), or prosthesis such as a fixed hybrid denture. Abutments are not always needed, but when placed are reported separately from the from the crown restoration.

Prefabricated Abutment (D6056): A manufactured component. The procedure includes modification and placement.

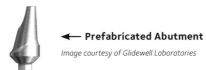

← **Prefabricated Abutment**

Image courtesy of Glidewell Laboratories

Custom Abutment (D6057): Created by a laboratory for a specific individual, usually if there are aesthetic concerns. The procedure includes placement. Custom abutments are custom cast by a laboratory or CAD/CAM milled.

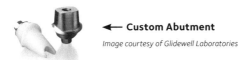

← **Custom Abutment**

Image courtesy of Glidewell Laboratories

Semi-precision Abutment – placement (D6191): One component part of the manufactured connection between a prosthesis and implant body. The procedure involves placement of this prefabricated abutment (also known as the "locator") onto the implant post.

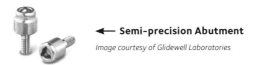

← **Semi-precision Abutment**

Image courtesy of Glidewell Laboratories

Note: Placement of the second component part of this connection (also known as the "keeper assembly") into the prosthesis is a separate procedure documented and reported with its own code **D6192 semi-precision attachment – placement**.

Connecting Bar – Implant Supported or Abutment Supported (D6055):
A device to help stabilize prostheses. Attaches to abutments or directly to the implants themselves to make the prosthesis more secure. Hader® and Dolder® are two types of connecting bars that can be designed to use other types of retentive mechanisms, such as semi-precision attachments. The entire bar is reported as a single unit; however, a supporting abutment (when present) would be documented for each implant that supports the connecting bar.

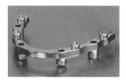

← **Connecting Bar – Implant Supported or Abutment Supported**

Image courtesy of Glidewell Laboratories

Implant Prostheses (Includes Single Crowns, Fixed Bridges, and Dentures)

There are two types of single unit implant crowns – abutment supported and implant supported. Selection of the appropriate crown procedure code is determined by the type of material used for the crown and the type of attachment.

Most of us are familiar with the type of material used (porcelain, metal, etc.). However, there is sometimes confusion over appropriate coding when there is more than one way to attach the restorative prosthesis to its supporting structure: via an intermediary abutment or directly by the implant.

Note: Both abutment supported and implant supported crowns may be cemented or screwed to the supporting structure, but neither of these options is a determining factor in code selection.

Abutment Supported Single Unit Crowns (D6058–D6064, D6094, and D6097): These are crowns that are attached to an abutment (D6056 or D6057), not directly to the implant post. The applicable abutment procedure code is submitted with the applicable single unit crown procedure code. These crowns obtain stability from the abutment. This is the most common type of implant crown.

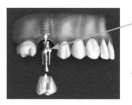

Abutment

Image courtesy of Glidewell Laboratories

Implant Supported Single Unit Crowns (D6065–D6067 and D6082– D6088): Implant crowns are attached directly to the implant post (one-piece retained crown). *Even though a separate abutment may be used in the manufacturing process, it is delivered as an integral part of the one-piece implant supported crown.* Typically, single unit implant supported are screw retained and the access opening sealed with composite material. These crowns obtain stability directly from the implant.

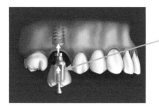

No abutment

Image courtesy of Glidewell Laboratories

Implant Supported Fixed Partial Dentures (Implant Bridges)

There are two types of implant retainer crowns: abutment supported and implant supported. Retainer crowns will have one or more pontics attached, the total number of pontics being determined (and reported separately with their applicable code) by the edentulous space being bridged. Selection of the appropriate retainer crown procedure code is based on the same criteria used for single implant crowns: the type of material used and the method of attachment.

Note: Both abutment supported and implant supported retainer crowns may be cemented or screwed to the supporting structure, but neither of these options is a determining factor in code selection.

Abutment Supported Retainer Crowns (D6068–D6074 and D6194– D6195): These are retainer crowns that are attached to an abutment (D6056 or D6057), not directly to the implant post. The applicable abutment procedure code is submitted with the applicable retainer crown procedure code.

Implant Supported Retainer Crowns (D6075–D6077, D6098–D6099, and D6120–D6123): Implant retainer crowns are attached directly to the implant post. *No abutment is used with this type of crown.*

Implant/Abutment Supported Dentures

There are two types of implant or abutment supported dentures: removable and fixed (also known as hybrid). Implant dentures, unlike single unit crowns and retainer crowns, are not determined by the type of attachment system.

Denture procedure code selection is determined by two factors:

- Is the denture replacing a full or partial complement of teeth?
- Will the patient be able to remove the denture by themselves, or is assistance needed from the dentist or dental staff?

If the patient is able to remove the denture by themselves, it is a removable implant denture. If the patient is unable to remove the denture and requires the assistance of dentist or dental staff, then the denture is a fixed implant denture.

Although a fixed implant bridge and fixed implant denture appear similar, the denture's supporting implant locations do not have a specific relationship to the missing natural teeth. This is why a fixed implant denture is referred to as a "hybrid" denture.

Implant/Abutment Supported Removable Dentures: Overdentures are supported by implants; the patient is able to remove them. These dentures typically have prefabricated abutments placed, a connecting bar, and a precision or semi-precision attachment. (Note: these components are not included in the denture and should all be submitted as separate procedures.) Codes for removable complete dentures are D6110 and D6111; codes for removable partials are D6112 and D6113.

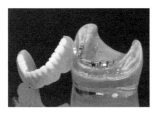

← **Implant/abutment supported removable dentures**

Image courtesy of Zest Dental Solutions

Implant/Abutment Supported Fixed (Hybrid) Dentures: Implant dentures that the patient cannot remove and are either screwed directly on the implant or connected via abutments. (Note: abutments are not included in the denture and when used should be submitted as separate procedures.) The implant supported dentures are heavily advertised as an "All-on-4®." Yet, there can be more implants. In addition to All-on-4®, another common name for implant supported dentures is hybrid denture. Codes for fixed complete dentures (dentures that replace all missing teeth) are D6114 and D6115. Typically, four to eight implants are utilized and are not in absolute tooth positions. Codes for fixed partials are D6116 and D6117.

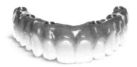

⟵ **Hybrid dentures**

Image courtesy of Glidewell Laboratories

Changes to This Category

The only changes in CDT 2023 are the addition of four new codes, prompted in part by changes in other categories of service. There are no deletions, revisions, or editorial changes. All four new codes allow for comprehensive patient record keeping and proper dental claims submissions.

The following code was added to close the coding gap arising from prior revision to **D6100 surgical removal of implant body**, where "by report" was removed from that code's nomenclature:

> **D6105   removal of implant body not requiring bone removal or flap elevation**

This new code was added to address removal of an implant body that is not surgical in nature. Prior to D6100's revision, the narrative "by report" would enable the provider to document whether the implant was removed surgically or non-surgically (i.e., does not require bone removal or flap elevation).

The following two codes were added as a result of revisions to the guided tissue regeneration (GTR) codes in the Periodontics category. Revisions to D4266 and D4267 indicated that these codes would be applicable when the procedure is delivered to address periodontal defects around natural teeth and not peri-implant defects—and this created a created a coding gap when GTR procedures are delivered to address peri-implantitis and at time of implant placement. D6106 and D6107 are reported per implant.

> **D6106   guided tissue regeneration – resorbable barrier, per implant**
> This procedure does not include flap entry and closure, or, when indicated, wound debridement, osseous contouring, bone replacement grafts, and placement of biologic materials to aid in osseous regeneration. This procedure is used for peri-implant defects and during implant placement.
>
> **D6107   guided tissue regeneration – non-resorbable barrier, per implant**
> This procedure does not include flap entry and closure, or, when indicated, wound debridement, osseous contouring, bone replacement grafts, and placement of biologic materials to aid in osseous regeneration. This procedure is used for peri-implant defects and during implant placement.

Notes: The D4266 and D4267 revisions also resulted in new codes for GTR procedures pertaining to edentulous areas, and these codes are found in the Oral and Maxillofacial Surgery category.

D6107 is a procedure that involves placement of a non-resorbable barrier. Removal of the non-resorbable barrier is reported with the following code in the Periodontics category, also added in CDT 2023:

D4286   removal of non-resorbable barrier

D4286 may be reported by any dentist who removes the barrier, including the dentist who placed it during the D6107 procedure.

The fourth CDT 2023 addition closes the coding gap when a restorative material used to close an access opening of a screw-retained implant supported prosthesis is replaced. This is a per implant code:

D6197   replacement of restorative material used to close an access opening of a screw-retained implant supported prosthesis, per implant

This procedure is not part of the initial implant restoration placement procedure. When delivered, it involves removal of any remaining restorative materials in the screw-retained implant access opening. Typically composite restorative material is placed, shaped, and cured, based on material directions and the restoration is polished.

Current codes D6080, D6090, or D6199 do not adequately describe this procedure. Placement of retentive aspects could be added as part of this procedure.

Abutment vs. Retainer

When implant procedures were first introduced in CDT-1 (effective January 1, 1990), confusion arose over the term abutment, a word with different meanings within the Implants category of service and within the Prosthodontics category of service. In the Implant category, "abutment" was associated with the piece that connected the implant body with the restorative prosthesis. In Prosthodontics, the term was used to describe a supporting (anchor) tooth in a fixed bridge.

The current and continuing usage for the term "abutment" applies only to the piece that connects the implant body with the restorative prosthesis. "Retainer" is the term solely used to describe the anchor tooth (natural or prosthetic) for a fixed partial denture.

CPT Codes Applicable to Implant Procedures

Claims against a patient's medical benefit plan use the AMA's Current Procedural Terminology (CPT) procedure codes and submit to the medical carrier via the 1500 (CMS-1500) medical claim form. Keep in mind there are no CDT codes that exactly match CPT codes regarding implant restorations. Medical carriers may benefit for diagnostics, the surgical implant placement and necessary bone grafting, but the final restorative prosthesis is typically never a benefit. When submitting to a patient's medical carrier, keep in mind there must be a diagnosis code for medical reimbursement of any procedure; typically there will be several. Proper selection of ICD-10-CM codes will establish medical necessity of the implant procedure and is critical to successful billing and reimbursement.

A sample of CPT codes for implant placement and bone grafting are in the tables that follow. The complete CPT code set, including modifiers, and instructions on their proper use is in a manual published annually by the AMA (e.g., *CPT© 2023 Professional Edition*). Claims filed with a patient's medical benefit plan must use the CPT codes from the version in effect on the date of service.

Surgical Placement and Removal of Dental Implants	
Code	**Nomenclature**
20670	Removal of implant, superficial
20680	Removal of implant, deep
21248	Reconstruction of maxilla/mandible endosteal implant, partial (1–3 per jaw)
21249	Reconstruction of maxilla/mandible endosteal implant, complete (4–6 per jaw)
21085	Diagnostic/surgical stent

Bone Grafts	
Code	**Nomenclature**
21210	Graft, bone, nasal, maxillary, or malar areas (includes obtaining graft)
21215	Graft, bone, mandibular areas (includes obtaining graft)
0232T	Platelet rich plasma
41899	Nonspecific code (Used for guided tissue regeneration)

Clinical Coding Scenario #1:
Abutment Supported Porcelain Implant Crown Tooth #7

The patient has a long history of dental treatment on #7 that began when hit by a ball in her mouth when she was 14 years old. The affected tooth (#7) received a root canal, post and core, and crown at the time of the accident. At age 22, she received retreatment of the root canal, apicoectomy, a new post and core, and a new crown procedures.

The patient recently fractured off the clinical crown and post and the remaining root has an unfavorable prognosis and therefore is non restorable. The adjacent teeth are perfectly healthy with no restorations, nor do they need restorations, so the dentist and patient agree on a single tooth abutment supported implant crown (aka "flipper").

What codes would document the services for each part of the treatment plan?

Part 1: Extraction of #7 with Ridge Preservation and Insertion of a "Flipper"

D7210 **extraction, erupted tooth requiring removal of bone and/or sectioning of tooth, and including elevation of mucoperiosteal flap if indicated**

D7953 **bone replacement graft for ridge preservation — per site**

Notes:

- Bone in this area is thin, therefore it is imperative that the ridge be preserved.

- This procedure is also referred to as "socket preservation," with the placement in the extraction site at the time of the extraction to preserve the size and shape of the bone.

- The D7953 procedure does not include placement of a barrier membrane to prevent tissue from invading the bone graft site, and there is no separate code for a membrane with ridge preservation. D7956 is used to document placement of the barrier membrane.

Continued on next page

D7956 guided tissue regeneration, edentulous area – resorbable barrier, per site

This procedure does not include flap entry and closure, or, when indicated, wound debridement, osseous contouring, bone replacement grafts, and placement of biologic materials to aid in osseous regeneration. This procedure may be used for ridge augmentation, sinus lift procedures, and after tooth extraction.

D5820 interim partial denture (including retentive/clasping materials, rests, and teeth), maxillary

Note: D5820 is the "flipper" procedure.

Part 2: Implant Placement Surgery, Interim Implant Abutment Placement, and Interim Implant Crown

The patient was unhappy with the removable appliance and wanted a tooth as soon as possible. The dentist decided to place an interim abutment along with an interim implant crown. After placement of the surgical implant, the dentist customized an interim abutment with composite and placed an interim crown.

Note: The implant post is surgically placed and followed the interim procedures.

D6010 surgical placement of implant body: endosteal implant

D6051 interim implant abutment placement

D6085 interim implant crown

Part 3: Final Restoration – Custom Abutment and Abutment Supported Porcelain Crown

Note: In this case, esthetics were a concern. A custom abutment was placed due to angulation concerns and final material chosen was porcelain since the patient has a high smile line. The existing interim abutment was removed and the final prosthesis was placed.

D6198 remove interim implant component

D6057 custom fabricated abutment – includes placement

D6058 abutment supported porcelain/ceramic crown

Clinical Coding Scenario #2:
Implant Supported Mandibular Denture for an Edentulous Patient

The patient has worn a complete mandibular denture for over ten years with an occasional reline. The most recent reline was two years ago. Before this there were no problems with fit or retention, but since the last reline the patient has been using an adhesive to glue in the denture with limited success. The patient is also edentulous on the maxillary but is happy with her denture. The patient had previously declined a recommendation to replace the denture with implants and fabricate an overdenture that would be placed on the implants. Now the patient has agreed to implant treatment.

What codes would be used to document services delivered as the treatment progressed?

Initial Services

Since the patient has been edentulous for over ten years, a cone beam CT scan was necessary to evaluate the mandibular jaw bone dimensions. This enables an assessment to determine whether bone augmentation is needed prior to implant placement. A surgical guide was made and used during radiographic exposure for treatment planning and will be used again during implant placement.

> **D0365** **cone beam CT capture and interpretation with field of view of one full dental arch – mandible**
>
> **D6190** **radiographic/surgical implant index, by report**

Implant Post Placement

The cone beam image revealed there was enough bone to place two implants in positions of teeth #22 and #27.

> **D6010** **surgical placement of implant body: endosteal implant**

Note: Report D6010 twice as two implant bodies were placed, one for #22 and the second for #27.

Continued on next page

Second Stage Surgery and Placement of the Restorative Prosthesis

The patient will continue to wear her existing denture as the implants heal. After the implants have successfully integrated, the next step is to begin the restorative treatment. Second stage surgery is followed by placement of semi-precision abutments. A newly fabricated mandibular complete overdenture is inserted with the semi-precision attachments in the denture.

These procedures are documented as follows:

D6011 surgical access to an implant body (second stage surgery)

Note: Report D6011 twice as the procedure is required for each of the two implant bodies placed.

D6191 semi-precision abutment – placement

Note: Report D6191 twice as the procedure is required for each of the two implant bodies placed.

D6111 implant/abutment supported removable denture for edentulous arch – mandibular

Note: This code is used for removable complete dentures that are either directly supported by the implant body, or by the abutments placed on the implant body.

D6192 semi-precision attachment – placement

Note: Report D6192 twice since this procedure involves the luting of the initial semi-precision attachment to the removable denture.

Replacement of Semi-Precision Attachment Replaceable Component

The patient is made aware that it is normal for the attachment's replaceable components to wear over time and will periodically need replacement. This future procedure is documented with the following CDT Code:

D6091 replacement of replaceable part of semi-precision or precision attachment of implant/abutment supported prosthesis, per attachment

Clinical Coding Scenario #3:

Implant Supported Maxillary Fixed Complete Denture

The patient in scenario two was so happy with the results of her lower denture she would now like implants on her maxilla. The final prostheses for this arch will be an abutment supported fixed complete denture.

What codes would be used to document services delivered as the treatment progressed?

Initial Services

Since the patient has low sinuses, a cone beam scan was necessary to evaluate their exact location as well as the jaw bone dimensions. This enables an assessment to determine whether sinus elevation and bone augmentation is needed prior to implant placement. A surgical guide was made and used during radiographic exposure for treatment planning and will be used again during implant placement.

D6190 **radiographic/surgical implant index, by report**

D0366 **cone beam CT capture and interpretation with field of view of one full dental arch – maxilla, with or without cranium**

Implant Post Placement and Sinus Elevation

The restorative dentist would like six implants placed since the final restoration will be a fixed denture. The cone beam image revealed there was enough bone in areas of teeth #7 and #10, however sinus elevation will be needed in areas of #3, #5, #12, and #14. The patient's existing denture will be utilized after implant placement and sinus elevation.

D7951 **sinus augmentation with bone or bone substitutes via a lateral open approach**

or

D7952 **sinus augmentation via a vertical approach**

Note: The appropriate sinus augmentation procedure is determined by the dentist's clinical judgment. Report the appropriate sinus elevation twice – once on the right side and once on the left, and both these procedures include obtaining the bone or bone substitutes.

D6010 **surgical placement of implant body: endosteal implant**

Note: Report D6010 six times since six implant bodies were placed, one for #3, #5, #7, #10, #12, and #14. *Continued on next page*

Second Stage Surgery and Placement Interim Prosthesis and Final Prosthetic

After three to six months of osseointegration, implants are uncovered, and an interim prosthesis is fabricated. An interim prosthesis was fabricated to evaluate the patient's esthetic and functional needs as well as soft tissue healing and assist with design of the definitive prosthesis. After healing is complete a newly fabricated implant supported fixed complete denture is inserted.

These procedures are documented as follows:

D6011   surgical access to an implant body (second stage surgery)

Note: Report D6011 six times as the procedure is required for each of the six implant bodies placed.

D6119   implant/abutment supported interim fixed denture for edentulous arch – maxillary

Note: D6119 is used during the healing prior to fabrication and placement of permanent prosthetic.

D6114   implant/abutment supported fixed denture for edentulous arch – maxillary

Note: This code is used for fixed complete dentures that are either directly supported by the implant body, or by the abutments placed on the implant body.

Clinical Coding Scenario #4:
Implant-borne Prosthesis

A patient with a fully edentulous mandible is ready to receive an implant/abutment supported overdenture. The oral surgeon performs the first stage surgery to place the implant fixtures. After osseointegration, the surgeon performs a second stage surgery and places prefabricated abutments before referring for completion of the prosthesis.

D6010 surgical placement of implant body: endosteal implant

D6011 surgical access to an implant body (second stage implant surgery)

D6056 prefabricated abutment – includes modification and placement

Modification of a prefabricated abutment may be necessary.

Note: The patient's record and claim submissions must report the number of implant bodies placed (D6010 procedure) and the number of prefabricated abutments placed (D6056 procedure).

The same patient presents with fully osseointegrated implant fixtures and is ready to receive the removable mandibular denture supported by the abutments on the implants. This denture will be retained with semi-precision attachments. The applicable CDT codes for placing the prosthesis in this case are:

D6191 semi-precision abutment – placement
This procedure is the initial placement, or replacement, of a semi-precision abutment on the implant body.

D6192 semi-precision attachment – placement
This procedure involves the luting of the initial, or replacement, semi-precision attachment to the removable prosthesis.

Notes:

- D6191 is reported for each semi-precision abutment and D6192 is reported for each semi-precision attachment that is placed within the overdenture and required to retain the prosthesis.

- For procedure D6192, the terms housing and keeper are synonyms for the term attachment.

D6111 implant/abutment supported removable denture for edentulous arch – mandibular

Continued on next page

Note: D6111 applies if the prosthesis placed is newly fabricated. However, if the patient has an existing denture that will be modified to be supported by the new attachments, the procedure to report is D5875 modification of removable prosthesis following implant surgery.

A few years later, the patient states that the overdenture feels loose, and the dentist determines that the appropriate course of action is to replace worn components of the attachments as well as reline the prosthesis for patient comfort – all done in-office. The applicable CDT codes for this later encounter are:

D6091 **replacement of replaceable part of semi-precision or precision attachment of implant/abutment supported prosthesis, per attachment**

D5731 **reline complete mandibular denture (direct)**

Clinical Coding Scenario #5:
Removal of a Broken Implant Retaining Screw

Five years ago, a dentist replaced tooth #19 with an implant post that successfully osseointegrated, and an implant supported crown. The patient came in for an emergency since he felt "something was loose." The radiograph image shows the post is still osseointegrated with no bone loss. However, the implant retaining screw is broken in the apical third of the implant chamber. The dentist was not able to retrieve the screw with a Cavitron®. In order to successfully retrieve the broken screw, the dentist had to purchase a screw retrieval kit.

How do you code for this visit?

D0140 **limited oral evaluation – problem focused**

D0220 **intraoral – periapical first radiographic image**

D6096 **remove broken implant retaining screw**

This procedure assumes the implant retaining screw is broken and the fragments are remaining in the body of the implant as well as the implant retained crown. This code is only submitted when removing the screw cannot be performed using standard and conventional techniques for removal. It does not report tightening of an intact screw or routine removal. When submitting to a dental plan, always submit a narrative with any supporting documentation.

Clinical Coding Scenario #6:
Tightening of an Implant Screw

Two years ago, a dentist placed a screw retained porcelain fused to metal implant crown on tooth #12. Today the patient was returning for a cleaning, exam, and four bitewings. The patient had no concerns in her mouth, but the hygienist noticed that the implant screw was loose and needed to be tightened. After the prophy was completed, four bitewing radiographs were taken. The dentist performed a periodic exam, which showed that the screw was slightly loose, and proceeded to tighten the implant screw.

How would you code for this visit?

    D1110   **prophylaxis – adult**

    D0274   **bitewings – four radiographic images**

    D0120   **periodic oral evaluation – established patient**

There is no separate code for tightening an implant retaining screw. This service may be reported with the code D6199 accompanied by a detailed narrative.

Note: The Code Maintenance Committee considers tightening loose screws as inclusive to the implant maintenance procedure (D6080), which was not performed in this scenario. D6080 can be used to document tightening an implant screw only if the fixed prosthesis was removed, inspected, cleansed, and reinserted.

Clinical Coding Scenario #7:

Cantilever Implant

The patient desperately wants implants. Upon review of the cone beam image, the proposed treatment is one surgical implant on tooth #5 with implant crown on #5 and a pontic on #4 cantilevering tooth #4 off tooth #5.

What code reports this structure that will be placed to replace teeth #4 and #5?

D6010   surgical placement of implant body: endosteal implant

(tooth #5)

D6076   implant supported retainer for FPD – porcelain fused to high noble alloys

(tooth #5)

D6240   pontic – porcelain fused to high noble metal

(tooth #4)

A porcelain fused to high noble metal cantilever (fixed) bridge on a natural tooth would be submitted with the same pontic code, D6240, plus **D6750 retainer crown – porcelain fused to high noble metal**.

Remember that pontic codes in the Prosthodontics, fixed category are used with all bridges placed on natural teeth or implants. All pontic codes (D6205–D6253) can be used with either an abutment or implant supported bridge. Be sure the implant crown retainer material is consistent with the pontic material.

Clinical Coding Scenario #8:

Implant/Abutment Supported Interim Fixed Denture for Edentulous Arch – Maxilla

A patient is completely edentulous on his upper jaw and he chooses implants as an option. The implants will not be in relative tooth positions since the surgeon will place the implants where the ridge is sufficient. The final prosthesis will be a complete abutment supported fixed denture (a hybrid prosthesis) placed on pre-fabricated abutments. The dentist will be placing abutments and an interim fixed denture for this patient on the day of surgery so the patient doesn't have to go without teeth.

How do you code for the different prostheses in this scenario?

D6010   surgical placement of implant body: endosteal implant

(Repeat for the number of implants placed)

D6056   prefabricated abutment – includes modification and placement

(Repeat for the number of abutments placed)

D6119   implant/abutment supported interim fixed denture for edentulous arch – maxillary

D6114   implant/abutment supported fixed denture for edentulous arch – maxillary

Clinical Coding Scenario #9:
Implant Overdenture – Mandibular

A 45-year-old patient has worn a complete mandibular denture for five years since she lost her teeth due to periodontal disease. She would like a more stable denture. Since her finances are limited, she opted for an overdenture which will be supported by two mini-implants in location of teeth #22 and #27. She will utilize her current denture as a temporary denture while the implants heal, but ultimately she wants a new overdenture.

What codes should the dentist submit for the mini implants and the overdenture?

D6013   surgical placement of mini implant

(teeth #22 and #27)

D6111   implant/abutment supported removable denture for edentulous arch – mandibular

(mandibular implant overdenture)

D6192   semi-precision attachment – placement

(teeth #22 and #27)

Note: D6192 is the correct code for luting of the semi-precision attachment keeper assembly in the denture.

Clinical Coding Scenario #10:
Cervitec Gel Application around an Implant to Treat Gingivitis

A dentist placed an implant and implant supported crown on tooth #6 five years ago. The implant is stable and radiographs show no bone loss around the implant fixture. The patient has very good oral hygiene. However, every time the patient presents for periodontal maintenance, the tissue around the implant is inflamed. The dentist recently took a course and learned about a product she can apply to the tissue to treat this type of tissue inflammation around the implant. She purchased the material and will apply the gel on the gingival tissue and the implant restoration.

How would you code this procedure?

D6199   unspecified implant procedure, by report

Currently, there is no CDT code to support application of the material that reduces tissue inflammation.

Clinical Coding Scenario #11:
Implant Removal

Two years ago, a dentist in another state placed an implant post and implant supported crown on tooth #14. Unfortunately, the patient admitted she began smoking again and has since developed diabetes. The implants have developed peri-implantitis and are extremely loose. The dentist needs to remove the implant crowns and the implant posts, as well as place a bone graft material.

How would you code these procedures?

This procedure does not require bone removal nor flap elevation since the failed implant is so loose. Due to the mobility and lack of bone structure, the dentist is able to remove the implant non-surgically by simply rotating the implant out of the bone with forceps.

D6105 **removal of implant body not requiring bone removal or flap elevation**

D7953 **bone replacement graft for ridge preservation – per site**

The treatment notes and documentation in the patient's record should include the location of the removed implant and a description of the procedure performed. Even though this procedure is not by report, it may still be helpful to the carrier to note on the claim when the implant was initially placed, as well as attach a radiographic image.

Currently there is no CDT code to remove the implant crown and it would be considered inclusive to D6105. However, if there are complex issues, use **D6199 unspecified implant procedure, by report**.

Clinical Coding Scenario #12:
Submerging a Fractured Implant

A new patient comes to your office with a fractured implant #23. The implant post was placed three years ago and restored with an implant supported crown. The dentist gives the patient all her options and they come to a mutual decision to bury the implant rather than remove it with a trephine since the jaw bone is so thin. Then a fixed partial denture will be fabricated. The dentist opens the area, grinds down the head of the implant, decontaminates the remaining screw channel with Peridex™, and places a connective tissue graft to reduce the height of the pontic on the proposed fixed partial denture.

How would you code these procedures?

D6199   unspecified implant procedure, by report

Note: Currently there is no CDT code to report "burial" of the implant. Describe the procedure with a clear and concise narrative. The narrative should include the location of the implant and the description of the procedure performed. If submitting a claim to a dental carrier, it is also helpful to include when the implant was initially placed, as well as a radiographic image.

D4273   autogenous connective tissue graft procedure (including donor and recipient surgical sites) first tooth, implant, or edentulous tooth position in graft

or

D4275   non-autogenous connective tissue graft (including recipient site and donor material) first tooth, implant, or edentulous tooth position in graft

Clinical Coding Scenario #13:
Cement Removal around the Implant Crown

A patient presents with pain around her #10 implant. The pain has persisted since the crown was put on. After the original dentist (the one that placed the crown on the implant) couldn't help her, the surgeon that placed the implant referred her to your practice. The patient brings her treatment records with all her radiographs, so the dentist knows which implant system was used. The dentists observes cement around the implant crown causing bone loss.

Since it is an anterior tooth in an esthetic area, the dentist does not want to cut any gingival tissue. She chooses to remove the crown and abutment. The dentist drills through the crown, then locates the screw holding the crown onto the implant, removes the crown, cleans the cement, and screws it all back together. This eliminates the patient's pain and most likely stops the bone loss.

How would you code this procedure?

> **D6080** implant maintenance procedures when prostheses are removed and reinserted, including cleansing of the prostheses and abutments

Note: You cannot submit D6092 re-cement or re-bond implant/abutment supported crown since this procedure is an inherent part of the D6080 procedure.

Note: Third-party payer reimbursement for this or any other procedure reported with a CDT code depends upon a dental benefit plan's coverage provisions, and the provisions of any participating provider contract in effect.

Additional procedures that may be performed to remove excess cement include:

> **D6081** scaling and debridement in the presence of inflammation or mucositis of a single implant, including cleaning of the implant surfaces, without flap entry and closure

The following code is utilized when a bony defect has occurred, and the implant surface is debrided and cleaned. It includes flap entry and closure.

> **D6101** debridement of a peri-implant defect or defects surrounding a single implant, and surface cleaning of the exposed implant surfaces, including flap entry and closure

Continued on next page

This next code is utilized when a bony defect has occurred, and the implant surface is debrided, cleaned and the dentist performs osseous contouring of the peri-implant defect. It includes flap entry and closure.

D6102 **debridement and osseous contouring of a peri-implant defect or defects surrounding a single implant and includes surface cleaning of the exposed implant surfaces, including flap entry and closure**

Clinical Coding Scenario #14:
Changing Healing Abutments

A dentist placed full sized implants on teeth #8 and #9 one month ago and the implants are successfully integrating. A week ago the dentist performed second stage surgery and placed two healing caps (gingival contours) with a cuff height of 2 mm. However, when the patient returned for suture removal, it was clear the collar of the healing caps that had been placed were too short. The gingival tissue has already overgrown. The dentist had misjudged the tissue depth and therefore needed to place healing caps with an increased cuff height. The dentist had already performed second stage surgery and was not sure of the code.

How would you code this procedure?

D6011 **surgical access to an implant body (second stage implant surgery)**
This procedure, also known as second stage implant surgery, involves removal of tissue that covers the implant body so that a fixture of any type can be placed, or an existing fixture be replaced with another.

Per its descriptor, this procedure includes replacement of an existing fixture, so D6011 is used again to report the service delivered to both implants. Even though this code should be used to document and report replacing the healing caps there are dental benefit plans with coverage provisions that only reimburse once per implant.

Clinical Coding Scenario #15:
Essix Retainer as a Temporary

A 74-year-old patient has existing crowns on all her maxillary teeth, many of which have been treated endodontically. Unfortunately, tooth #9 has a fracture and the dentist needs to remove it and place an implant. Since esthetics are a concern, the dentist would like to use an Essix retainer as a temporary while the implant is healing. Even though an Essix retainer is traditionally used for orthodontic retention, the dentist is not using it as a retainer so she doubts it would be appropriate to use the orthodontic code.

How would you code this temporary procedure?

There is no existing code that specifically describes an Essix retainer but there are codes that might describe this situation.

D5899 unspecified removable prosthodontic procedure, by report
Used for a procedure that is not adequately described by a codes. Describe the procedure.

D5820 interim partial denture (including retentive/clasping materials, rests, and teeth), maxillary

Note: D5820 is often used to report a "flipper," which includes an Essix retainer.

Clinical Coding Scenario #16:
Implant Crown Repair

A patient presented to a dental office for a periodic cleaning and exam visit. The patient's chief complaint was that they felt like they may have a crack in one of their molars that they would like the dentist to look at. An oral examination revealed the implant crown on #30 had a chip in the porcelain on the distal occlusal and had become a food trap. Treatment options presented to the patient were to repair the chip on the existing crown with a bonded resin or to have a whole new crown and custom abutment fabricated. The patient chose to have it repaired for now. The repair procedure's steps included porcelain etching (e.g., Clearfil SE™), a flowable composite (e.g., SureFill® SDR), and a light-cured resin (e.g., QuiXX®).

How would you code this procedure?

D6090 repair implant supported prosthesis, by report
> This procedure involves the repair or replacement of any part of the implant supported prosthesis.

Be sure to include brief narrative, including the original date of placement and a description of the repair, when reporting D6090 on a claim.

Clinical Coding Scenario #17:
Replacement of Clips on Hader Bar

A patient currently wears a lower implant supported overdenture. Implants are in positions #22 and #27 with a Hader bar connecting them. After many years of wear, it is now evident that the plastic clips in the metal housings require replacement.

What is the proper code for replacement of plastic clips on a Hader Bar?

D6091 replacement of replaceable part of semi-precision or precision attachment of implant/abutment supported prosthesis, per attachment

Note: A clip is a replaceable part and therefore the code D6091 describes the procedure.

Note: Submit this code per clip (per attachment) not per visit.

Clinical Coding Scenario #18:
Covering Implant Screw Holes

A patient presents who had three implants placed and restored with implant crowns that are screw retained on #2, #3, and #4 by another dental office. Two of the screw holes have lost the composites covering them, and the dentist needs to replace the missing composites to cover the screw access hole. Would it be acceptable to use **D2391 resin-based composite – one surface, posterior** for these implants or is there a more appropriate code?

The correct code is:

> **D6197** **replacement of restorative material used to close an access opening of a screw-retained implant supported prosthesis, per implant**

Note: The D6197 is per implant, so if two of the implants needed closing of the access opening, this code should be reported twice on a claim and in the patient's dental record (also noting where the implant(s) are located).

Clinical Coding Scenario #19:
Implant/Abutment Supported Mandibular Fixed Complete Denture with Connecting Bar

My patient is edentulous in the mandible and recently had four implants placed in the areas of #20, #22, #27, and #29. Prefabricated abutments will be placed on each implant. To enhance the denture retention, it was decided to use a Hader bar, which is a connecting bar.

How would you code this procedure?

> **D6056** **prefabricated abutment – includes modification and placement**

(on #20, #22, #27, and #29)

> **D6055** **connecting bar – implant supported or abutment supported**
>
> **D6115** **implant/abutment supported fixed denture for edentulous arch – mandibular**

Note: The connector bar should be reported just once, regardless of the number of abutments/implants to which it is attached. If this connector bar was attached to fixed partial denture retainer crown or coping, see CDT code D6920.

Clinical Coding Scenario #20:
Cleaning of Removable Implant Dentures

We have several patients that we placed implant/abutment supported complete removable dentures (D6110 and D6111). I recommend to these patients they come in every six months so I can clean and inspect the denture.

What procedure code would be used to report cleaning of the dentures?

There are two procedure codes for cleaning complete dentures and two for partial dentures:

D9932 **cleaning and inspection of removable complete denture, maxillary**

D9933 **cleaning and inspection of removable complete denture, mandibular**

Note: If the dentures were partial removable (D6112 or D6113), use

D9934 **cleaning and inspection of removable partial denture, maxillary**

D9935 **cleaning and inspection of removable partial denture, mandibular**

The descriptor for each of these four codes states "this procedure does not include any adjustments." Also keep in mind the procedures (and codes) are applicable to prostheses that are either abutment supported or directly supported by an implant post.

If the cleaning procedure involves prostheses removal, cleaning of the prosthesis and abutments, and then reinsertion, the following code is reported (per prosthesis):

D6080 **implant maintenance procedures when prostheses are removed and reinserted, including cleansing of prostheses and abutments**
This procedure includes active debriding of the implant(s) and examination of all aspects of the implant system(s), including the occlusion and stability of the superstructure. The patient is also instructed in thorough daily cleansing of the implant(s). This is not a per implant code, and is indicated for implant-supported fixed prostheses.

Clinical Coding Scenario #21:
Fixed Implant Partial Denture

My patient just relocated jobs and moved to my state. This was a rather sudden move, so she didn't have time to finish her implant treatment. I received the treatment records from her previous dentist and spoke to him directly. He informed me he recently extracted teeth #12 and #14 (noting also that tooth #13 had been extracted years ago) as well as surgically placed implants in areas of #12 and #14 with bone graft and a non-resorbable barrier around the implant #12. The final prosthetic treatment plan was to restore the two implants with a fixed implant partial denture.

How would you code the following procedures?

Visit #1:

Prior to fabricating the fixed implant partial denture I sent her to a local periodontist to remove the non-resorbable barrier. The code used was:

D4286   removal of non-resorbable barrier

Visit #2:

The patient then came back to my office for the fixed implant supported partial denture. The codes used to document these procedures were:

D6075   implant supported retainer for ceramic FPD (tooth #12)

D6245   pontic – porcelain/ceramic (tooth #13)

D6075   implant supported retainer for ceramic FPD (tooth #14)

Clinical Coding Scenario #22:
Bone Graft at the Time of Implant Placement with Barrier

While placing an implant body on tooth #19, a few threads were exposed, so a bone graft and membrane were also necessary to cover the exposed threads.

How would you code these procedures?

> **D6010** **surgical placement of implant body: endosteal implant** (tooth #19)

> **D6104** **bone graft at the time of implant placement** (tooth #19)

Note: The bone graft procedure (D6104) does not include placement of a barrier, which is a separate procedure documented with one of the following codes, determined by the type of barrier involved.

> **D6106** **guided tissue regeneration – resorbable barrier, per implant**
> This procedure does not include flap entry and closure, or, when indicated, wound debridement, osseous contouring, bone replacement grafts, and placement of biologic materials to aid in osseous regeneration. This procedure is used for peri-implant defects and during implant placement.

> **D6107** **guided tissue regeneration – non-resorbable barrier, per implant**
> This procedure does not include flap entry and closure, or, when indicated, wound debridement, osseous contouring, bone replacement grafts, and placement of biologic materials to aid in osseous regeneration. This procedure is used for peri-implant defects and during implant placement.

Note: When a non-resorbable barrier is placed during the D6107 procedure, removal is a separate procedure documented at that time with **D4286 removal of non-resorbable barrier**.

Coding Q&A

1. *My patient does not have implant coverage but does have crown coverage. Would I be able to use the code D2740 instead of D6065 to report an implant supported porcelain/ceramic crown?*

    No. If implants are not a covered benefit under the patient's benefits, reporting D2740 is misrepresenting a service to gain insurance reimbursement. You must report the procedure performed (D6065) regardless of insurance reimbursement. This statement also applies for retainer crowns. Reporting implant retainer crowns (D6075) as retainer crowns on natural teeth (D6740) to gain insurance reimbursement is also misrepresenting a service.

    Note: Even though you may be submitting the implant crowns appropriately, occasionally benefit plans may reimburse the implant crown as an alternate benefit of a natural tooth crown. An alternative benefit is typically subject to the same limitations, such as time, as the standard prosthodontic service.

2. *I submitted the following codes on a claim to my patient's dental insurance carrier for two implant procedures for tooth #12:*

    D6056   prefabricated abutment – includes modification and placement

    D6066   implant supported crown – porcelain fused to high noble alloys

    The carrier has not reimbursed the procedures, stating, "There is a coding error. A prefabricated abutment and an implant supported crown may not be reported together. Please resubmit with the appropriate codes." What do I do?

    The insurance carrier is correct as there is an inconsistency. When reporting an implant abutment (either D6056 or D6057), the crown code must indicate that support and retention is through the abutment. In this case, assuming an abutment was placed, the correct crown code is **D6059 abutment supported porcelain fused to metal crown (high noble metal)**. Code D6066 is for reporting a crown that is directly supported by the implant post (i.e., an abutment is neither required nor present).

3. *What is the difference between a temporary anchorage device (TAD) reported with codes D7292, D7293, or D7294 (as applicable) and a mini implant reported with code D6013?*

    Although both TADs and mini implants look similar, a TAD is typically smaller, has an area for orthodontic wire, is used for orthodontic anchorage or as part of orthodontic treatment, and is removed after a period of time. A mini implant (D6013) is not typically removed and usually supports a removable denture.

4. *A patient is having endosteal implants placed for a complete implant supported denture. The dentist will fabricate a stent-like appliance for the surgeon to be sure the implants are placed exactly where the dentist needs them. Would the appliance be documented as* **D5982 surgical stent**, **D5988 surgical splint**, *or* **D6190 radiographic/surgical implant index, by report**?

The correct code for this appliance, which is a guide and not a stent, is:

D6190   radiographic/surgical implant index, by report

An appliance, designed to relate osteotomy or fixture position to existing anatomic structures, to be utilized during radiographic exposure for treatment planning and/or during osteotomy creation for fixture installation.

D5982 surgical stent is not correct because a stent is an appliance that applies pressure to soft tissues to facilitate healing and prevent collapse of soft tissue.

D5988 surgical splint is not correct as it uses existing teeth and/or alveolar processes as points of anchorage to assist in stabilization and immobilization of broken bones during healing.

5. *I noticed there are no pontic codes in the CDT Code's Implant Services category. When reporting a fixed partial denture placed on implants, how do I report the pontic?*

Pontic codes, found in the Fixed Prosthodontic category of the CDT Code, can be used with all bridges whether the bridge is on natural teeth or implants. All pontic codes (D6205–D6253) can be used with either an abutment or implant supported bridge. Be sure the implant's pontic material is consistent with the implant retainer material.

6. *I placed an implant on tooth #30 two years ago. The patient has since developed peri-implantitis. There is radiographic evidence of bone loss only on the mesial aspect, so I am confident this can successfully be treated with bone grafting and a resorbable barrier. Would the osseous surgery procedure be documented with D4261, the bone graft documented with D4263, and the guided tissue resorbable barrier with D4266?*

No, the D426x procedure codes are not appropriate for documenting surgical repairs, bone grafting, and barriers in conjunction with implants. The correct codes in this situation are:

D6102   debridement and osseous contouring of a peri-implant defect or defects surrounding a single implant and includes surface cleaning of exposed implant surfaces, including flap entry and closure

D6103 **bone graft for repair of peri-implant defect – does not include flap entry and closure**

D6106 **guided tissue regeneration – resorbable barrier, per implant**
This procedure does not include flap entry and closure, or, when indicated, wound debridement, osseous contouring, bone replacement grafts, and placement of biologic materials to aid in osseous regeneration. This procedure is used for peri-implant defects and during implant placement.

7. *What code should I use to document placement of an implant abutment?*

There is no placement procedure code. As seen in the following current codes and their nomenclatures, implant abutment procedures include placement:

D6056 **prefabricated abutment – includes modification and placement**

D6057 **custom fabricated abutment – includes placement**

8. *We have several patients that have implant supported mandibular complete dentures. However, they have natural teeth in their maxillary arch. What procedure code would be used to report cleaning of the implants, and can this code be submitted with a prophy (D1110) and a periodic oral evaluation (D0120)?*

The answer depends on whether or not the prosthesis placed on the implants is removed.

If the prosthesis is not removed, cleaning both the natural teeth and implant bodies may be reported with the applicable prophylaxis code. The CDT code descriptors for both D1110 and D1120 indicate that these procedures apply to both natural dentition and implants placed within that dentition:

D1110 **prophylaxis – adult**
Removal of plaque, calculus and stains from tooth structures and implants in the permanent and transitional dentition. It is intended to control local irritational factors.

D1120 **prophylaxis – child**
Removal of plaque, calculus and stains from tooth structures and implants in the primary and transitional dentition. It is intended to control local irritational factors.

However, if the prosthesis is removed, the following code is reported:

D6080 **implant maintenance procedures when prostheses are removed and reinserted, including cleansing of prostheses and abutments**

This procedure includes active debriding of the implant(s) and examination of all aspects of the implant system(s), including the occlusion and stability of the superstructure. The patient is also instructed in thorough daily cleansing of the implant(s). This is not a per implant code, and is indicated for implant supported fixed prostheses.

An implant maintenance procedure can be delivered and submitted for the same date of service that the patient receives a prophylaxis or periodontal maintenance because the implant maintenance procedure does not include services rendered to the patient's natural teeth. A periodic oral evaluation can also be submitted on this date of service.

However, when both the D6080 and D1110 are performed on the same date of service, some dental benefit plan limitations and exclusions provisions may, for claim adjudication, consider D6080 to be inclusive in the D1110 (or D4910) and D0120 procedure and not provide additional reimbursement.

9. *I placed interim crowns on three implants to allow time for healing, which should take about six months. There are interim crowns in the Restorative category of service, but what about reporting the interim implant crown procedure?*

The appropriate CDT code for this procedure is:

D6085 **interim implant crown**

Placed when a period of healing is necessary prior to fabrication and placement of the definitive prosthesis.

This procedure is similar to other interim codes (e.g., D2799 interim crown...) in that there is neither a requirement that the interim implant crown be used for a specific time period, nor prohibition on use if the final impression for the permanent implant crown has been taken. Keep in mind, a benefits plan may not cover this procedure or make the code inclusive of the final prosthesis. Report D6085 for each interim crown placed.

10. *A patient presents with a complete lower denture made 11 months ago at another dental office. She is unhappy with the fit and now realizes she should have had the implants her dentist recommended. The treatment plan consists of two mini implants and two Zest LOCATOR®s on an overdenture. Is there any way to still use her existing denture after we place the implants and locator attachments?*

Yes, the existing denture can be used. This is a retrofitting procedure where the internal surface of the existing denture is modified to accommodate the retentive elements. The code is:

D5875   modification of removable prosthesis following implant surgery
Attachment assemblies are reported using separate codes.

Surgical implants are coded as **D6013 surgical placement of mini implant** and the two locators on the overdenture are coded as **D5862 precision attachment, by report**. A Zest LOCATOR® is just one example of a precision attachment.

Any relines are reported separately.

11. *I placed a prefabricated abutment (D6056) and an abutment supported porcelain fused to metal crown (high noble metal) (D6059). Six months later, the patient presented with the implant crown in his hand. I took a radiographic image which showed no problems with the implant fixture or abutment, so I cemented the implant crown back in his mouth. Is there a code for this procedure?*

Yes, the code you would use is:

D6092   re-cement or re-bond implant/abutment supported crown

Note: If this were an implant/abutment supported fixed partial denture, the correct code would be D6093.

12. *My patient comes in every three months for periodontal maintenance (D4910). She has all her teeth with the exception of implants on teeth #2 and #4 which I placed one year ago. A restorative dentist has since placed the abutments and abutment supported crowns. She noticed bleeding around the implants after the implant crowns were placed so she came to my office to have them evaluated. I took a radiographic image and noticed that around both of her implants, the gingival tissue was inflamed due to excess cement from the implant crown placement. However, there were no threads exposed and no bone loss present. I need to scale and debride around the implants; should I use the code D4346?*

No. For scaling and debridement of the implants, use D6081. You would submit it twice – once for #2 and also for #4 since this is a per implant code.

D6081   scaling and debridement in the presence of inflammation or mucositis of a single implant, including cleaning of the implant surfaces, without flap entry and closure
This procedure is not performed in conjunction with D1110, D4910, or D4346.

13. *My patient has an implant on tooth #7 which was placed four years ago. The implant is well integrated with the bone and the patient is happy with the esthetics of the crown. However, there is now slight recession present on the buccal and I plan on performing a connective tissue graft. But, I can't find a code in the implant section. What code would I use?*

The correct soft tissue graft codes are located in the Periodontics section, and the code you choose depends on if you are performing an autogenous or non-autogenous connective tissue graft:

> **D4273** **autogenous connective tissue graft procedure (including donor and recipient surgical sites) first tooth, implant or edentulous tooth position in graft**
>
> **D4275** **non-autogenous connective tissue graft (including recipient site and donor material) first tooth, implant, or edentulous tooth position in graft**

14. **D6010 surgical placement of an implant body: endosteal implant**, *as well as placement of other implant body types (e.g., eposteal; mini), does not include placement of a healing cap. The implant has osseointegrated and is ready to be uncovered. What code would be used for placement of a healing cap? Can I also bill for the healing cap itself?*

Surgical exposure of the implant is called "uncovering" or "second stage surgery," and is reported separately as D6011. The descriptor of **D6011 surgical access to an implant body (second stage implant surgery)** states:

> "This procedure, also known as second stage implant surgery, involves removal of tissue that covers the implant body so that a fixture of any type can be placed, or an existing fixture be replaced with another. Examples of fixtures include but are not limited to healing caps, abutments shaped to help contour the gingival margins or the final restorative prosthesis."

Note: A healing cap is not reported separately, nor is a separate fee charged for the healing cap.

Note: Some benefit plans consider the D6011 procedure to be "inclusive" under D6010 with no separate reimbursement.

15. Is an interim abutment the same as a healing cap?

No. An interim implant abutment is used while awaiting definitive treatment during a healing phase and is ultimately replaced by either **D6056 prefabricated abutment – includes modification and placement** or **D6057 custom fabricated abutment – includes placement**. A healing cap is placed at the time of second stage surgery and just maintains an access opening to the implant body prior to the restorative phase of implant treatment.

Note: Two CDT codes are used for interim implant abutments. One for placement (**D6051 interim implant abutment placement**) and one for removal (**D6198 remove interim implant component**).

16. Is there a code for an immediate implant placement?

There is no distinction in the surgical implant placement codes. They can be submitted whether the implant is placed at the time of tooth extraction or post-extraction.

17. I just placed a UCLA-type single crown, which is screw retained, and I am using a composite to seal the access opening. What are the codes for the crown and the composite material placed?

There is no separate code for a UCLA-type crown. These are implant supported crowns (D6065–D6088). There is no separate code for closure of the access opening with composite material at the time of initial placement.

18. My patient is edentulous on the mandibular arch and would like a definitive prosthesis as soon as possible, so I am going to use the Trefoil™ system. What is the code for the Trefoil™ bar?

The Trefoil™ bar is a pre-manufactured titanium bar with a unique retention mechanism that can be adjusted to compensate for inherent deviations from the ideal implant position and enable the passive fit of the definitive prosthesis. This is a type of a connecting bar and therefore the code is D6055.

19. My patient has transitional dentition with primary tooth H remaining as well as permanent teeth #9, #10, #12, etc. present. However, there is a congenitally missing canine (#11). The patient's orthodontist had moved tooth #10 to the vacant position of #11. I determined that the appropriate treatment for this patient is to extract H and then place an implant and fixture in the congenitally missing tooth space. On the claim I reported the implant as a replacement for the missing canine (#11). The payer rejected the claim on the grounds that there is a tooth in position #11. How should I address this denial?

Tooth #11 is the appropriate number to report as this is the congenitally missing tooth that is now the implant supported prosthesis. According to the ADA claim form completion instructions, tooth numbers are reported on the basis of morphology, not anatomical position. The denial should be appealed, with the resubmitted claim including a supporting narrative and images (etc.) so that there is a paper trail that accurately reflects the patient's dental records and history of services provided.

20. *When coding a screw retained full contour implant supported zirconia crown, what is the proper CDT code?*

Zirconia is a ceramic and therefore the appropriate code is:

D6065 implant supported porcelain/ceramic crown

21. *I placed an implant and screw retained crown on #14. The patient has all remaining teeth except for #15. The implant is osseointegrated but has an open contact between the dental implant crown and #13, which is a natural tooth. My concern is that food is beginning to get impacted and this can lead to peri-implantitis. I easily removed the crown, placed a healing abutment, and sent the crown back to the lab to add porcelain. How do I code for this procedure?*

D6090 repair implant supported prosthesis, by report
This procedure involves the repair or replacement of any part of the implant supported prosthesis.

Be sure to include brief narrative, including the original date of placement and a description of the repair, when reporting D6090 on a claim.

22. *I took a course and I am about to restore my first case of an "All-on-4®" lower arch. What is the correct code?*

An "All-on-4®" denture is a trademark name given to a denture permanently attached to a jaw by four implants, hence the "four" in "All-on-4®." Note that over the years the number of implants placed has changed and is not necessarily four, but the name is catchy, so it stuck. In this case, the correct code is **D6115 implant/abutment supported fixed denture for edentulous arch – mandibular**.

If you are performing an "All-on-4®" in the maxilla the CDT code would be:

D6114 implant/abutment supported fixed denture for edentulous arch – maxillary

23. *I will be restoring my patient's upper arch with an "All-on 4®" denture. I will be extracting remaining teeth, performing alveoloplasty, taking a cone beam image, placing full body implants and prefabricated abutments, modifying her existing denture as well as many other procedures. Since the patient does not have implant coverage with her current dental plan, how should I code these procedures on a claim for reimbursement?*

You must utilize the proper CDT codes for the procedures you perform whether or not the dental benefit plan provides coverage. Keep in mind even if a patient doesn't have implant coverage, they still have coverage for extractions and some carriers may pay an alternate benefit (e.g., reimburse for a natural tooth borne denture in place of the implant denture).

24. *If a patient needs a prefabricated abutment, does the implant surgeon or the restorative dentist submit the D6056?*

The practitioner who actually places the abutment submits the claim for this procedure (D6056). This person could be either the oral surgeon or the restorative dentist, depending on the circumstances.

25. *What code do I use for a prophy on a patient who has all her natural permanent teeth except for one that has been replaced with a healthy implant?*

The D1110 descriptor indicates that the procedure is applicable to removal of plaque, calculus and stains from natural tooth structures and implants.

D1110 prophylaxis – adult
> Removal of plaque, calculus and stains from tooth structures and implants in the permanent and transitional dentition. It is intended to control local irritational factors.

26. *If a dentist uses technology to mill an abutment with an implant crown or cements a prefabricated abutment into the implant crown outside the mouth, can he charge the patient for D6056 prefabricated abutment as well as the implant crown prior to delivery?*

If the crown and abutment is attached directly to the implant body as one piece (that is, the abutment is an integral part of the crown), the abutment is not reported separately and the appropriate crown code would be an implant supported crown.

27. *What is the CDT code for replacement of O-rings?*

The correct code is **D6091 replacement of replaceable part of semi-precision or precision attachment of implant/abutment supported prosthesis, per attachment**.

Note: This code is reported per attachment replaced, meaning it is reported for each O-ring that is replaced and not per denture.

28. *I just purchased the Osstell IDx system to check stability after the implant I placed on tooth #18. It provides the accurate, consistent, and objective information needed regarding the stability of the implant. Regardless of the system I use, what is the correct CDT code?*

Implant stability is inclusive to the global fee of the implant placement; therefore there is no separate CDT code. It is not a separate procedure, more of a step during the treatment.

29. *I will be fabricating a full arch hybrid zirconia bridge on the maxilla. How do I code for this full arch (#3–#14) zirconia bridge with abutments on 5 implants, which are placed in what appear to be sites of teeth #3, #6, #8, #11, and #14 (I am guessing since I cannot be exact with the location of the corresponding teeth)? My final prosthesis resembles a complete denture with holes in it for the attachment screws.*

D6056   prefabricated abutment – includes modification and placement

Report 5 times (once each for tooth # 3, #6, #8, #11, and #14)

D6114   implant/abutment supported fixed denture for edentulous arch – maxillary

For the zirconia fixed bridge.

30. *I recently graduated from dental school and opened my own practice, so I decided to contract with all PPO plans to help direct patients to my newly opened practice. I calculated my expenses when performing implant restorations and noticed that my negotiated fee is lower than what I had expected. Does the contracted fee typically include the lab fees or am I allowed to charge an additional fee for my lab expenses on implant restorations?*

Similar to other restorations such as crowns, fixed partial dentures, and dentures, the lab fees are included and cannot be billed to the patients.

31. *My patient is ready to restore the implant placed by an oral surgeon 4 months ago on tooth #30. I decided to use a prefabricated abutment and an abutment supported porcelain fused to metal crown. Today I am taking my impressions and then submitting to the patients benefit carrier. I will be submitting D6056 and D6059, but I can't find a CDT code for the lab analog? What CDT code should I use?*

There is no separate CDT code for lab analog; this is included in the global fee for the implant restoration.

32. *Would it be possible charge a global fee for an "All-on-4®" treatment since most dental carriers do not reimburse this?*

No, you must report the components and procedures separately with the appropriate CDT code. There are times when certain procedures, such as the oral evaluation, diagnostic procedures, are covered under the patient's benefit plan. There are also times that some of the procedures, such as the implant supported denture itself, are reimbursed as an alternate benefit of a denture that is not supported by implants. Lastly, be sure to submit all codes to the carrier since the carrier contract may dictate (subject to applicable state or federal law) the fee charged to the patient, even though it is not a covered benefit.

33. *After I place an implant on my patient I typically see them once a month after surgical placement to evaluate the gingival tissue and implant integration. The visit includes an evaluation of the surgical site as well as taking a PA of the area. What code should I use for the post-op/follow up visit procedures?*

> **D0171   re-evaluation – post-operative office visit**
>
> **D0220   intraoral – periapical first radiographic image**

Typically, when billed to carrier, these procedures are part of the global fee for the implant itself and will not be reimbursed.

34. *Are there any helpful tips when I submit implant restorations such as an implant crown D6058 to a carrier?*

There is no universal requirement since each carrier requests different information. Carriers typically request pre and post op radiographs, the date of the implant placement, that the claim date coincides with the date of seating the crown, and that you record the missing teeth in the arch. The carrier will then reimburse for the procedure based on the patient's plan limitations and exclusions.

35. *I need to remove an implant on #29 (placed by another dentist) that is fractured due to the patient's bruxism habit and lack of compliance on wearing his night-guard. The implant is fully engaged in bone. I laid a surgical flap and used a trephine bur to remove the implant. What code do I use to submit the procedure?*

D6100   surgical removal of implant body

The treatment notes and documentation in the patient's record should include the location of the removed implant and a description of the procedure performed. Even though this procedure is not by report, it may still be helpful to the carrier to put on the claim when the implant was initially placed, as well as to provide a radiographic image.

36. *I am reading CDT 2023 and I see three unique implant types (endosteal, eposteal and transosteal). Can you briefly explain the difference?*

Endosteal implant (D6010): In this type of implant, the tooth roots are replaced by screws or cylinders that are usually made of titanium or ceramic material. The implant is surgically drilled into the jawbone, thus the implant lies completely within the jawbone and it protrudes through the gum to hold the replacement tooth. It is by far the most commonly used dental implant.

Eposteal implant (D6040): Also known as a subperiosteal implant, this type consists of a metal framework that is firmly secured on the jawbone, but the framework itself is under the gum line. Metal posts are attached to this framework and they project outwards above the gum line through the metal frame to hold the replacement tooth. This is not a common procedure performed today.

Transosteal implant (D6050): The procedure involves attaching a metal plate at the bottom of the jawbone, with screws running through the jawbone, and the posts embedded within the gum tissue. An incision is made below the chin to fix the plate with screws and posts on top, to attach the artificial teeth. These implants that can be fitted only to the lower jawbone are generally not recommended as the surgical procedure is complicated and extensive.

Summary

Coding for implants may appear challenging, but accurate coding helps ensure proper claim adjudication and reimbursement in accordance with dental benefit plan coverage provisions. However, it can be straightforward once you learn the basics. It's important to document the material used to fabricate the prosthesis, and it must match the lab prescription. Some coding rules of thumb are in the following charts:

When the Final Prosthesis Is an Implant Crown or a Fixed Bridge

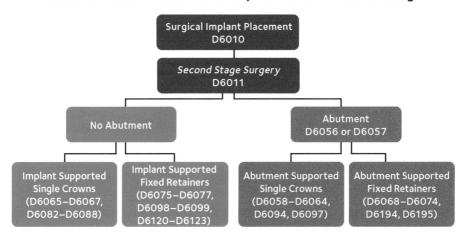

When the Final Prosthesis is a Removable or Fixed Implant Denture

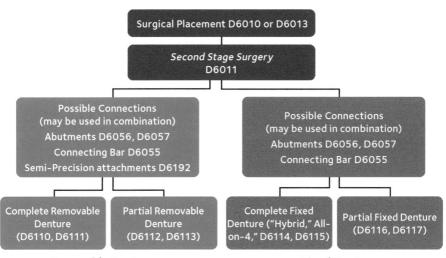

Chapter 8: D6000–D6199 Implant Services

Reimbursement for surgical implant placement and restorations varies among dental benefit plans. Often when the surgical implant is not a benefit, the implant restorations are reimbursed as an alternative benefit. Even if a dental benefit plan does have implant coverage or has an implant rider, there still may be limitations and may not mean the plan includes benefits for implant maintenance related procedures. Pre-authorizing implants is highly recommended and may be a requirement of some patients' plans. A written estimate for the total cost of treatment – regardless of insurance coverage – should be presented, signed by the patient, and retained in the patient's file.

Contributor Biography

Linda Vidone, D.M.D., is the Chief Clinical Officer/V.P. Clinical Management at Delta Dental of Massachusetts. She has 20 years of dental experience in clinical private practice, as dental school faculty, and in the dental benefits industry. Dr. Vidone, a board-certified dental consultant, is a hands-on leader in the dental insurance industry, setting clinical policies and performing routine claim review while staying abreast of innovations in oral health care. She shares her unique knowledge of being on both sides of the claim form while lecturing nationwide on all aspects of dental benefits, dental coding, claim accuracy, utilization management, and utilization review.

A graduate of Boston University School of Dental Medicine, Dr. Vidone holds a D.M.D. and C.A.G.S. in General Dentistry and Periodontology. She is currently a member of the Delta Dental Plan Association Policy Committee. She is a board member of the American Association of Dental Consultants and also serves as Chair of the Certification Committee. She is on National Association of Dental Plans Code workgroup and is a voting member of the American Dental Association's Code Maintenance Committee, where she represents American Health Insurance Plans. She also maintains a private practice in periodontology in Brookline, Massachusetts.

By Teresa Duncan, M.S.

Introduction

Fixed prosthodontics replace missing teeth using fabricated materials that are cemented onto existing natural teeth or roots. It is important to remember that the codes for pontics listed in this category of service are used when documenting both tooth borne fixed denture procedures and for pontics that are part of an implant borne denture.

Clinicians must take into account the patient's oral health habits along with existing restorations in order to determine if a fixed prosthetic is the best choice. When treatment planning for fixed prosthodontics, it is important to remember that multiple appointments and procedures are usually required, and it is advisable to inform the patient of the number of visits required.

Patients are often confused by the terminology used when discussing fixed prosthodontics. A treatment coordinator may be referring to a fixed partial denture between teeth #13 and #15, but the patient may not understand that this is the same as fixed bridgework. It is helpful to have visual aids and even tangible examples on hand. Consider adding models, videos, and images to your case presentation tools. Often the only time the patient has even seen a bridge or fixed partial denture is right before it is cemented into his or her mouth.

From the beginning, your team should use the same language when discussing the components of fixed prosthodontics. They should also keep in mind that although most fixed prosthodontics are cemented permanently, there can be situations in which the practitioner will choose to do so temporarily.

Key Definitions and Concepts

Abutment: When discussing fixed prosthodontics, the term used to describe the part of a tooth upon which the retainer will seat. There may be times when additional buildup material is needed in order to properly seat a retainer. Such build-up procedures are reported with CDT codes from the Restorative category.

Cantilever bridge: A fixed partial denture (bridge) in which a stabilizing retainer is not present on one end.

Connector bar: A device attached to fixed partial denture retainer or coping which serves to stabilize and anchor a removable overdenture prosthesis.

Fixed partial denture: A laboratory fabricated prosthetic that replaces missing teeth or empty tooth spaces. It is meant to stabilize the bite and maintain arch integrity. This means that it prevents teeth from shifting and changing the patient's bite, which can lead to future required treatment. Also referred to as fixed bridgework or a bridge.

Pontic: An artificial tooth created to take the place of a missing tooth. It will be attached to retainers. There is no supporting tooth or root below it. It may rest against but is not meant to be supported by the soft tissue. As bone resorbs, the soft tissue may pull away from the pontic.

Retainer: As defined by the American College of Prosthodontics, a retainer is "any type of device used for the stabilization or retention of a prosthesis." The Prosthodontics, fixed category of service has codes for retainer inlays, onlays, and crowns. A fixed partial denture would be comprised of two retainers and one or more pontics as needed for the prosthesis.

The following "ADA Glossary of Clinical Dental Terms" definition (**emphasis added**) has affected the wording of code nomenclatures in this category of service.

Interim: (a) A restoration or prosthesis designed for use over a limited period of time; (b) A procedure that whose outcome is, by intent, subject to change arising from subsequent delivery of another procedure. The "interim" period of time for a restoration, a prosthesis or a procedure, **is determined by the clinical and professional judgment of the dentist**.

This definition has resulted in past code revisions where the term *provisional* was replaced with *interim*. Although the terms are similar, *interim* more accurately describes the intent of the procedure.

There are also continuing term changes seen in code descriptors. The terms *male* and *female* were removed from the descriptors in this category because not all component pieces fit together in this way. Using the term *set* or *pair of components* more accurately describes a two-part fixture.

The Prosthodontics, fixed category has evolved to incorporate codes for procedures for prostheses fabricated from a variety of materials. For example, code additions and editorial changes enable reporting of prostheses whose fabrication include titanium and titanium alloys – as well as high noble, noble, and base alloys. These materials, described in the Classification of Metals table within the CDT Manual's *Classification of Materials,* are parsed on the basis of biocompatibility, not cost. Previously, offices had no choice but to bill D6999 with an explanation of the difference in materials and charges.

Note: The CDT 2023 Manual's *Classification of Materials* definition of Porcelain/Ceramic has been revised to accommodate reporting of prostheses fabricated by 3D printing.

Changes to This Category

There are no changes of any type within this category of service as published in CDT 2023.

.

Clinical Coding Scenario #1:
Cantilever Bridge

A patient presents with tooth #27 missing and the dentist learned that this tooth has been missing for under a year. The dentist also observed that teeth #26 and #28 appeared to be in good condition. Upon further evaluation, the dentist determined that tooth #26 would not provide enough retention for a Maryland bridge and was reluctant to incorporate a virgin tooth in the prosthetic.

The patient was presented the information regarding Maryland bridge replacement and cantilever bridge replacement, with the doctor recommending a cantilever bridge off tooth #28 to preserve #26's tooth structure. Porcelain fused to high noble metal was the recommended material for this fixed prosthesis. The patient reviewed the treatment plan and opted for the cantilever bridge procedure.

What codes are used to document and report this procedure?

Tooth #28 is a retainer, and the applicable code is:

D6750   retainer crown – porcelain fused to high noble metal

Note: Retainers, for coding purposes, are differentiated by their material.

The pontic code for a "cantilever" bridge is the same as a conventional bridge, which for tooth #27 would be:

D6240   pontic – porcelain fused to high noble metal

As with the retainers, pontics may be made of different material.

Refer to CDT 2023 for the full list of applicable codes based on the prosthetic's material.

Clinical Coding Scenario #2:
Maryland Bridge

A patient suffered an accident that damaged the dentition as follows:

- Two teeth were lost – #23 and #24

- One tooth was broken – #26

The doctor determined that #26 could not be restored and required extraction.

The initial treatment plan involved implants, which the patient declined due to cost. An alternative treatment plan was accepted. This alternative involved a Maryland bridge, as this would preserve the remaining teeth and retain the option of implant in the future. The Maryland bridge consisted of a resin bonded porcelain-fused-to-metal (noble) bridge from teeth #22 to #27 with #25 acting as a pier.

What codes are used to document and report this procedure?

Teeth #22, #25, and #27 become retainers and the applicable code for each is:

D6545   retainer – cast metal for resin bonded fixed prosthesis

The pontic codes for a Maryland bridge are the same as a conventional bridge, which for teeth #23, #24, and #26 is (reported for each):

D6242   pontic – porcelain fused to noble metal

Note: Resin bonded bridge retainers (often referred to as wings) are differentiated by their material:

- All cast metal or porcelain fused to metal bridges would utilize the D6545 code noted above.

- The porcelain/ceramic retainer code (D6548) could only be used with a porcelain/ceramic pontic.

- Should the retainer be fabricated out of resin/composite, the applicable CDT code is **D6549 resin retainer – for resin bonded fixed prosthesis**.

Clinical Coding Scenario #3:
Three-Unit Fixed Partial Denture (Bridge) for Teeth #28–#30

The patient presented with missing tooth #29 due to extraction at an oral surgery office and wished to replace this tooth. A treatment plan was presented that offered the following options: fixed prosthetic; removable prosthetic; or implant placement and restoration. The patient chose a fixed prosthetic incorporating teeth #28 and #30 for retainers.

Informed consent was obtained, and the patient returned for a tooth preparation appointment and a cementation appointment.

How would you code this scenario's treatment plan?

Tooth #28	**D6752**	**retainer crown – porcelain fused to noble metal**
Tooth #29	**D6242**	**pontic – porcelain fused to noble metal**
Tooth #30	**D6752**	**retainer crown – porcelain fused to noble metal**

Clinical Coding Scenario #4:
Three-Unit Fixed Partial Denture (Bridge) for Teeth #12–#14 with Buildup on Molar Tooth

The patient presented with an existing fixed partial denture that needed to be replaced, and the dentist also determined that a gingivectomy would be necessary. The patient was presented the treatment plan and gave informed consent. Upon removal of the existing prosthetic, the treating dentist decided that a buildup was needed to properly restore the molar tooth.

How would you code this scenario's initial treatment plan?

The initial treatment plan was for a replacement fixed partial denture involving teeth #12–#14, and the doctor decided to use porcelain fused to noble metal based on soft tissue and material selection criteria. This plan was documented with the following codes:

Tooth #12	**D4212**	**gingivectomy or gingivoplasty to allow access for restorative procedure, per tooth**
Tooth #12	**D6752**	**retainer crown – porcelain fused to noble metal**
Tooth #13	**D6242**	**pontic – porcelain fused to noble metal**
Tooth #14	**D6752**	**retainer crown – porcelain fused to noble metal**

A flap of gingiva was prohibiting proper preparation of the tooth for the retainer crown so D4212 was appropriate in this situation.

Removal of existing decay during delivery of the D4212 procedure necessitated the addition of buildup material, and the dentist informed the patient of the change in treatment.

When the treatment plan changed to include the buildup, the code for this additional procedure (below) was added:

Tooth #14	**D2950**	**core buildup, including any pins when required**

It is important to note that this code is located in the CDT Code's "Restorative" category of service.

Clinical Coding Scenario #5:
Fractured Tooth and Infection

A patient presents with painful and fractured tooth #5. The doctor took a radiograph that imaged the entire tooth as part of the focused oral evaluation. A two-phase treatment plan was presented and accepted. Descriptions of each phase, and applicable coding, follow.

How would you code each phase in this scenario?

First Phase

- Evaluation and diagnosis
- Extraction of #5 – no need to remove bone
- Impression of the extraction area and adjacent hard and soft tissues
- Creation and placement of a temporary fixed partial denture for healing and space maintenance

Codes for first phase procedures:

	D0140	**limited oral evaluation – problem focused**
	D0220	**intraoral – periapical first radiographic image**
Tooth #4:	**D6793**	**interim retainer crown – further treatment or completion of diagnosis necessary prior to final impression**
Tooth #5:	**D7140**	**extraction, erupted tooth or exposed root (elevation and/or forceps removal)**
Tooth #5:	**D6253**	**interim pontic – further treatment or completion of diagnosis necessary prior to final impression**
Tooth #6:	**D6793**	**interim retainer crown – further treatment or completion of diagnosis necessary prior to final impression**

Second Phase

- Place permanent, porcelain/ceramic, fixed partial denture

Codes for second phase procedures:

Tooth #4:	**D6740**	**retainer crown – porcelain/ceramic**
Tooth #5:	**D6245**	**pontic – porcelain/ceramic**
Tooth #6:	**D6740**	**retainer crown – porcelain/ceramic**

Clinical Coding Scenario #6:
The Replacement of the Missing Tooth

During a comprehensive evaluation, which included an intraoral radiographic survey of the whole mouth, the patient stated that she would like to replace tooth #14 which had been "missing for years." A comprehensive set of intraoral images were also obtained. The dentist recommended the following three treatment plan options:

- a fixed partial denture (recommended by the dentist)

- an implant placement and restoration

- the option to do nothing

The patient elected to proceed with the fixed partial denture. The patient and doctor both agreed to a titanium alloy as the patient complained of extreme sensitivity in previous restorations. Costs were presented to the patient who signed and agreed to the fact that the full cost would be the responsibility of the patient due to a "missing tooth clause" in the patient's dental benefit plan. After informed consent was obtained, second and third appointments for the denture procedures were scheduled.

How would you code this scenario?

Visit #1: Initial Appointment

The patient presented for a comprehensive evaluation and had radiographs as well as intraoral images taken and reviewed.

D0150 **comprehensive oral evaluation – new or established patient**

D0210 **intraoral – comprehensive series of radiographic images**

D0350 **2D oral/facial photographic image obtained intra-orally or extra-orally**

Visit #2: Restoration

Tooth #13: **D6753** **retainer crown – porcelain fused to titanium and titanium alloys**

Tooth #14: **D6243** **pontic – porcelain fused to titanium and titanium alloys**

Tooth #15: **D6753** **retainer crown – porcelain fused to titanium and titanium alloys**   *Continued on next page*

Visit #3: Cementation of Fixed Partial Denture

The patient presented for cementation of the fixed partial denture. After the new margins were verified and the patient stated they were happy, the doctor took a final bitewing radiograph to verify the margins were accurate.

D0270 bitewing – single radiographic image

Clinical Coding Scenario #7:
Re-cementation of Fixed Partial Denture

A patient presented with his bridge for teeth #29–#31 in his hand. He stated it had come out over the weekend, and also complained of sensitivity in the area.

A limited evaluation was completed, and the provider prescribed two periapical radiographs before re-cementation to assess health and stability of the teeth. The radiographs showed no periapical infections and confirmed the visual determination that no active caries was present. After removing cement from the bridgework, it was re-cemented with no incident. The patient was told to return in two weeks for assessment of bridge health and the sensitivity complaint.

How would you code this scenario?

Visit #1: Initial Appointment

D0140 limited oral evaluation – problem focused

D0220 intraoral – periapical first radiographic image

D0230 intraoral – periapical each additional radiographic image

D6930 re-cement or re-bond fixed partial denture

It is appropriate to document D0140 as the provider had to assess the situation before prescribing radiographs and treatment. However, some carriers may have benefit clauses that will preclude payment of the evaluation due to frequency limitations for that procedure, or as a non-covered service in the benefit plan or participating provider contract.

Visit #2: Post-operative Appointment

D0171 re-evaluation – post-operative office visit

Clinical Coding Scenario #8:
Fixed Partial Denture for a Child

During a periodic evaluation and prophylaxis visit, it was determined that a child could benefit from a space maintainer for primary tooth C. The primary tooth had been shed earlier than anticipated. A panoramic radiograph revealed that eruption would not occur for some time. The parent was given the option of a removable or fixed space maintainer. The parent's concern was function and aesthetics.

It was decided that a more permanent space maintainer was necessary. The patient presented for treatment with no issues. The final appointment included cementation and oral instructions. The parent was advised to call the provider with any issues.

How would you code this scenario?

Visit #1: Initial Appointment

D0120   periodic oral evaluation – established patient

D1120   prophylaxis – child

D0330   panoramic radiographic image

Visit #2: Operative Appointment

D6985   pediatric partial denture, fixed

Visit #3: Post-operative Appointment

There is no separate procedure code for the cementation as it is an integral part of the denture procedure.

D1330   oral hygiene instructions

Clinical Coding Scenario #9:
Removal of a Fixed Partial Denture Followed by Interim Prosthetic

A patient presented with a damaged fixed partial denture for teeth #13–#16. #14 is the pontic tooth. After evaluation, the doctor observed that tooth #16 was sound with no open margins or any radiographic issues. Tooth #13 had fractured porcelain on the lingual and buccal, and tooth #15 had open lingual margins. Recommended immediate treatment included sectioning the existing fixed prosthetic and placement of an interim prosthesis.

Note: The doctor and the patient agreed that an implant should eventually replace tooth #14 and that teeth #s 13 and 15 would require separate crowns. However, the patient was not ready to start treatment and indicated it would be "at least a year" before she could schedule.

How would you code this scenario?

Visit #1: Initial Appointment

D0140 limited oral evaluation – problem focused

D0220 intraoral – periapical first radiographic image

D0230 intraoral – periapical each additional radiographic image

Visit #2: Treatment

D9120 fixed partial denture sectioning

(between #15 and #16)

D6793 interim retainer crown – further treatment or completion of diagnosis necessary prior to final impression

(#13 and #15)

D6253 interim pontic – further treatment or completion of diagnosis necessary prior to final impression

(#14)

Visit #3: Interim Placement of Fixed Partial Denture

The patient presented for temporary cementation of the interim prosthetic. After the new margins were verified and the patient stated she was happy, the doctor took a final bitewing radiograph to verify the margins were accurate. The patient agreed to return for her continuing care appointment to monitor any changes.

D0270 bitewing – single radiographic image

Clinical Coding Scenario #10:
Repair of a Fixed Partial Denture for Cosmetic Reasons

An existing patient presented with porcelain missing from pontic #3. An existing fixed partial denture included teeth #2–#4. The bridge was placed five years ago. After an evaluation and radiographic examination, the bridge was deemed to be functional with a good long-term prognosis. The doctor and patient agreed that a repair of the pontic would be made. The dentist planned to use material that could be bonded to the porcelain after etching and preparation of the surface.

How would you code this scenario?

Visit #1: Initial Appointment

D0140 **limited oral evaluation – problem focused**

D0220 **intraoral – periapical first radiographic image**

D0230 **intraoral – periapical each additional radiographic image**

Visit #2: Treatment

D6980 **fixed partial denture repair necessitated by restorative material failure**

Clinical Coding Scenario #11:
Removal of Implant Followed by Impression for a Fixed Partial Denture

An existing patient has requested to remove implant #13 due to discomfort. This happened during a hygiene appointment. She stated that "it just doesn't feel right." After several discussions of the benefits and risks, the doctor agreed to remove the implant. The doctor recommended bone grafting to further preserve bone height.

How would you code this scenario?

Visit #1: Initial Appointment

D0120 periodic oral evaluation – established patient

D1110 prophylaxis – adult

D0220 intraoral – periapical first radiographic image

Visit #2: Initial Treatment

D6100 surgical removal of implant body

D7953 bone replacement graft for ridge preservation – per site

Visit #3: Re-evaluation

The patient returned after three weeks for a re-evaluation of the site.

D0171 re-evaluation – post-operative office visit

The site was deemed to be healthy and the doctor recommended that they proceed with treatment. Treatment costs were reviewed again with the patient. Informed consent was obtained for the fixed partial denture to replace tooth #13.

Continued on next page

The definitive prosthesis consisted of two porcelain fused to high noble metal retainer crowns and a single porcelain fused to high noble metal pontic. More than one visit was required for the impression, temporary denture, and cementation of the definitive fixed partial denture.

Tooth #12:   **D6750   retainer crown – porcelain fused to high noble metal**

Tooth #13:   **D6240   pontic – porcelain fused to high noble metal**

Tooth #14:   **D6750   retainer crown – porcelain fused to high noble metal**

Post Definitive Prosthesis Follow-up

The patient presented on a later date and stated they were happy with the outcome. The dentist determined that the bite was accurate and a final bitewing radiograph was taken to verify that the margins were accurate.

D0270   bitewing – single radiographic image

Clinical Coding Scenario #12:
Fixed Partial Denture with Extra-coronal or Intra-coronal Attachment

Patient presented for a comprehensive evaluation with a concern regarding an existing fixed partial denture spanning #3–#6. The patient was unhappy with the fit and the bite. She estimates that the bridge is "well over 15 years old." Comprehensive radiographs were taken along with intra-oral images.

The doctor suggested the use of an attachment to better distribute occlusal forces. Tooth #4 had enough tooth structure to accommodate an intra-coronal precision attachment. Fabrication of a four-unit bridge with the intra-coronal attachment set placed on the distal of #4 and mesial of #3 was approved with the patient. Informed consent was obtained from the patient.

Visit #1: Comprehensive evaluation

D0150 comprehensive oral evaluation – new or established patient

D0210 intraoral – comprehensive series of radiographic images

D0350 2D oral/facial photographic image obtained intra-orally or extra-orally

Definitive Prosthesis Treatment Visit(s)

The definitive prosthesis consisted of two porcelain fused to high noble metal retainer crowns, one precision attachment, and two porcelain fused to high noble metal pontics. More than one visit was required for the impression, temporary denture, and cementation of the definitive fixed partial denture.

Tooth #3: **D6750 retainer crown – porcelain fused to high noble metal**

Tooth #3: **D6950 precision attachment**

Tooth #4: **D6240 pontic – porcelain fused to high noble metal**

Tooth #5: **D6240 pontic – porcelain fused to high noble metal**

Tooth #6: **D6750 retainer crown – porcelain fused to high noble metal**

Post Definitive Prosthesis Follow-up Appointment

The patient presented on a later date and stated they were happy with their "new bite." The prosthetic was slightly adjusted and a radiograph was taken to verify margins.

D0270 bitewing – single radiographic image

Coding Q&A

1. *Should I present a treatment plan for an implant if my recommendation is to place a fixed partial denture?*

   Yes, you should always present all available options to the patient. The patient must be aware of all the options available to restore their oral condition. However, you can present a recommended treatment.

2. *We placed a pediatric partial denture on a child but it has come loose. Is there a re-cementation code for this prosthetic?*

   The code **D6930 re-cement or re-bond fixed partial denture** is appropriate. The age of the patient is not a determining factor when using this code.

3. *We have had to temporarily cement fixed bridgework. Is there a separate code for that?*

   Sometimes a fixed partial denture is temporarily cemented so that the clinician can observe the oral condition for a time period. If the fixed partial denture is intended to be the permanent restoration, then there is not a separate code. You are simply delaying the permanent delivery. You may want to use code **D6999 unspecified fixed prosthodontic procedure, by report** to request reimbursement. This will require a narrative and supporting images.

4. *Our patient presented with a multi-unit bridge that had come out. It is a large bridge with five pontics in addition to the retainers. Can we charge the re-cement fee for multiple teeth?*

   Existing code **D6930 re-cement or re-bond fixed partial denture** is per prosthetic. The number of units is not a factor.

5. *I'd like to place a post and core buildup in a tooth that previously had endodontic therapy as this tooth will serve as the abutment for a fixed bridge retainer. Are the post and build-up codes found in this category or in Endodontics?*

   Neither. The post and core procedure codes are actually found in the CDT Code's Restorative category of service.

   D2952   post and core in addition to crown, indirectly fabricated

   D2954   prefabricated post and core in addition to crown

   There is no post and core buildup code that is specific to only crowns or only fixed partial dentures.

6. *I would like to place a temporary bridge while a site is healing. We are planning to treat adjacent teeth but would like to preserve the tooth space in the meantime. What code should I use?*

   You are referring to an interim fixed partial denture, which means the interim retainer crowns are documented with code D6793, and the interim pontic(s) with code D6253 (for each interim pontic in the temporary bridge).

7. *I plan to use a precision attachment. Do I bill for the male and female component separately?*

   No. The full CDT Code entry for a precision attachment is:

   D6950   precision attachment
   >A pair of components constitutes one precision attachment that is separate from the prosthesis.

   The precision attachment procedure involves placement of a pair of components, previously described as "male and female" and should be reported for each pair placed on the fixed prosthesis. Using the term "pair of components" more accurately describes the two-part attachment fixture.

8. *We are placing a fixed partial denture made from a porcelain fused to a titanium alloy. Should I use the high noble code for the retainer crowns and the pontic?*

   There is no reason to use a procedure code that does not correctly reflect the material used. Since both the retainer crowns and pontics are porcelain fused to a titanium alloy, the applicable codes are:

   D6753   retainer crown – porcelain fused to titanium and titanium alloys

   D6243   pontic – porcelain fused to titanium and titanium alloys

9. *Should I pass the laboratory costs through to the patient?*

   The full fee for a procedure includes all associated costs, which would include laboratory charges, milling expenses, and any minor occlusal adjustments made at the seat appointment. Always review the full code entry (nomenclature and descriptor) to understand the procedure's scope, and any specific procedures that would be reported separately. Please be aware that third-party claim adjudication policies, and provisions of your participating provider contract (if one is in force), affect reimbursement of reported procedures.

10. *I was told by a carrier that the patient has a missing tooth clause. What does that mean, and why does it matter in this category?*

A missing tooth clause means that benefits are not available to replace a tooth that was missing prior to the date of service. If your patient agrees to replace a missing tooth with a fixed partial denture, then the full cost will be the patient's responsibility. Always advise the patient if this is the case so that they can plan their financial obligations.

11. *We took impressions for a fixed partial denture and provided the patient with a temporary bridge. The patient has not replied to any of our requests for a cementation appointment. Can we collect on the full amount of the prosthetic? We have already paid the laboratory bill.*

You may seek compensation for costs incurred, although there is no specific CDT code for an incomplete procedure. When there is no specific CDT code, consider a "999" unspecified procedure code such as **D6999 unspecified fixed prosthodontic procedure, by report**.

This will require a narrative and supporting images. In addition, you will need to evaluate your materials and labor costs and decide on an appropriate fee. Documentation of your attempts to reach the patient should be entered into the clinical record to represent the treatment timeline. The patient's record should document the preparation of teeth to receive the prosthesis and any temporary or interim restoration provided to the patient.

12. *Are there general guidelines for third-party-requested documentation for procedures within this category?*

Every plan will have its own set of requirements, but in general the radiographs and intraoral images should be of clear diagnostic quality and labeled for orientation. A common requirement is a full set of radiographs or panoramic image that shows both arches. Radiographs and intraoral images should be current (within 12–24 months according to the carrier guidelines). Replacement of an existing fixed prosthetic may also require radiographs showing any open margins, breakages, or missing tooth structure (upon removal of structure).

13. *I'm finding that carriers now frequently request the reason for extraction along with the date. How do I document this if we don't have access to their dental records?*

It's difficult to provide an exact date if the patient does not provide records. Ask the patient if they have any memory of the reason and date of the extraction. Your clinical notes should reflect the answer the patient provides. Direct quotes can be entered to help establish history. Examples of this would be:

- Patient states that tooth #3 was extracted due to an infection. She does not remember the exact date but states that "it must have been over 10 years ago."

- Patient stated "I fell down some stairs in college and knocked my two front teeth loose [pointed to #8 and #9] then they had to pull them." Patient estimates that it was "over 20 years ago, at least."

14. *If a patient presents with pain and we remove a fixed partial denture as a result, can we charge for the evaluation?*

Yes. A limited evaluation and/or diagnostic images are needed for a diagnosis and plan of action. Some plan designs will not benefit for the evaluation if definitive treatment is performed on the same day. Remember to always code for what you did rather than what can be paid.

15. *Are interim fixed partial dentures used often in children?*

Yes. It's common for a dentist to place one while the child's jaw and dentition mature. At that point the doctor may recommend a fixed partial denture or other method of tooth replacement.

16. *We'd like to replace a patient's flipper for tooth #20 with a fixed partial denture. The carrier is not covering it due to the frequency limitation for prosthetics. Why does this apply if there are two different methods used?*

It's possible that the flipper was placed within the last five years. A common carrier clause pertaining to fixed or removable prosthetics will prevent reimbursement if the interim prosthetic is in place for more than a year after placement. The carriers can consider this to be the permanent prosthetic after that period of time. Always let the patient know about their treatment costs prior to treatment.

17. *We often provide a flipper after an anterior extraction. Can that impact benefit payment for the fixed partial denture?*

    Many plans will provide benefits for the flipper but then deny benefits for the fixed partial denture (bridge). The patient should be informed that their carrier may apply benefits to the lower cost procedure since that claim will be processed prior to the fixed partial denture date of service.

18. *I'd like to add a bar to stabilize a bridge spanning #11– #13. Is there a code for that?*

    Yes, connecter bars would be coded as D6920. Its descriptor states: A device attached to fixed partial denture retainer or coping which serves to stabilize and anchor a removable overdenture prosthesis.

Summary

Always use the CDT version in effect on the date of service (e.g., CDT 2023) to select the appropriate code for the procedure delivered.

The selection of a fixed prosthodontics code should be made with the following items in mind:

- Material used in restoration
- Is it to replace a missing tooth or tooth space?
- Is the end result meant to be part of a permanent placement?
- Diagnostic procedures are separate from fixed prosthodontic codes
- Any soft tissue preparation is separate from the fixed prosthodontic code

In some situations, a fixed prosthetic is part of an implant case. Specifically, the pontic codes for a fixed partial denture that is supported by implants are found in the Prosthodontics, fixed category. There are no pontic codes that are specific to implant restoration cases.

If you cannot find an appropriate code for your procedure use:

D6999   unspecified fixed prosthodontic procedure, by report

When using a "by report" code, remember to include a diagnosis, description of procedure, and prognosis. Include any supporting documentation such as radiographs and intraoral images. Clear and current documentation will always be needed for communications with carriers.

Contributor Biography

Teresa Duncan, M.S., is the president of Odyssey Management, Inc. She lectures nationally on the topics of insurance administration; case and financial presentations; and practice manager skill improvement. These topics are also tackled on her podcasts and in her book. She may be reached via her website at *www.OdysseyMgmt.com*. Her website contains many management and insurance articles, as well as complimentary webinars.

By James E. Mercer, D.D.S.

Introduction

Oral and maxillofacial surgery is a broad area. It encompasses not only the discipline of oral surgery, but also that of implant services, radiologic imaging, trauma, facial cosmetic procedures and anesthesia services. Some of the procedures are medical in nature and need to be submitted to medical carriers along with ICD-10-CM codes. However, there are still many procedures that are purely dental in nature.

Key Definitions and Concepts

Autogenous graft: A graft that is taken from one part of a patient's body and transferred to another.

Anesthesia definitions: A patient's level of consciousness is determined by the anesthesia provider's documentation of a patient's level of consciousness and is not dependent upon the route of administration of anesthesia.

Deep sedation: A drug-induced depression of consciousness during which patients cannot be easily aroused but respond purposefully following repeated or painful stimulation. The ability to independently maintain ventilator function may be impaired. Patients may require assistance in maintaining a patent airway. Cardiovascular function is usually maintained.

General anesthesia: A drug-induced loss of consciousness during which patients are not arousable. The ability to maintain ventilator function is often impaired. Cardiovascular function may be impaired.

Minimal sedation: A minimally depressed level of consciousness that retains the patient's ability to independently and continuously maintain an airway and respond normally to tactile stimulation and verbal command. Ventilatory and cardiovascular functions are unaffected.

Moderate sedation: A drug-induced depression of consciousness during which patients respond purposefully to verbal commands either alone or accompanied by light tactile stimulation. Spontaneous ventilation is adequate. Cardiovascular function is usually maintained.

Anxiolysis: The diminution or elimination of anxiety.

Provisional: Formed or preformed for temporary purposes or used over a limited period.

Soft tissue impacted tooth: Occlusal surface of the tooth is covered by soft tissue.

Partial bone impacted tooth: Part of the crown is covered by bone.

Full bone impacted tooth: Most or all of the crown is covered by bone.

Changes to This Category

There are three additions and one revision to this category in CDT 2023. The additions fill gaps by describing surgical procedures that had not been previously described in the CDT code set. The revision was made to add more clarity to the nomenclature and descriptor.

The additions are:

D7509 marsupialization of odontogenic cyst
Surgical decompression of a large cystic lesion by creating a long-term open pocket or pouch.

D7956 guided tissue regeneration, edentulous area – resorbable barrier, per site
This procedure does not include flap entry and closure, or, when indicated, wound debridement, osseous contouring, bone replacement grafts, and placement of biologic materials to aid in osseous regeneration. This procedure may be used for ridge augmentation, sinus lift procedures, and after tooth extraction.

D7957 guided tissue regeneration, edentulous area – non-resorbable barrier, per site
This procedure does not include flap entry and closure, or, when indicated, wound debridement, osseous contouring, bone replacement grafts, and placement of biologic materials to aid in osseous regeneration. This procedure may be used for ridge augmentation, sinus lift procedures, and after tooth extraction.

The revision is:

D7251 coronectomy – intentional partial tooth removal, impacted teeth only
Intentional partial tooth removal is performed when a neurovascular complication is likely if the entire impacted tooth is removed.

Clinical Coding Scenario #1:
Connective Tissue Grafts — Autogenous and Non–autogenous

A 55-year-old male who is a patient of record presented to an oral surgeon's office six years after placement of two separate implants for teeth #12 and #13. The exam revealed loss of 3 mm of attached gingiva on the buccal aspect of the implants. X-rays revealed minimal bone loss on the implants. There was one thread on each implant exposed. Along with debridement of the area, the treatment plan consisted of placing a connective tissue graft on the buccal of both implants.

How would you code for the autogenous grafts?

D4273 **autogenous connective tissue graft procedure (including donor and recipient surgical sites) first tooth, implant or edentulous tooth position in graft**

D4283 **autogenous connective tissue graft procedure (including donor and recipient surgical sites) — each additional contiguous implant in same graft site**

Note: D4273 is the code used when the procedure involves two surgical sites, donor and recipient. The recipient site has a split thickness incision and the connective tissue is from a separate donor site leaving an epithelized flap for closure. D4283 is used to code for additional sites adjacent to the first site.

If using a non–autogenous connective graft, the procedures are coded as follows:

D4275 **non-autogenous connective tissue graft (including recipient site and donor material) first tooth, implant or edentulous tooth position in graft**

D4285 **non-autogenous connective tissue graft procedure (including recipient surgical site and donor material) — each additional contiguous tooth, implant and edentulous tooth position in the same graft site**

Clinical Coding Scenario #2:
Harvesting Bone and Hard Tissue Grafting

Two years following an ATV accident, the patient was still dealing with the after effects of the comminuted fracture of his anterior maxilla. A traumatic defect and oronasal fistula, not much different from a congenital alveolar cleft, still existed.

The patient's oral surgeon recommended closure of the fistula and reconstruction of the bony deficit prior to prosthetic reconstruction. The doctor planned to do this as an in office procedure utilizing an autogenous bone graft from the tibia.

What codes would be used to document these procedures?

Two codes would be used to document the planned services to be delivered in the doctor's office:

D7955 repair of maxillofacial soft tissue and/or hard tissue defect
Reconstruction of surgical, traumatic, or congenital defects of the facial bones, including the mandible, may utilize graft materials in conjunction with soft tissue procedures to repair and restore the facial bones to form and function. This does not include obtaining the graft and these procedures may require multiple surgical approaches. This procedure does not include edentulous maxilla and mandibular reconstructions for prosthetic considerations.

D7295 harvest of bone for use in autogenous grafting procedure
Reported in addition to those autogenous graft placement procedures that do not include harvesting of bone.

Note: The harvesting code D7295 provides a means to report the separate procedure of obtaining osseous material for the purpose of grafting to a distant site. It enables documentation of the harvesting procedure when the grafting procedure (e.g., D4263; D7953; D7955) does not include obtaining bone to be grafted.

Clinical Coding Scenario #3:
Implant Placement with Inadequate Bone Volume

A 36-year-old female patient presents for placement of an implant in the mandibular right posterior. Tooth #30 had been extracted two years ago. There is inadequate bone volume in the site where the implant will be placed and ridge augmentation is required.

How do you code for the graft?

D7950   **osseous, osteoperiosteal, or cartilage graft of the mandible or maxilla – autogenous or nonautogenous, by report**
This procedure is for ridge augmentation or reconstruction to increase height, width and/or volume of residual alveolar ridge. It includes obtaining graft material. Placement of a barrier membrane, if used, should be reported separately.

How do you code for the barrier membrane if used?

For a resorbable membrane you would use:

D6106   **guided tissue regeneration – resorbable barrier, per implant**
This procedure does not include flap entry and closure, or, when indicated, wound debridement, osseous contouring, bone replacement grafts, and placement of biologic materials to aid in osseous regeneration. This procedure is used for peri-implant defects and during implant placement.

Or if a non-resorbable membrane is placed you would use:

D6107   **guided tissue regeneration – non-resorbable barrier, per implant**
This procedure does not include flap entry and closure, or, when indicated, wound debridement, osseous contouring, bone replacement grafts, and placement of biologic materials to aid in osseous regeneration. This procedure is used for peri-implant defects and during implant placement.

D6107   **does not include the removal of the non-resorbable barrier. How do I code for its removal at a later date?**

D4286   **removal of non-resorbable barrier**

Clinical Coding Scenario #4:
Extractions and Immediate Placement of Implants for an Implant Supported Denture

The patient in this scenario requires extraction of teeth #22 and #27 and immediate placement of two implants. The procedure includes developing a flap, removing the teeth, and placing the implants. A mucoperiosteal flap was used to access the area of the extractions and implant sites and the teeth were removed by elevation.

Can I use D7210 for the extractions since I utilized a mucoperiosteal flap or should I use D7140 along with another code for the flap?

The correct code for the extractions would be:

D7140 extraction, erupted tooth or exposed root (elevation and/or forceps removal)
> Includes routine removal of tooth structure, minor smoothing of socket bone, and closure, as necessary.

To use D7210 for an erupted tooth you must either remove bone, section the tooth or both. Elevating the flap may be part of the procedure but not required for the use of D7210. Elevation of a flap alone for an erupted tooth does not merit use of D7210.

In this case, when you use D7140 for the extractions and D6010 for each of the implants placed, no flap code would be used since the flap is part of the implant placement.

Clinical Coding Scenario #5:
Zygomatic Implants

A 65-year-old female is referred for evaluation for maxillary implants. The patient has a severely atrophic maxilla posteriorly and a history of failed bilateral maxillary sinus augmentation. After obtaining a cone beam CT of the maxilla and comprehensive evaluation, the treatment plan is to place four implants in the anterior region and one zygomatic implant on each side of the maxilla to support a maxillary fixed complete denture.

How do you code for the implants?

D6010 surgical placement of implant body: endosteal implant

Report D6010 four times – once for each of the anterior implants.

D7994 surgical placement: zygomatic implant
An implant placed in the zygomatic bone and exiting though the maxillary mucosal tissue providing support and attachment of a maxillary dental prosthesis.

Report D7994 two times – once for each of the zygomatic implants.

Previously, the code **D6199 unspecified implant procedure, by report** would have been used for documenting the two zygomatic implant procedures.

Clinical Coding Scenario #6:
Autogenous Bone Graft

A 45-year-old male presents for extraction of non-restorable tooth #5 and placement of an implant at a later date. An autogenous bone graft is placed with a membrane at the time of extraction to increase the bone volume and preserve ridge integrity at the future implant site.

After coding for the extraction, how do you code for the graft and membrane portion of the procedure?

D7953 bone replacement graft for ridge preservation – per site
Graft is placed in an extraction site or implant removal site at the time of the extraction or removal to preserve ridge integrity (e.g., clinically indicated in preparation for implant reconstruction or where alveolar contour is critical to planned prosthetic reconstruction). Does not include obtaining graft material. Membrane, if used should be reported separately.

D7295 harvest of bone for use in autogenous grafting procedure
Reported in addition to those autogenous graft placement procedures that do not include harvesting of bone.

D7956 guided tissue regeneration, edentulous area – resorbable barrier, per site
This procedure does not include flap entry and closure, or, when indicated, wound debridement, osseous contouring, bone replacement grafts, and placement of biologic materials to aid in osseous regeneration. This procedure may be used for ridge augmentation, sinus lift procedures, and after tooth extraction.

or

D7957 guided tissue regeneration, edentulous area – non-resorbable barrier, per site
This procedure does not include flap entry and closure, or, when indicated, wound debridement, osseous contouring, bone replacement grafts, and placement of biologic materials to aid in osseous regeneration. This procedure may be used for ridge augmentation, sinus lift procedures, and after tooth extraction.

Continued on next page

D7957 does not include the removal of the non-resorbable barrier. How do I code for its removal at a later date?

D4286   removal of non-resorbable barrier

But – If at the time of surgery, it is determined there is adequate bone apically for the implant to be placed at the time of extraction with bone grafting, how would you code for this procedure if the implant is placed at the same time of the extraction and the graft?

D6010   surgical placement of implant body: endosteal implant

D6104   bone graft at time of implant placement
Placement of a barrier membrane, or biologic materials to aid in osseous regeneration are reported separately.

D7295   harvest of bone for use in autogenous grafting procedure
Reported in addition to those autogenous graft placement procedures that do not include harvesting of bone.

And – If a barrier membrane were placed at the time of grafting and implant placement, the following codes may be used depending on the type of membrane.

D6106   guided tissue regeneration – resorbable barrier, per implant
This procedure does not include flap entry and closure, or, when indicated, wound debridement, osseous contouring, bone replacement grafts, and placement of biologic materials to aid in osseous regeneration. This procedure is used for peri-implant defects and during implant placement.

or

D6107   guided tissue regeneration – non-resorbable barrier, per implant
This procedure does not include flap entry and closure, or, when indicated, wound debridement, osseous contouring, bone replacement grafts, and placement of biologic materials to aid in osseous regeneration. This procedure is used for peri-implant defects and during implant placement.

D6107 does not include the removal of the non-resorbable barrier. How do I code for its removal at a later date?

D4286   removal of non-resorbable barrier

Clinical Coding Scenario #7:
Possible Orbital Fracture

A 23-year-old male presents to the office after being punched in the face the night before. He has severe periorbital swelling of the left eye. The surgeon is unable to perform an adequate clinical exam and does not have a CBCT in the office. But she does have a cephalometric x-ray machine capable of taking a flat plate extra-oral film. She takes a Waters view film to rule out an orbital fracture.

How do you code for this diagnostic imaging procedure?

> **D0250   extra-oral – 2D projection radiographic image created using a stationary radiation source, and detector**

D0250 covers a class of images which can be obtained utilizing a flat plate radiographic image to view aspects of the skull and facial bones when a CBCT scan is not available.

Clinical Coding Scenario #8:
Extraction of Full Bony Impacted Teeth

A 20-year-old male presents to the oral surgeon's office for extraction of full bony impacted teeth #1, #16, #17 and #32. The procedure was performed utilizing deep IV sedation. The procedure lasted 53 minutes.

How would you code for the deep sedation anesthesia procedure?

D9222   deep sedation/general anesthesia – first 15 minutes

(Report D9222 once for minutes one through 15.)

D9223   deep sedation/general anesthesia – each subsequent 15 minute increment

(Report D9223 three times for the additional 38 minutes (16 through 53). D9223 documents each additional full or partial 15-minute increment.)

What code would be reported if 53 minutes of moderate IV sedation were appropriate?

D9239   intravenous moderate (conscious) sedation/analgesia – first 15 minutes

(Report D9239 once for minutes one through 15.)

D9243   intravenous moderate (conscious) sedation/analgesia – each subsequent 15 minute increment

(Report D9243 for the additional 38 minutes (16 through 53). D9223 documents each additional full or partial 15-minute increment.)

What code would be reported if the extraction procedure could be performed with non-IV conscious sedation?

D9248   non-intravenous conscious sedation

This procedure would be reported once as it is not time-based.

Clinical Coding Scenario #9:
Extraction of Full Bony Impacted Tooth and Periodontal Defect

A 32-year-old male presents for extraction of a full bony impacted horizontal tooth #17. On exam, the patient has an increased probing depth and osseous defect on the distal of tooth #18 with bone loss to the mid root of tooth #18. The treatment plan is to extract tooth #17 and perform a bone graft at the time of extraction to regenerate the bone on distal aspect of tooth #18.

How do you code for the procedure?

D7240 **removal of impacted tooth – completely bony**
Most or all of crown is covered by bone; requires mucoperiosteal flap elevation and bone removal.

D4263 **bone replacement graft – retained natural tooth – first site in quadrant**
This procedure involves the use of grafts to stimulate periodontal regeneration when the disease process has led to a deformity of the bone. This procedure does not include flap entry and closure, wound debridement, osseous contouring, or the placement of biologic materials to aid in osseous tissue regeneration or barrier membranes. Other separate procedures delivered concurrently are documented with their own codes. Not to be reported for an edentulous space or an extraction site.

Use of D7953 for the graft would be the incorrect code since the purpose of the graft is not ridge preservation of the extraction socket of tooth #17. The purpose of the delivered procedure (D4263) is to stimulate periodontal regeneration on the distal of tooth #18.

If additional biologic materials are used the following code would also be appropriate:

D4265 **biologic materials to aid in soft and osseous tissue regeneration, per site**

If a barrier membrane was used, the following codes may be used depending on the type of membrane.

Continued on next page

D4266 guided tissue regeneration, natural teeth – resorbable barrier, per site

This procedure does not include flap entry and closure, or, when indicated, wound debridement, osseous contouring, bone replacement grafts, and placement of biologic materials to aid in osseous regeneration. This procedure can be used for periodontal defects around natural teeth.

or

D4267 guided tissue regeneration, natural teeth – non-resorbable barrier, per site

This procedure does not include flap entry and closure, or, when indicated, wound debridement, osseous contouring, bone replacement grafts, and placement of biologic materials to aid in osseous regeneration. This procedure can be used for periodontal defects around natural teeth

D4267 does not include the removal of the non-resorbable barrier. How do I code for its removal at a later date?

D4286 removal of non-resorbable barrier

Clinical Coding Scenario #10:
Extraction of Fully Impacted Tooth and Exposure of an Unerupted Adjacent Tooth

A 17-year-old male is referred by his orthodontist for removal of impacted tooth #32 with most of the crown covered by bone and exposure of partially impacted tooth #31. Extraction of tooth #32 and exposure of tooth #31 requires a modified mucoperiosteal flap design and additional bone removal around tooth #32 vs. removal of only tooth #32.

How do you code for the procedures?

D7240 removal of impacted tooth – completely bony

Most or all of crown is covered by bone; requires mucoperiosteal flap elevation and bone removal.

D7280 exposure of an unerupted tooth

An incision is made and the tissue is reflected and bone is removed as necessary to expose the crown of an impacted tooth not intended to be extracted.

Continued on next page

The orthodontist also requested an eruption appliance be attached to the exposed tooth #31. How do you code for placement of the eruption appliance?

> **D7283**   **placement of device to facilitate eruption of the impacted tooth**
> Placement of an attachment on an unerupted tooth, after its exposure, to aid in its eruption. Report the surgical exposure separately using D7280.

Clinical Coding Scenario #11:
Extraction of Impacted Tooth and Marsupialization of an Odontogenic Cyst

A 17-year-old male is referred for removal of a large cyst associated with impacted tooth #17. The cyst extends from the inferior border of the mandible involving the inferior alveolar canal up into the left mandibular ramus. Because of the large size of the cyst and involvement of the inferior alveolar canal, the surgical plan is to remove tooth #17 and suture the cystic lining of the cavity to the oral mucosa creating an opening from the bony cavity to the oral cavity. This will allow the cyst to remain decompressed and the bone to fill in the defect.

How do I code for this procedure?

> **D7240**   **removal of impacted tooth – completely bony**
> Most or all of crown is covered by bone; requires mucoperiosteal flap elevation and bone removal.

> **D7509**   **marsupialization of odontogenic cyst**
> Surgical decompression of a large cystic lesion by creating a long-term open pocket or pouch.

Clinical Coding Scenario #12:
Removal of Non-vital Bone (Two Different Cases)

Patient A

Patient A, a 55-year-old male, is referred for evaluation of pain in the area of a previously extracted tooth #31. Examination reveals exposed loose bone lingual to where tooth #31 had been extracted. There is no swelling or signs of acute infection at the time of presentation. The patient tells you tooth #31 was extracted five weeks prior to your exam due to infection and non-restorability. The initial plan is to provide local wound care and removal of the loose bone.

How would you code for this the removal of the loose bone?

D7550 **partial ostectomy/sequestrectomy for removal of non-vital bone**
Removal of loose or sloughed-off dead bone caused by infection or reduced blood supply.

Patient B

Patient B, a 65-year-old female complaining of jaw pain, is referred for evaluation of a large area of mandibular exposed bone 9 weeks after extraction of tooth #31. She has a history of treatment with oral bisphosphonates for osteoporosis. There is no history of radiation therapy to the area. On examination of the mandible, there is obvious loose exposed bone. Part of the treatment plan is to remove the loose bony sequestra to eliminate the source of soft tissue irritation.

How would you code for the removal of the loose bone?

D7550 **partial ostectomy/sequestrectomy for removal of non-vital bone**
Removal of loose or sloughed-off dead bone caused by infection or reduced blood supply.

Since the treatment may be more extensive than the first case described above and not completely described by D7550, you may consider using the following code.

D7999 **unspecified oral surgery procedure, by report**
Used for a procedure that is not adequately described by a code. Describe the procedure.

This is a "by report" code that may be used when no other code adequately describes the procedure you performed. You should include a narrative describing the procedure with the claim form.

Clinical Coding Scenario #13:
Orthognathic Surgery Planning

An oral and maxillofacial surgery office recently installed a cone beam radiography machine. It was used to treatment plan some anticipated orthognathic surgery for a patient. Following image capture, several axial and lateral views were constructed to plan the surgery. A panoramic view was also produced to send to the patient's orthodontist.

After consultation with the orthodontist, the surgeon constructed a 3D virtual model, which they viewed together on the computer, to properly locate a temporary implant to anchor the orthodontic appliance. The virtual model could be manipulated on the screen to allow them to visualize other anatomical structures in the area and their relationship to the teeth to determine the ideal location to place the implant.

A transmucosal endosseous implant was placed as a temporary fixation device for the patient's braces. The temporary implant will be removed when orthodontic treatment is completed.

How could you code for procedures delivered during the initial treatment planning visit (includes initial scan, coronal and sagittal views, and panoramic view)?

D0367   cone beam CT capture and interpretation with field of view of both jaws; with or without cranium

This code enables documenting a specific type of cone beam image capture and reconstruction. The procedure includes two-dimensional sectional (tomographic) views from the axial (coronal or frontal) and lateral (sagittal) planes, as well as the panoramic view.

How could you code the subsequent virtual treatment simulation (3D virtual model)?

D0393   virtual treatment simulation using 3D image volume or surface scan
Virtual simulation of treatment including, but not limited to, dental implant placement, prosthetic reconstruction, orthognathic surgery and orthodontic tooth movement.

The 3D virtual model is a three-dimensional image reconstructed from data acquired during the initial treatment planning visit.

Continued on next page

How could you code the temporary implant placement procedure that required a surgical flap?

D7293   placement of temporary anchorage device requiring flap

Temporary implants represent a new kind of technology. The correct code to use for this type of implant depends upon whether it will be used for fixation or an interim restoration. In this case, the implant is being used as a fixation device for orthodontics, so the correct code comes from the CDT Code's Oral & Maxillofacial Surgery category.

Note: If the temporary implant does not require a surgical flap, the correct code would be **D7294 placement of temporary anchorage device without flap**.

How do you code the temporary implant removal procedure when placement required a surgical flap?

D7299   removal of temporary anchorage device, requiring flap

Clinical Coding Scenario #14:
Treating a Traumatic Wound and Fabrication of an Athletic Mouthguard

An eight-year-old patient arrived at the oral and maxillofacial surgeon's office literally screaming. The doctor understood why when he saw the patient who was injured during a baseball game. A headfirst slide had resulted in a lower lip full of gravel and a chin raspberry in the making.

An intramuscular injection of 40 mg of ketamine provided a reasonable amount of sedation and allowed sufficient time to completely debride the wound, followed by placing sutures in the cut in the patient's lip. No teeth were broken. The doctor recommended a mouthguard for future protection against dental trauma and orofacial injury.

What codes would be used to document and report procedures delivered during this visit?

The CDT code for a parenteral sedative is:

D9248 non-intravenous conscious sedation

Note: It is not appropriate to report delivery of the parenteral sedative with **D9610 therapeutic parenteral drug, single administration** as the CDT Code's entry for this procedure states that it does not include delivery of sedative agents.

There is not a code for traumatic wound debridement, but **D7999 unspecified oral surgery procedure, by report** could be used for that procedure.

Suture placement is reported with a code based on the size of the wound:

D7910 suture of recent small wounds up to 5 cm

The code to use when making a mouthguard is:

D9941 fabrication of athletic mouthguard

Clinical Coding Scenario #15
Submergence of an Erupted Tooth

A 75-year-old male is referred for evaluation of pain in the right mandible. A painful, non-restorable tooth #30 is present and all other teeth in the quadrant are asymptomatic. There is a history of oral squamous cell carcinoma treated with surgery and radiation therapy. The right mandible was within the field of radiation. Because of the risk of radiation related osteonecrosis tooth #30 received non-surgical endodontic treatment and then the coronal tooth structure was removed (amputated crown).

How do you code for the submergence of the tooth portion of the treatment?

D3921   decoronation or submergence of an erupted tooth
Intentional removal of coronal tooth structure for preservation of the root and surrounding bone.

Clinical Coding Scenario #16:
Coronectomy (Two Different Cases)

An oral and maxillofacial surgeon completed consultations with two patients, both of whom faced similar complications.

Patient A

Patient A, a 38-year-old male, presents with chronic pericoronitis associated with a deep mesio-angular impaction of tooth #32. There is gingival inflammation and substantial bone loss surrounding the crown. The root of the tooth extends well past the inferior alveolar nerve canal and it is the dentist's opinion that removal of the entire tooth is a substantial risk to the nerve.

Patient B

Patient B, a 19-year-old female, presents for evaluation and treatment of a dentigerous cyst, associated with an impacted supernumerary tooth in the area of #20, displaced inferiorly and encroaching on the left mental foramen. After evaluation and examination, the dentist determines that total removal of the supernumerary tooth risks injury to the inferior alveolar nerve.

What procedure codes would be used to document the services delivered today and planned for a future date?

Each patient's record would have the same procedure codes.

For today's consultation:

D9310   consultation – diagnostic service provided by dentist or physician other than requesting dentist or physician

For the planned procedure:

D7251   coronectomy – intentional partial tooth removal, impacted teeth only
Intentional partial tooth removal is performed when a neurovascular complication is likely if the entire impacted tooth is removed.

Note: D7251 enables documentation of intentional partial tooth removal that is performed when a neurovascular complication is likely if the entire impacted tooth is removed. The procedure avoids complications involving the inferior alveolar nerve and the lingual nerve.

Clinical Coding Scenario #17:
Oroantral Fistula

A 23-year-old male is referred to the oral surgeon for evaluation of a partial boney impacted tooth #1. A clinical exam reveals pain on palpation. A panoramic image shows that the roots are in close proximity to the sinus and that there is no cystic lesion present. The procedure for the extraction of #1 is reviewed including risks and alternate treatments. The patient elects to have the tooth removed utilizing general anesthesia.

The patient returns for the surgery. After extracting the tooth, a large oroantral opening is noted and a mucoperiosteal flap is elevated with a buccal releasing incision to obtain primary closure. The procedure takes 20 minutes and the patient heals without incident.

How do you code for procedures related to the surgery encounter?

D7230 removal of impacted tooth – partially bony
Part of crown covered by bone; requires mucoperiosteal flap elevation and bone removal.

D7261 primary closure of a sinus perforation
Subsequent to surgical removal of tooth, exposure of sinus requiring repair, or immediate closure of oroantral or oronasal communication in absence of fistulous tract.

D9222 deep sedation/general anesthesia – first 15 minutes

D9223 deep sedation/general anesthesia – each subsequent 15 minute increment

Note: D9223 is reported once since the entire anesthesia time is 20 minutes.

If during the extraction there was no oroantral opening but the patient returned a few weeks later with an oroantral opening with a fistulous tract but no signs of infection, and the oroantral opening was closed at this subsequent visit with a primary closure, what would be the correct code for the closure procedure?

D7260 oroantral fistula closure
Excision of fistulous tract between maxillary sinus and oral cavity and closure by advancement flap.

Clinical Coding Scenario #18:
TMD Therapy

You have been treating a 32-year-old female who previously presented with complaints of several years of headaches, facial pain and "popping" in her left TMJ with occasional locking. Her treatment plan includes but is not limited to a splint for her temporomandibular joint dysfunction and in-office physical therapy.

How do you code for the splint device and physical therapy?

D7880 occlusal orthotic device, by report
Presently includes splints provided for the treatment of temporomandibular joint dysfunction.

D9130 temporomandibular joint dysfunction – non-invasive physical therapies
Therapy including but not limited to massage, diathermy, ultrasound, or cold application to provide relief from muscle spasms, inflammation or pain, intending to improve freedom of motion and joint function. This should be reported on a per session basis.

You feel an MRI is needed to further evaluate the soft tissue of the joint. The mandible needs to be in a specific position at the time of the MRI and a device is used to position the mandible for the MRI.

How do you code for the positioning device?

If the occlusal orthotic device is used that is also being used in her ongoing treatment, then no additional code is needed. If you construct an additional device to position the jaw for the MRI, then you may use:

D7899 unspecified TMD therapy, by report
Used for procedure that is not adequately described by a code. Describe procedure.

As therapy continues, the occlusal orthotic device needs adjustment. How do I code for the adjustment?

D7881 occlusal orthotic device adjustment

Clinical Coding Scenario #19:
Hyperplastic Tissue Excision

A 77-year-old male presents with ill-fitting dentures and requests new dentures. You determine that prior to constructing new dentures, he will require excision of some excess tissue in the maxilla related to irritation from his current dentures.

How would you code for the excision in the maxilla using a laser vs. excision using a scalpel?

Codes are procedure based rather than instrument based. Therefore, in this scenario, the same code is used for either instrumentation.

D7970 excision of hyperplastic tissue – per arch

Clinical Coding Scenario #20:
Non-opioid Post-operative Pain Management

A 17-year-old female is referred for extraction of painful impacted teeth #1, #16, #17, and #32. During the consultation, the patient's mother expresses concern about her daughter receiving opioids as part of the post-operative pain management protocol. To address this concern, following the manufacturer's instructions, the surgeon plans to infiltrate bupivacaine liposome injectable suspension at the surgical sites at the end of the procedure.

How would you code for the bupivacaine liposome injectable suspension?

D9613 infiltration of sustained release therapeutic drug, per quadrant
Infiltration of a sustained release pharmacologic agent for long acting surgical site pain control. Not for local anesthesia purposes.

Note: This procedure is reported four times and the four quadrants treated are identified by entering the applicable area of the oral cavity on the claim. Also, D9613's nomenclature explicitly states that the service is delivered and reported "per quadrant."

Clinical Coding Scenario #21:
Using a 3D Printer as Part of a Patient's Restoration Process

A 32-year-old female is referred for restoration of missing teeth #7, #8, #9, and #10 with implants. The dentist incorporates a 3D printer into his digital workflow for fabrication of his surgical guides. How do I code for this new step leading up to the implant placement?

One of the following codes may be used for documenting the referred patient's clinical oral evaluation. The code reported must be supported by your documentation in the patient's chart.

D0140 limited oral evaluation – problem focused
An evaluation limited to a specific oral health problem or complaint.

This may require interpretation of information acquired through additional diagnostic procedures. Report additional diagnostic procedures separately. Definitive procedures may be required on the same date as evaluation.

Typically, patients receiving this type of evaluation present with a specific problem or dental emergencies, trauma, acute infections, etc.

D0160 detailed and extensive oral evaluation – problem focused, by report
A detailed and extensive problem focused evaluation entails extensive diagnostic and cognitive modalities based on the findings of a comprehensive oral evaluation. Integration of more extensive diagnostic modalities to develop a treatment plan for a specific problem is required. The condition requiring this type of evaluation should be described and documented.

Examples of conditions requiring this type of evaluation may include dentofacial anomalies, complicated perio-prosthetic conditions, complex temporomandibular dysfunction, facial pain of unknown origin, conditions requiring multi-disciplinary consultation, etc.

If an intraoral digital scanner was used to obtain the desired intraoral structures the following code may be used:

D0801 3D dental surface scan – direct

Continued on next page

The following code may be reported for the diagnostic cast:

D0470 diagnostic cast
Also known as diagnostic models or study models.

The following codes may be used to report the CBCT. The selection of the code depends on the field of view and if the procedure includes image capture and interpretation (D0366–D0367) or if image capture is separate from interpretation (D0382–D0383):

D0366 cone beam CT capture and interpretation with field of view of one full dental arch – maxilla, with or without cranium

D0367 cone beam CT capture and interpretation with field of view of both jaws; with or without cranium

D0382 cone beam CT image capture with field of view of one full dental arch – maxilla, with or without cranium

D0383 cone beam CT image capture with field of view of both jaws, with or without cranium

The following code may be used to report the merging of the CBCT data and the digital cast information. It also includes the virtual planning of the surgical guide and implant positions:

D0393 virtual treatment simulation using 3D image volume or surface scan
Virtual simulation of treatment including, but not limited to, dental implant placement, prosthetic reconstruction, orthognathic surgery and orthodontic tooth movement.

The following code may be used when the surgeon fabricates the guide. The code is "by report" so it may be used to report different types of guides. It is important to include a detailed description of the guide when submitting the code.

D6190 radiographic/surgical implant index, by report
An appliance, designed to relate osteotomy or fixture position to existing anatomic structures, to be utilized during radiographic exposure for treatment planning and/or during osteotomy creation for fixture installation.

Clinical Coding Scenario #22:
Extraction for a Patient with Cardiovascular Disease Who Takes Anti-platelet Agents

A 72-year-old man presents for extraction of non-restorable teeth #29, #30, and #31. Review of his medical history reveals a history of cardiovascular disease. He is currently taking two anti-platelet agents. In consultation with the patient's physician, the surgery will be performed while continuing the antiplatelet agents. Bleeding will be controlled with local hemostatic measures including intra-socket wound dressing.

Is there a code available to describe the use of the intra-socket dressing?

D7922 **placement of intra-socket biological dressing to aid in hemostasis or clot stabilization, per site**
This procedure can be performed at time and/or after extraction to aid in hemostasis. The socket is packed with a hemostatic agent to aid in hemostasis and or clot stabilization.

Coding Q&A

1. *A patient presents to the office for a follow up treatment for bruxing and an adjustment was made to his occlusal guard.*

   What is the correct code?

   D9943   occlusal guard adjustment

---

2. *How do I code for constructing, adjusting, repairing or relining a custom sleep apnea appliance?*

   The correct procedure code for constructing the appliance is:

   D9947   custom sleep apnea appliance fabrication and placement

   The correct procedure code for adjusting the appliance is:

   D9948   adjustment of custom sleep apnea appliance

   The correct procedure code for repairing the appliance is:

   D9949   repair of custom sleep apnea appliance

   The correct code for relining the appliance is:

   D9953   reline custom sleep apnea appliance (indirect)
   Resurface dentition side of appliance with new soft or hard base material as required to restore original form and function.

---

3. *An immediate implant and a provisional crown was placed in the #8 position. What is the proper code for the crown?*

   D6085   interim implant crown

---

4. *A 75-year-old male with severe cardiac disease, including a history of aortic valve replacement, presents to the office for evaluation of his remaining dentition for extraction. The surgeon gives the patient antibiotics to be taken at home one hour prior to the scheduled appointment for his extractions. Due to the severity of his cardiac condition, the surgeon contacted the patient's cardiologist to discuss the planned procedure.*

   How do you code for the medication and the phone consultation with the cardiologist?

   D9630   drugs or medicaments dispensed in the office for home use

   D9311   consultation with a medical health care professional

5. *A 19-year-old patient presents for their initial visit. After reviewing their past medical history, it is noted that the patient admits to vaping. During the visit, you have a detailed conversation with the patient about the risks and adverse effects this may have on oral and systemic health. The patient indicates they would like to stop vaping, and methods of cessation are discussed in detail. Is there a code for this counseling?*

The proper code to use is:

D1321 counseling for the control and prevention of adverse oral, behavioral, and systemic health effects associated with high-risk substance use
Counseling services may include patient education about adverse oral, behavioral, and systemic effects associated with high-risk substance use and administration routes. This includes ingesting, injecting, inhaling and vaping. Substances used in a high-risk manner may include but are not limited to alcohol, opioids, nicotine, cannabis, methamphetamine and other pharmaceuticals or chemicals.

6. *I was forwarded a panoramic radiographic image, which I did not capture, for interpretation and a report. How do I code for my interpretation of the image?*

D0391 interpretation of diagnostic image by a practitioner not associated with the capture of the image, including report

7. *A patient needed an extraction, and it turned into a very difficult procedure. The doctor removed most of the tooth, but was unable to remove the entire root and the patient was referred to an oral surgeon immediately. Is there a code for a partial extraction?*

There are no partial extraction codes available. To report this procedure, use code **D7999 unspecified oral surgery procedure, by report**.

8. *I was not able to complete the extraction of an erupted tooth as the crown separated from its roots, and my attempts to remove them were unsuccessful. How should I document this incomplete extraction?*

There is a no code for an incomplete extraction of an erupted tooth, therefore CDT code **D7999 unspecified oral surgery procedure, by report** would be used to document what was completed. Details of what occurred would be in the report's narrative.

9. *When an erupted tooth extraction is incomplete what procedure is reported when another dentist is extracting only the residual roots?*

D7140 if the separated root is exposed and can be extracted with forceps or elevation. If removal requires cutting soft or bony tissue, it is the D7250 procedure.

10. *The patient has been to another dentist who attempted to extract a tooth, but did not successfully remove all structure and roots remain. What is the applicable procedure and its code to document only removal of the residual roots?*

It depends. If the residual root can be extracted using an elevator and forceps, the applicable procedure is D7140, as this code's nomenclature states the procedure is applicable to extraction of the entire tooth or only the root, or both. However, if removal of the residual root requires cutting tissue (soft and bone), the applicable procedure and its code is D7250.

11. *I removed a portion of the patient's fractured tooth, but not the entire tooth, to provide immediate relief of pain. How should I report this procedure?*

There is no code that specifically refers to removal of a portion of a fractured tooth to relieve pain. When there is no procedure code whose nomenclature and descriptor reflect the service provided, an "unspecified...procedure, by report" code may be considered (e.g., D7999 unspecified oral surgery procedure, by report).

12. *I am an oral surgeon and extracted a fully erupted tooth. My extractions are usually documented with CDT code D7210.*

For this patient, however, there was no need for any of the surgical actions listed in this code's nomenclature and descriptor. Is D7210 appropriate to document the service, or should I consider D7140?

Selection of the appropriate code comes through consideration of the full code entries, as follows:

D7140 **extraction, erupted tooth or exposed root (elevation and/or forceps removal)**
Includes routine removal of tooth structure, minor smoothing of socket bone, and closure, as necessary.

D7210 **extraction of erupted tooth requiring removal of bone and/or sectioning of tooth, and including elevation of mucoperiosteal flap if indicated**
Includes related cutting of gingiva and bone, removal of tooth structure, minor smoothing of socket bone and closure.

As you did not perform any of the actions listed in the D7210 entry, D7140 is the only applicable CDT code to document and report the service.

13. *When extracting an erupted tooth, what procedure is reported when: a) the crown and root are extracted in one piece; or b) during the course of the procedure the crown and root separate and are extracted individually?*

There are separate codes for each scenario –

a. D7140 is reported when a dentist completes the erupted tooth extraction procedure and the crown and root are extracted in one piece.

b. D7210 is reported when the crown and root separated during the extraction procedure (for any reason) and both were removed, with the removal of the root tip requiring bone removal.

14. *According to its descriptor code,* **D7241 removal of impacted tooth – completely bony, with unusual surgical complications** *can be used for a completely impacted tooth with an "aberrant tooth position." Would a completely impacted wisdom tooth that is radiographically very close to the mandibular nerve justify use of this procedure code?*

Perhaps. The dentist serving the patient is in the best position to determine whether the observed clinical condition of the patient's dentition and the procedure provided matches a dental procedure code (e.g., D7241). Radiographic images may not provide enough visual information to determine the extent of bony coverage, aberrant tooth position or other unusual circumstances.

Should a dentist determine that a specific code does not adequately apply to the service rendered, it is recommended that the service be reported using an "unspecified procedure, by report" code (e.g., **D7999 unspecified oral surgery procedure, by report**).

15. *I have used D3427 in the past for exploration and repair of root resorption. I see that D3427 has been deleted. What code do I use now?*

There are now six code options for documenting root resorption procedures. Three are for surgical repair, and three are for exploration without repair or apicoectomy:

Repair codes:

D3471 **surgical repair of root resorption – anterior**
For surgery on root of anterior tooth. Does not include placement of restoration.

D3472 **surgical repair of root resorption – premolar**
For surgery on root of premolar tooth. Does not include placement of restoration.

D3473 **surgical repair of root resorption – molar**
For surgery on root of molar tooth. Does not include placement of restoration.

Exploration without repair:

D3501 **surgical exposure of root surface without apicoectomy or repair of root resorption – anterior**
Exposure of root surface followed by observation and surgical closure of the exposed area. Not to be used for or in conjunction with apicoectomy or repair of root resorption.

D3502 **surgical exposure of root surface without apicoectomy or repair of root resorption – premolar**
Exposure of root surface followed by observation and surgical closure of the exposed area. Not to be used for or in conjunction with apicoectomy or repair of root resorption.

D3503 **surgical exposure of root surface without apicoectomy or repair of root resorption – molar**
Exposure of root surface followed by observation and surgical closure of the exposed area. Not to be used for or in conjunction with apicoectomy or repair of root resorption.

16. Which soft tissue biopsy code should I use?

There are three codes for soft tissue biopsies, differentiated by the depth and structural integrity of the tissue sample.

D7286 **incisional biopsy of oral tissue – soft tissue**
For partial removal of an architecturally intact specimen only. This procedure is not used at the same time as codes for apicoectomy/periradicular curettage. This procedure does not entail an excision.

D7287 **exfoliative cytological sample collection**
For collection of non-transepithelial cytology sample via mild scraping of the oral mucosa.

D7288 **brush biopsy – transepithelial sample collection**
For collection of oral disaggregated transepithelial cells via rotational brushing of the oral mucosa.

Code D7286 would be used for incisional tissue samples that maintain the original structure. Codes D7287 and D7288 are used for cell sampling biopsies that do not maintain tissue architecture.

17. *What is the appropriate code for reporting a supra-crestal fiberotomy?*

    The appropriate procedure code is:

    D7291 transseptal fiberotomy/supra crestal fiberotomy, by report

18. *What is a fibroma and how would removal be reported?*

    A fibroma is a benign tumor composed of fibrous or connective tissue, and the available procedure codes are:

    D7410 excision of benign lesion up to 1.25 cm

    D7411 excision of benign lesion greater than 1.25 cm

19. *How do I code removal of mandibular tori?*

    If the bony elevations are located lingually **D7473 removal of torus mandibularis** may be reported by quadrant.

20. *What is a torus/exostosis and how would removal be reported?*

    A torus/exostosis is a benign overgrowth of bone forming an elevation or protuberance of bone. They can form in the patient's palate, lingual or lateral aspect of the maxilla or mandible.

    Available procedure codes include:

    D7471 removal of lateral exostosis (maxilla or mandible)

    D7472 removal of torus palatinus

    D7473 removal of torus mandibularis

21. *What is the difference between the bone graft procedures reported with the following CDT codes?*

    D4263 bone replacement graft – retained natural tooth first site in quadrant

    Report when the bone graft is performed to stimulate periodontal regeneration when the disease process has led to a deformity of the bone around an existing tooth.

    D7950 osseous, osteoperiosteal, or cartilage graft of the mandible or maxilla – autogenous or nonautogenous, by report

    Report when the graft is used for ridge augmentation or reconstruction of an edentulous area of a ridge.

    D7953 bone replacement graft for ridge preservation – per site

Report when the bone graft is placed in an extraction site or implant removal site at the time of the extraction or removal to preserve ridge integrity.

D6104 bone graft at the time of implant placement

Report when the graft is placed in conjunction with implant placement.

D7955 repair of maxillofacial soft tissue and/or hard tissue defect

Report when reconstructing surgical, traumatic, or congenital defects of the facial bones, including the mandible to restore form and function. This procedure code should not be used for grafting the mandible or maxilla for prosthetic considerations.

22. *Can I use D7922 in place of D7956 or D7957? What is the difference between these procedure codes?*

Although each code may be used following an extraction they are used for different purposes. They are not interchangeable.

D7922 placement of intra-socket biological dressing to aid in hemostasis or clot stabilization, per site

This procedure can be performed at time and/or after extraction to aid in hemostasis. The socket is packed with a hemostatic agent to aid in hemostasis and or clot stabilization.

As the code states, the purpose of the dressing is to aid clot stabilization or hemostasis at the time of or after an extraction.

D7956 guided tissue regeneration, edentulous area – resorbable barrier, per site

This procedure does not include flap entry and closure, or, when indicated, wound debridement, osseous contouring, bone replacement grafts, and placement of biologic materials to aid in osseous regeneration. This procedure may be used for ridge augmentation, sinus lift procedures, and after tooth extraction.

D7957 guided tissue regeneration, edentulous area – non-resorbable barrier, per site

This procedure does not include flap entry and closure, or, when indicated, wound debridement, osseous contouring, bone replacement grafts, and placement of biologic materials to aid in osseous regeneration. This procedure may be used for ridge augmentation, sinus lift procedures, and after tooth extraction.

These codes have a very different purpose. The barrier membrane codes are used when the objective is to delay soft tissue growth into a graft or surgical site.

23. *How can I report a sinus lift procedure?*

There are discrete codes available for the two different approaches:

D7951 **sinus augmentation with bone or bone substitutes via a lateral open approach**

D7952 **sinus augmentation via a vertical approach**

24. *I performed a sinus augmentation via a vertical approach and placed an implant in the augmentation site on the same visit. How do I code for these procedures delivered at the same time?*

The correct procedure codes are:

D7952 **sinus augmentation via a vertical approach**

D6010 **surgical placement of implant body: endosteal implant**

25. *I performed a sinus augmentation via a lateral open approach. There was enough bone to stabilize the implant, so I placed an implant in the augmentation site on the same visit. How do I code for these procedures delivered at the same time?*

The correct procedure codes are:

D7951 **sinus augmentation with bone or bone substitutes via a lateral open approach**

D6010 **surgical placement of implant body: endosteal implant**

Obtaining the bone or bone substitute is included in procedure code D7951. If a barrier membrane is used it should be reported separately.

26. *Can D7921 and D4265 be used together when performing a sinus augmentation via an open approach?*

Yes, in certain circumstances. An example would be when you use platelet-rich plasma and bone morphogenetic protein (or other biologic material) for a sinus augmentation via an open approach.

The correct procedure codes to use are:

D7951 **sinus augmentation with bone or bone substitutes via a lateral open approach**

D7921 **collection and application of autologous blood concentrate product**

D4265 **biologic materials to aid in soft and osseous tissue regeneration, per site**

Obtaining the bone or bone substitute is included in procedure code D7951. If a barrier membrane is used it should be reported separately.

27. *What is an operculectomy, and how would it be coded?*

In dentistry, an operculum is a small flap of tissue surrounding or partially covering the back molars, and "ectomy" is a suffix referring to the removal of something. Therefore, an operculectomy is the surgical removal of a flap of tissue surrounding a partially erupted or impacted tooth.

The available procedure code is:

D7971 excision of pericoronal gingiva
Removal of inflammatory or hypertrophied tissues surrounding partially erupted/impacted teeth.

28. *The dentist performed a frenectomy on a child that had been diagnosed with ankyloglossia. What is ankyloglossia and how would treatment be documented?*

Ankyloglossia, more commonly referred to as "tongue tied," is a condition in which the lingual frenum is short and attached to the tip of the tongue, making normal speech difficult.

The available procedure code is:

D7962 lingual frenectomy (frenulectomy)

29. *A patient presents with a small sialolith in his right Wartons duct. Utilizing non-surgical manipulation, which included dilatation and manual manipulation, the stone was removed. How would you code for the removal of the stone?*

The correct procedure code is:

D7979 non-surgical sialolithotomy

30. *A restorative dentist refers a patient to your office for evaluation and removal of a broken retaining screw in an implant that you placed two years prior. You are able to remove the screw without damaging the implant. What would the proper code for this procedure be?*

Use the following code to correctly document this procedure:

D6096 remove broken implant retaining screw

31. *I am working with a maxillofacial prosthodontist and I have been using* **D6199 unspecified implant procedure, by report** *when placing craniofacial implants. Is that the correct code to use?*

The proper code to use is:

D7993 surgical placement of craniofacial implant — extra oral
Surgical placement of a craniofacial implant to aid in retention of an auricular, nasal, or orbital prosthesis.

32. *An orthodontist refers a patient to the oral surgeon because he would like to accelerate orthodontic movement, and by modifying the alveolus, enable teeth to move into areas with limited bone. You determine that a corticotomy would be the appropriate treatment to enable the desired orthodontic movement. How would you code for this procedure?*

The proper code(s) for this procedure depends on the number and location of teeth involved and would be either:

D7296   corticotomy – one to three teeth or tooth spaces, per quadrant

or

D7297   corticotomy – four or more teeth or tooth spaces, per quadrant

Note: When the involved teeth cross the mid-line, two quadrant codes must be reported.

33. *I am treating a patient for xerostomia. Is there a way to code for my assessment of the salivary flow?*

D0419   assessment of salivary flow by measurement
This procedure is for identification of low salivary flow in patients at risk for hyposalivation and xerostomia, as well as effectiveness of pharmacological agents used to stimulate saliva production.

34. *Can I use D7283 in conjunction with surgical exposure code D7280 even if no orthodontics is involved?*

D7283   placement of device to facilitate eruption of impacted tooth
Placement of an attachment on an unerupted tooth, after its exposure, to aid in its eruption. Report the surgical exposure separately using D7280.

The word "attachment" in the descriptor indicates that this procedure can be delivered when the dentist determines it is clinically necessary (e.g., not limited to placement for orthodontic purposes).

An example where this code would be reported is when an attachment is placed after surgical exposure of a mesially impacted permanent first molar that is trapped by the deciduous second molar. The attachment is designed to "unlock" the permanent first molar and allow normal eruption. No orthodontics are being done and may never be done to achieve eruption.

Summary

Oral and maxillofacial surgery cases use codes from many different categories of service, as well as from the CPT medical codes, and require a step-by-step approach to coding. With time, practice and patience, it will get easier to code for what you do.

Contributor Biography

James E. Mercer, D.D.S., is a board-certified oral and maxillofacial surgeon practicing in Columbia, SC since 1988. He is a graduate of Vanderbilt University and The Ohio State University College of Dentistry. He completed a one-year general practice residency, a two-year research fellowship, and his four-year specialty training in Oral and Maxillofacial Surgery at the Medical College of Georgia at Augusta University.

Dr. Mercer is a past chairman of the ADA's Council on Dental Benefit Programs and has been active in code maintenance nationally since 2003. He continues to be active in the tripartite and is currently a member of the American Association of Oral and Maxillofacial Surgeon's Committee on Health Care Policy, Coding, and Reimbursement representing them on the Code Maintenance Committee, the Dental Quality Alliance, and the SNODENT Maintenance Committee.

Chapter 11: D8000–D8999
Orthodontics

By Randall C. Markarian, D.M.D., M.S.

Introduction

Orthodontics is a unique CDT Code category of service when compared with others published in the CDT manual. This is due to the lower number of procedure codes and because a single code is used describe a procedure that involves a multi-visit and possibly multi-year treatment. It is advantageous for the dentist to understand the Orthodontics codes, even though there are only a few, so that they may choose the appropriate code to describe the service that they are providing. It is also important to note that even though the orthodontic treatment can be defined with a single code, codes from outside the orthodontic category are necessary to document all of the procedures that are performed, especially diagnostic procedures such as a comprehensive oral evaluation (D0150), panoramic radiograph (D0330), and diagnostic models (D0470).

Orthodontic treatment is a complex, dentist-guided process that alters the structure of the dentofacial complex requiring a comprehensive clinical examination including: pre-treatment diagnostic records such as radiographs, photos, and models; diagnosis and treatment planning; informed consent; supervision of the treatment; remediation and re-assessment of the therapy; retention; and retrospective evaluation by the treating dentist.

Terminology used in the orthodontic codes can be somewhat different than what is used in other areas of dentistry. For example, understanding the definition of terms like adolescent dentition, limited treatment, and comprehensive treatment influences the selection of the code used to document the procedure. A review of relevant terminology is the appropriate place to start.

Key Definitions and Concepts

Primary dentition: The stage during which the deciduous (or "baby") teeth erupt and are present. Typically, orthodontic treatment does not begin prior to complete eruption of the primary dentition and the permanent first molars are usually in the process of erupting or have fully erupted. The age of a patient can vary based on development, but usually ranges from ages five to eight.

Transitional dentition: This stage, also referred to as the mixed dentition, begins with the eruption of the first molars and is while the patient has both primary teeth remaining and permanent teeth erupting. The transitional dentition ends with the exfoliation of the final remaining primary tooth. The age of a patient in the transitional dentition will vary, but typically age ranges are from six to twelve years old.

Adolescent dentition: The stage where primary teeth are exfoliated and permanent teeth are in the process of erupting or have fully erupted, with the exception of the third molars. The patient is still in a growing phase, and dramatic changes to the oral-maxillofacial complex typically occur during this time. Adolescent dentition typically occurs during ages eleven to eighteen, depending upon the sex of the patient as males and females mature at different rates.

Adult dentition: This final stage is the full permanent dentition with little or no patient growth remaining. Third molars, if present, are usually erupted unless there is lack of space for eruption or the teeth are malposed.

Limited orthodontic treatment: The category of orthodontic treatment that involves a specific, defined, and limited scope. Examples would be a single tooth in crossbite or a tooth that needs guidance during eruption. Limited treatment does not involve the entire dentition and can be done at any of the stages of dental development.

Codes exist for each stage of development:

- D8010 for the primary dentition
- D8020 for the transitional dentition
- D8030 for the adolescent dentition
- D8040 for the adult dentition

Limited orthodontic treatment could involve palatal expansion or be a simple singular tooth movement with a retainer. Typically, limited coding can be used to report treatment utilizing simpler appliances and movements that are directed at addressing a specific problem for the patient.

Comprehensive orthodontic treatment: These treatments are the most complicated that the orthodontist can provide to a patient, and they must include careful diagnosis and treatment planning with complete and detailed orthodontic records. It involves correction of all of the patient's dentofacial issues including any skeletal, muscular, and dental alignment and occlusion issues. Comprehensive treatment can be provided during the transitional (D8070), adolescent (D8080), or permanent (D8090) dentition stage of dental development. These treatments may include a multi-disciplinary approach and involve treatment or consultation with other dental or medical providers such as oral surgeons and periodontists.

Changes to This Category

For CDT 2023's Orthodontic category there is one revision to the "preamble" that precedes all the procedure codes. The revision is:

D8000–D8999

All of the following orthodontic treatment codes may be used more than once for the treatment of a particular patient depending on the particular circumstance. A patient may require more than one interceptive procedure or more than one limited or comprehensive procedure depending on their particular problems.

The revision in the "preamble" is intended to clarify that both limited and comprehensive codes may be used more than one time during a patient's lifetime and that is consistent with orthodontic treatment guidelines. For example, a patient presenting for a Phase I orthodontic treatment may require a treatment that is considered comprehensive and a second comprehensive treatment for their Phase II treatment later.

There are no additions, revisions, or deletions to any procedure code entry in the Orthodontics category.

However, there are changes in other of the CDT categories that affect orthodontic coding. These changes are primarily related to 3D digital workflow including dental and facial scans and 3D virtual treatment simulations. Many orthodontists utilize 3D scanning on patients and should incorporate these codes into their coding protocol. These changes are:

D0393 virtual tTreatment simulation using 3D image volume or surface scan
The use of 3D image volumes forVirtual simulation of treatment including, but not limited to, dental implant placement, prosthetic reconstruction, orthognathic surgery and orthodontic tooth movement.

D0801 3D dental surface scan – direct

D0802 3D dental surface scan – indirect
A surface scan of a diagnostic cast.

D0803 3D facial surface scan – direct

D0804 3D facial surface scan – indirect
A surface scan of constructed facial features.

Clinical Coding Scenario #1:
Claim for Diagnostic Services Necessary for Treatment Planning

Preparation of an orthodontic case treatment plan requires an understanding of the patient's clinical condition, information that a dentist acquired through several diagnostic procedures. The diagnostic procedures usually performed include:

- A comprehensive patient examination
- Panoramic, cephalometric, and photographic images
- Diagnostic study models

How would you code a claim for these diagnostic procedures?

Applicable codes in this scenario are found in the Diagnostics category of service:

D0150   comprehensive oral evaluation – new or established patient

D0330   panoramic radiographic image

D0340   2D cephalometric radiographic image – acquisition, measurement and analysis

D0350   2D oral/facial photographic images obtained intra-orally or extra-orally

D0470   diagnostic casts

Offices that utilize an intraoral scanner for 3D image capture of the patient's dentition for diagnostic models and for 3D virtual treatment simulation should also use these applicable codes:

D0801   3D dental surface scan – direct

D0393   virtual simulation using 3D image volume or surface scan

Notes:

Information acquired through these diagnostic procedures must be documented in the patient's record and may also be reported on a claim regardless of whether the third-party payer will provide reimbursement for these services.

The orthodontic treatment plan then prepared would include the applicable procedure codes from the Orthodontics category of service. If your office also provides a consultation that service is reported with **D9450 case presentation, subsequent to detailed and extensive treatment planning**. Many offices overlook this very important part of reporting treatment planning.

Clinical Coding Scenario #2:
Coding All Aspects of an Orthodontic Case – Comprehensive Treatment of the Adolescent Dentition

A 14-year-old patient with adolescent dentition is now undergoing comprehensive orthodontic treatment that will last approximately two years. The appropriate code for comprehensive treatment is **D8080 comprehensive orthodontic treatment of the adolescent dentition**, but that is not the only CDT code applicable to this case.

Which CDT codes must be included in the patient's record and on claim submissions so that all necessary services are documented?

Procedures and Codes for Diagnosing the Patient's Condition

An oral evaluation and diagnosis is necessary in order to develop an appropriate treatment plan, and the applicable CDT codes for these services are found in the Diagnostic category of service. Although they are not listed in the Orthodontics category, diagnostic procedures and their codes may be delivered and reported by any licensed dentist.

Procedures and codes that are typical for diagnosing a patient's condition are:

D0150 **comprehensive oral evaluation – new or established patient**

D0330 **panoramic radiographic image**

D0340 **2D cephalometric radiographic image – acquisition, measurement and analysis**

D0350 **2D oral/facial photographic image obtained intra-orally or extra-orally**

D0801 **3D dental surface scan – direct**

D0393 **virtual simulation using 3D image volume or surface scan**

D0470 **diagnostic casts**

D9450 **case presentation, subsequent to detailed and extensive treatment planning**

Continued on next page

Note: The findings from these procedures will lead to development of the appropriate orthodontic treatment plan. It is possible that the orthodontist may determine that treatment should not start immediately. In that case, there is a monitoring procedure that may also be performed and reported with its own unique code in the Orthodontics category.

D8660 pre-orthodontic treatment examination to monitor growth and development

Codes during Active Treatment

Even though orthodontic treatments are coded under an "umbrella code," such as D8080 in this case, there are other codes that should be used in conjunction to fully describe the services provided to the patient.

The overarching "umbrella" code for the type of orthodontic treatment for the patient in this scenario is:

D8080 comprehensive orthodontic treatment of the adolescent dentition

During the active orthodontic treatment, each visit would be coded using:

D8670 periodic orthodontic treatment visit

When the orthodontic treatment is complete and patient will receive retainers, the procedure is coded with:

D8680 orthodontic retention (removal of appliances, construction and placement of retainer(s))

All subsequent orthodontic retainer adjustments should be coded as:

D8681 removable orthodontic retainer adjustment

Many orthodontists will be confused by this coding since most third-party payers only pay a set lifetime maximum for an orthodontic treatment, and therefore, the additional coding does not affect the reimbursement received. Utilization of the CDT codes is not directly about billing and insurance as much as it is about documenting in the patient record the treatment that was provided to the patient.

Clinical Coding Scenario #3:
Multi-Phase Orthodontic Treatment

A 9-year-old boy presents for treatment. The patient has a moderate arch length discrepancy in the mandibular arch, with primary molars still present. Maxillary arch shows flared incisors with spacing and a significant overjet. Patient is treatment planned for a maxillary and mandibular 2x4 appliances to correct alignment and spacing, along with a mandibular lingual arch to retain the leeway space. Parents are informed that a future Phase II treatment will be necessary to fully correct all orthodontic issues.

How do you code for both phases of treatment in this scenario?

Coding for any orthodontic treatment should start by documenting what diagnostic procedures were performed prior to the treatment planning of the case. For Phase 1 the appropriate orthodontic treatment code would be **D8070 comprehensive orthodontic treatment of the transitional dentition**.

Many dentists are concerned that a comprehensive orthodontic treatment code can only be reported once in a patient's life as a dental benefit plan may have reimbursement limitations. There are however many times, as in this case, the patient will have two comprehensive treatments in order to achieve the treatment plan's outcomes. The code for the Phase II treatment depends on the patient's dentition at that time and would most likely be **D8080 comprehensive orthodontic treatment of the adolescent dentition**.

Note: It would also be appropriate to utilize the codes for **D8670 periodic orthodontic treatment visit, D8680 orthodontic retention (removal of appliances, construction and placement of retainer(s))**, and **D8681 removable orthodontic retainer adjustment** during and after both phases of treatment.

Clinical Coding Scenario #4:
Tongue Thrust Habit and Appliances

An eight-year-old patient has a tongue thrust habit that is causing a significant open bite. An appliance was recommended and placed to aid in resolving the habit.

How would you code this procedure?

Coding for appliances to stop harmful habits depends upon the design. For removable appliances the code is **D8210 removable appliance therapy**; for a fixed appliance, **D8220 fixed appliance therapy**.

Clinical Coding Scenario #5:
Removable Retainers to Stabilize Teeth

A patient has completed active treatment and is wearing removable retainers to stabilize the teeth. The retainers are becoming loose and require an appointment for the orthodontist to make adjustments to these appliances.

How would you code this visit?

This visit would be coded using **D8681 removable orthodontic retainer adjustment**.

Clinical Coding Scenario #6:
Class II Malocclusion and Severe Crowding

A 12-year-old patient presents with a Class II malocclusion and severe crowding. The patient just lost her last deciduous tooth. Parents want the teeth straightened and bite corrected. The case has been diagnosed and treatment planned for full upper and lower braces and extraction of all four first bicuspids.

How would you code this treatment?

This case would be coded as **D8080 comprehensive orthodontic treatment of the adolescent dentition** because the patient is still experiencing erupting teeth and growth.

Clinical Coding Scenario #7:
Orthodontic Recall Visits

After the initial orthodontic evaluation, many times orthodontists feel that orthodontic treatment should not begin at that time. They will set an appointment for the patient to return in the future to monitor their growth and development. They will then evaluate whether treatment should begin at that point.

What code should be used to report these visits to monitor the dentition?

D8660   pre-orthodontic treatment examination to monitor growth and development

Clinical Coding Scenario #8:
Discontinued Treatment and Removal of Braces

A ten-year-old patient's parents have decided that they would like to discontinue orthodontic treatment. As such, they also wish to have their child's braces removed.

How would you code for this scenario?

D8695   removal of fixed orthodontic appliances for reasons other than completion of treatment

Although it may not be needed, please consider requesting the parents sign a waiver of release for premature removal of braces.

The practice should make a decision about whether to provide retention based on the treatment progress made, and in conjunction with the patient's or parent's treatment wishes. In addition, the practice should ensure that the patient's results to-date are held should the decision be reversed and treatment continues

Clinical Coding Scenario #9:
Removal of Orthodontic Braces and Appliances in an Emergency Situation

A patient with braces has been struck in the face. Since it's an emergency, the patient is rushed to his general dentist. In order to assess and repair the damage, the dentist must remove the patient's braces and appliances.

How would you code for the removal of the patient's braces and appliances?

> **D8695** removal of fixed orthodontic appliances for reasons other than the completion of treatment

Note: D8695's CDT Code entry does not specify the type or specialty of the dentist who removes the appliance. As with all CDT codes, state licensure determines whether or not the dentist may deliver the procedure reported with a CDT code. As noted in this scenario, the removal was by a general practitioner. In the preceding scenario (#8) removal was by an orthodontist.

Clinical Coding Scenario #10:
Re-cementing a Loose Fixed Appliance

A patient presents with a palatal expander that has a band loose on one side. The only way to take care of the problem is to remove the expander, clean and repair the appliance, polish the teeth involved, and then re-cement the expander on the teeth.

How would you code for this treatment?

Since the loose appliance must be repaired before re-cementation, and the palatal expander is placed in the maxillary arch, you would use:

> **D8696** repair of orthodontic appliance – maxillary

Clinical Coding Scenario #11:

Repair and Complete Reattachment of a Mandibular Fixed Retainer

The patient presents with a mandibular bonded lingual retainer with one side of the retainer having come un-bonded. Due to a distortion of the retainer wire, the retainer must be removed, all adhesive cleaned off and teeth polished. Once the retainer's proper form is restored, the retainer is re-bonded.

How would you code for this procedure?

D8699 re-cement or re-bond fixed retainer – mandibular

Clinical Coding Scenario #12:
Remote Patient Encounter Utilizing Teledentistry

A patient with adolescent dentition is unable to come to the office to have their aligners checked and would like more aligners shipped to them. A videoconference examination and subsequent review of digital photos sent by the patient are utilized to determine whether the patient should advance to further aligner trays.

How would you code for this encounter?

D8670 periodic orthodontic treatment visit

D9996 teledentistry – asynchronous; information stored and forwarded to dentist for subsequent review
Reported in addition to other procedures (e.g., diagnostic) delivered to the patient on the date of service.

In a teledentistry encounter, both the applicable orthodontic procedure code and teledentistry code are documented in the patient record and recorded on a claim submission. In this case, the applicable orthodontic procedure (D8670) is reported along with asynchronous teledentistry code (D9996) as the photographs were forwarded to the orthodontist for review after the videoconference ended. If the images were transmitted in real-time, the applicable teledentistry code reported would be **D9995 teledentistry – synchronous; real-time encounter** instead of D9996.

The criterion for selection of the applicable teledentistry code is the CDT code's nomenclature and descriptor, regardless of the type of treatment modality or appliance that is being used to treat the patient. As noted above, the applicable teledentistry code is reported with the appropriate orthodontic procedure code.

There are limitations in use of teledentistry in orthodontics for reasons that include the difficulty in obtaining adequate quality photographs from patients to document their current condition, as well as being unable to accurately check the patient's occlusion remotely. Further, diagnostic information (e.g., images) captured remotely by a patient or person without professional training or licensure are unlikely to be of the same diagnostic quality as those captured in-office by appropriately trained staff.

Periodic orthodontic treatment visits utilizing teledentistry can, however, be useful for established patients who are away at college or for other extended periods and when the dentist has a familiarity with the patient's malocclusion and treatment.

Clinical Coding Scenario #13:
Crossbite with Lower Anterior Teeth

A nine-year-old patient's #8 tooth has erupted into crossbite with the lower anterior teeth. The parents are simply interested in getting the central incisor out of crossbite. Different treatment options were offered to the parents for correction of the problem. After the decision was made, treatment on the central incisor was initiated.

How would you code this treatment?

Since this is treating one specific issue or problem with no forethought to further treatment later on in the patient's development, this case is best reported using **D8020 limited orthodontic treatment of the transitional dentition**.

Clinical Coding Scenario #14:
Limited Orthodontic Treatment

An 8-year-old patient presents with an overjet of 12 mm and severe spacing between the permanent maxillary anterior teeth. None of the patient's remaining primary teeth are involved. After evaluation, the treatment plan determined to be the best is 2x4 bonding of the maxillary permanent incisors and the permanent first molars.

How would you code for this procedure?

With CDT 2022's deletion of the Interceptive Orthodontic codes, the best coding for Phase I treatment would be to determine the extent of the treatment. In this example, the treatment is a limited orthodontic treatment and should be coded using **D8020 limited orthodontic treatment of the transitional dentition**.

Coding Q&A

1. *Many offices now produce digital versus plaster study models for their cases. What code should be used to report digital study models (e.g., iTero® scans)?*

   Code **D0470 diagnostic casts** is used to report fabricating any type of orthodontic study models. CDT coding is intended to be procedure specific, not modality or technique specific. With the addition of the 3D surface scan codes, if one uses an intraoral scanner, then **D0801 3D dental surface scan – direct** would be applied along with the **D0470 diagnostic casts** code.

2. *What code or codes should be used to report multiple stages of orthodontic treatment?*

   It is appropriate to use limited coding for the initial phase of orthodontic treatment when treating only a portion of the dentition (e.g., treatment of crossbite with an expansion appliance). Interceptive treatments could also be coded as comprehensive if both arches are included, such as to allow for bite correction during this phase. These treatments are followed later in the patient's development with comprehensive treatment of the adolescent or adult dentition. As noted in the preamble to the Orthodontic codes, limited or comprehensive treatment codes may be used more than one time for the same individual.

3. *What code should be used to report treatment using clear aligners?*

   Treatments using clear aligner therapy would be the same codes that would be used for a treatment utilizing orthodontic brackets. Code selection is dependent on the nature of the treatment (limited or comprehensive) and the stage of dental development, rather than the type of appliance used.

4. *When should an orthodontic practice use* **D8999 unspecified orthodontic procedure, by report***?*

   This code should be used sparingly and only when the orthodontist determines that there is no other applicable CDT code. In most cases, another code can be found that will adequately and appropriately report the procedure performed. If the D8999 code is used, make certain that the claim is accompanied by a narrative report to describe the patient's condition, the need for treatment, and the treatment provided.

5. *Often when orthodontic cases are completed, the orthodontist may wish to put final touches on the case to perfect the result by slightly altering the shape of a tooth or teeth with enameloplasty. What code should be used?*

The code most often used to report enameloplasty is **D9971 odontoplasty – per tooth**.

···

6. *When space maintenance is part of an orthodontic case treatment plan, what procedure codes would be reported – passive appliance procedure codes in the Preventive category, or a limited orthodontic treatment code in the Orthodontics category?*

Selection of the appropriate code to report depends on whether the procedure involves passive space maintenance or active tooth movement. For passive space maintenance, a procedure code in the Preventive's passive appliance subcategory (e.g., D1510–D1527 or D1575) should be reported, with selection determined by the type of space maintainer (i.e., fixed or removable; unilateral or bi-lateral; distal shoe) placed. If the appliance will be used to actively regain (and then maintain) space that will allow for eruption of permanent teeth (e.g., by placement of a lingual holding arch or a Nance appliance), the appropriate procedure code would be from Orthodontics' limited orthodontic treatment subcategory (D8010–D8040) as appropriate based on the patient's dentition.

···

7. *A patient has been placed on recall appointments every six months to monitor growth and development and to determine the best time to start orthodontic treatment. How should these appointments be recorded?*

These appointments should be reported using **D8660 pre-orthodontic treatment examination to monitor growth and development**.

···

8. *I am using a remote dental monitoring app to check progress on my aligner cases. This software uses AI to determine whether the patient's teeth are tracking according to the plan. How do I code for this monitoring?*

This would be coded using **D9996 teledentistry – asynchronous; information stored and forwarded to dentist for subsequent review**, since the data is collected then transmitted to the doctor at a later time. Also, **D8670 periodic orthodontic treatment visit** would be used in conjunction with the teledentistry code.

9. *A patient has lost her retainer and it must be replaced. What code would you use?*

   Replacement of lost or broken retainers is coded using either **D8703 replacement of lost or broken retainer – maxillary** or **D8704 replacement of lost or broken retainer – mandibular**, depending on the arch involved.

10. *A patient comes in with three mandibular brackets off. Can I use code* **D8697 repair of orthodontic appliance - mandibular** *for that appointment to re-bond them?*

    No. That code is only for repairs to appliances on the mandibular arch such as an expander, a lip bumper, or other functional appliances. There is no specific CDT code for re-bonding brackets. The visit during which the re-bonding occurs would be documented with the following codes:

    D8670 periodic orthodontic treatment visit

    D8999 unspecified orthodontic procedure, by report

11. *A patient presents with a lower lingual bonded retainer that developed a sharp edge, irritating the tongue. How would I code a procedure of smoothing and burnishing that sharp edge?*

    Any repair of a fixed mandibular retainer without having to remove the retainer is coded **D8702 repair of fixed retainer, includes reattachment – mandibular**.

12. *At each appointment with an Invisalign® patient, I perform an intraoral scan and use software to compare whether the patient's teeth are in the position that they should be compared to the aligner stage they are in. How do I code for this?*

    The first code would be **D8670 periodic orthodontic treatment visit** to document the regular adjustment appointment. The second code would be **D0801 3D dental surface scan – direct**. That code includes interpretation of the scan which would describe the procedure being done to compare the predicted tooth position to actual.

13. *I am using a rapid palatal expander in conjunction with a complete set of braces. How do I code for the use of a fixed appliance like an RPE?*

    The RPE is part of a comprehensive treatment and there is no separate code for placement of this appliance. Its use is a component of the appropriate comprehensive orthodontic treatment code reported for treating the patient's dentition. There should be a notation of RPE use in the patient's dental record.

14. *A patient has completed orthodontic treatment and is in retainers and has no additional orthodontic benefit. When I adjust their retainer, how should I code for that?*

    You could code for the adjustment **D8681 removable orthodontic retainer adjustment** regardless of the patient's dental benefit status.

Summary

To properly code for the orthodontic procedures that are performed, the dentist must correctly identify the scope of the treatment and the appropriate stage of dental development while understanding that codes outside of the orthodontic section are necessary to fully describe all procedures provided. This is especially true of the pretreatment diagnostic workup. While the smaller number of codes in the orthodontic section may appear to simplify the coding process, it is easy to be confused and overlook all of the codes needed to properly document the full treatment.

Contributor Biography

Randall C. Markarian, D.M.D., M.S., has been practicing orthodontics in Swansea, Illinois since 1994. Dr. Markarian is a past chair of the Council on Dental Benefit Programs and the Code Maintenance Committee. He is currently chair of the American Association of Orthodontists Council on Orthodontic Benefits and the ADA Trustee representing the 8th district.

Chapter 12: D9000–D9999
Adjunctive General Services

By Charles D. Stewart, D.M.D.

Introduction

Many health professions including dentistry, medicine, and veterinary science accept that the word "adjunctive" refers to any treatment or service delivered in addition to a primary treatment, so that the combination of codes: a) increases the primary treatment's efficacy; or b) assists with completion or reporting of the primary treatment. Adjunctive treatment or therapy is generally an additional or secondary activity separate to, or in some way related to, the primary therapy. Adjunctive procedures can also be referred to as ancillary, supporting, accessory, and parallel procedures. The word "general" in the dental or medical context means not specialized or limited in range of subject, application, activity, and the like.

Differentiation between primary and secondary treatment as noted above is consistent with the current ADA Glossary definition of adjunctive: "A secondary treatment in addition to the primary therapy." The CDT Code's Adjunctive General Services category contains codes needed to document procedures or services that are performed on patients when an appropriate code is not found in any of the other eleven CDT Code categories.

This twelfth category contains a variety of codes for clinical services, such as anesthesia, sleep apnea appliances, and occlusal guards, and non-clinical services including case management, other administrative events such as cancelled or missed appointments, and even sales tax! This variety has led many to describe the Adjunctive General Services category as a catchall for procedures and services that don't quite fit in the other CDT Code categories.

The value, relevance, and use of codes in the Adjunctive category was demonstrated through increased utilization of the teledentistry codes during the COVID-19 pandemic that began in 2020. Response to the pandemic led to emergency regulations and publication of guidelines that directly impacted the practice of dentistry, what services were permitted, and how services can be provided to patients in need who received services in virtual (also known as remote) encounters. The ADA, along with dental benefit plans, provided guidance to dental providers on reporting services performed during this emergency, including the use of the two very important teledentistry codes in the Adjunctive category. Many dental benefit plans continue to provide some form of coverage for teledentistry encounters even during a control phase of the pandemic.

Key Definitions and Concepts

Anesthesia: A patient's level of consciousness is determined by the patient's response to the drugs or medications administered, not the route of the anesthetic agent administration. State dental licensing boards regulate the use of anesthesia techniques and license those who render this service. The ADA House of Delegates adopted and published anesthesia policy and guidelines, which are available at *ADA.org/anesthesiasedation*. There are several CDT codes for anesthesia procedures such as local, regional, block, moderate sedation, deep sedation, general anesthesia, etc.

Consultation: In a dental setting, a service or meeting provided by a dentist or other licensed dental professional where the dentist, patient, or other parties (e.g., another dentist, physician, or legal guardian) discuss the patient's dental needs, conditions, and proposed treatment modalities. The consultation is appropriate when the opinion or advice of a fellow practitioner is sought to evaluate or manage a specific problem or patient concern. A consultation could be performed in-person or by using a teledentistry model or methodology.

Medicament: Substance or combination of substances intended to be pharmacologically active, specially prepared to be prescribed, dispensed, applied or administered by authorized professional personnel to prevent or treat diseases in humans or animals. This can be an agent that promotes recovery from an injury or ailment. It can also be referred to in some cases as a medicine. It can be a substance used for medical treatment. In dentistry, medicaments can be placed in the mouth, in a tooth, in the jaws, in the gingiva, or dispensed by a licensed dental professional and may also be purchased as a prescription or an over-the-counter treatment. Medicaments may be indicated based on results of clinical examination and diagnostic procedure, which could be performed both in person and remotely via a teledentistry model.

Microabrasion: Mechanical and chemical removal of a small amount of tooth structure to eliminate superficial enamel discoloration defects. This process uses chemical solutions and or abrasive substances such as pumice to remove thin layers of tooth enamel in order to eliminate yellow, white, and brown spots, or stains and discolorations on the teeth. Microabrasion may be used as a step or process in a conservative, less invasive restorative treatment. It also may be a definitive stand-alone procedure and as such should be reported using the appropriate CDT code.

Obstructive sleep apnea (OSA): OSA syndrome is characterized by repeat episodes of upper airway obstruction due to the collapse of the upper airway during sleep. Medical management of the syndrome may include evaluation, sleep studies, weight loss, avoidance of stimulants (including caffeine), body position adjustment, oral appliances, and use of continuous positive airway pressure (CPAP) during sleep.

Palliative: Action that relieves pain and symptoms without dealing with the underlying disease or cause of the condition. The ADA Glossary definition of palliative is more concise: "Action that relieves pain but is not curative." (See discussion later in this chapter in regard to the revision of CDT code D9110.)

Parenteral: A technique of administration in which the drug bypasses the gastrointestinal (GI) tract. Examples of parenteral administration may include intramuscular (IM), intravenous (IV), intranasal (IN), submucosal (SM), subcutaneous (SC), or intraosseous (IO). Simply put, bypassing the gastrointestinal tract means the drug is not administered through the mouth or alimentary canal.

Special health care needs: Any physical, developmental, mental, sensory, behavioral, cognitive, or emotional impairment or limiting condition or incapacitation that requires medical management, health care intervention, and/or use of specialized services or programs. The condition may be congenital, developmental, or acquired through disease, trauma, or environmental cause and may impose limitations in performing daily self-maintenance activities or substantial limitations in a major life activity. Health care for individuals with special needs requires specialized knowledge, as well as increased awareness and attention, adaptation, and accommodative measures beyond what are considered routine. (This definition was developed by the American Academy of Pediatric Dentistry (AAPD) Council on Clinical Affairs.)

Teledentistry, asynchronous: Also known as "store-and-forward," or "capture-and-interpret," involves transmission of recorded health information to a dentist or dental professional, who uses the information to evaluate a patient's condition or render a service outside of a real-time or live interaction. Such transmitted information can include all forms of images, including but not limited to radiographs, photographs, video recordings, digital impressions, digital models, and photomicrographs of patients. Transmission is through a secure electronic communications system. CAD-CAM technology could be considered an asynchronous encounter with appliance fabrication, design, and treatment applications. This technology is currently used within dentistry in several practice areas such as: diagnostic, preventive, restorative, prosthetic, and orthodontic procedures.

Teledentistry, synchronous: Also referred to as live video or real-time interaction, synchronous teledentistry involves live, two-way communication and interaction between a person or persons (e.g., patient; dental, medical or health caregiver) at one physical location, and an overseeing supervising or consulting dentist or dental professional at another location. This type of interaction saw increased utilization during the mandatory closures and dental practice restrictions associated with the COVID-19 pandemic.

Changes to This Category

CDT 2023 contains revisions to two existing CDT codes and one code addition, described below.

The revisions are:

D9110 **palliative ~~(emergency)~~ treatment of dental pain~~-minor procedure,~~– per visit**
Treatment that relieves pain but is not curative; services provided do not have distinct procedure codes. ~~This is typically reported on a "per visit" basis for emergency treatment of dental pain.~~

The nomenclature revision clarifies the broad scope of the service documented with code D9110. By removing emergency from the nomenclature, the non-emergent palliative procedures can now be reported appropriately and accurately using this code. Deleting "minor procedure" eliminates confusing verbiage as currently there is no definition of what is a minor procedure that is widely accepted within the practice of dentistry. The descriptor revision provides clarity as it describes the situation as well as the procedure's scope and expected outcome.

D9450 **case presentation, subsequent to detailed and extensive treatment planning**
~~Established patient. Not performed on same day as evaluation.~~

The rationale for revisions to D9450 was provided by testimony from the ADA's Code Maintenance Committee's member organizations. This testimony noted that with modern diagnostic instruments, tools, intelligence, and programs it is possible to develop a treatment plan on the same day as the evaluation. Eliminating the descriptor's restrictive wording regarding timing is beneficial to the patient and professional as more (e.g., diagnosis, evaluation and treatment plan delivery) can be provided on the same date of service.

The addition is:

D9953 **reline custom sleep apnea appliance (indirect)**
Resurface dentition side of appliance with new soft or hard base material as required to restore original form and function.

This new code is a logical complement to CDT 2022's addition of the following suite of CDT codes:

D9947   custom sleep apnea appliance fabrication and placement

D9948   adjustment of custom sleep apnea appliance

D9949   repair of custom sleep apnea appliance

Appliances and prosthetics used in dentistry routinely require adjustments, repairs, and relines. The CMC determined that one code for an indirect sleep apnea reline procedure (assigned number "D9953") should be added to CDT. Only an indirect reline procedure is appropriate for a sleep apnea appliance as a direct reline is not be indicated and would not work due to the nature of the material used to fabricate the custom sleep apnea appliance.

Note:
Oral sleep appliances fabricated by a dentist had traditionally been reported using medical CPT codes and the claim was submitted to the patient's medical benefit plan. The suite of CDT sleep apnea appliance procedure codes affects this tradition. These CDT codes enable the dentist to report and document the sleep procedures in the electronic health record and to bill dental benefit plans, with payer reimbursement dependent on available dental benefits.

By establishing the suite of codes for sleep apnea appliances, the ADA recognizes the role that dentists play in the treatment of obstructive sleep apnea (OSA). The profession acknowledges and encourages that the diagnosis of OSA requires a physician-supervised sleep study (polysomnography) as well as a formal prescription to a dentist for the fabrication of an appliance.

OSA appliances can be broadly categorized as mandibular advancing and or positioning devices or as tongue retaining devices. The potential insurance benefit for these appliances have traditionally followed the categorization of them by Medicare as durable medical equipment (DME), and as such have not been considered dental devices in the past.

Clinical Coding Scenario #1:
Dental Emergency when Dentist is on Vacation

A patient calls the office and states they are having a dental emergency. The office staff informs the patient that their dentist is away on vacation and that there is a covering dentist taking calls and providing care. Staff schedules an appointment where the covering dentist will meet virtually with the patient via a secured connection using the Zoom™ conferencing application.

During the virtual encounter the dentist has the patient explain their history, symptoms, and issue of concern. Since the patient has video capability (e.g., mobile phone) the dentist asks the patient to move the camera so that the area of the mouth and condition that exists can be visualized. The patient opens their mouth and the dentist sees the oral cavity's teeth and surrounding soft tissues.

The covering dentist makes a diagnosis based on the visual and oral information gathered during this encounter, and then determines a course of treatment to address the patient's issues until the patient's dentist returns from vacation and can deliver definitive treatment of the concerns presented. The covering dentist also provides appropriate medications and advice based on the Zoom™ encounter.

How do you code this remote care?

   D9995 **teledentistry – synchronous; real-time encounter**

Note: D9995 is used since the entire encounter, including the dentist's viewing of the patient's oral cavity, is live and completed without interruption.

   D0140 **limited oral evaluation – problem focused**

or

   D0170 **re-evaluation – limited, problem focused (established patient, not post-operative visit)**

or

   D0171 **re-evaluation – post-operative office visit**

Note: Only one of these three evaluation codes should be reported in the electronic health record and on the dental claim form. The appropriate code is selected based on the history of the condition being presented. If it is the first experience of this issue, the D0140 is the proper code. If the condition involves a previously known, addressed, or treated condition, the re-evaluation code can be selected based on whether or not this is a post-operative encounter.

Continued on next page

It is of vital importance that the D9995 be listed on the dental claim form to identify it as a teledentistry claim. Several individual states have mandated special handling of claims identified as "telehealth" and such identification is afforded by using the D9995 or D9996 CDT codes, as applicable.

Many dental plans view these two codes as documenting the modality of service delivery, reported on a claim submission along with the diagnostic and treatment procedure codes for the actual services performed. All codes accurately reported enable calculation of reimbursements for available dental plan benefits. During the COVID-19 pandemic, several dental benefit plans extended special benefits for services performed via teledentistry.

Clinical Coding Scenario #2:
Anesthesia

A patient, referred by a general dentist, is scheduled for surgical removal of third molars. A text message with a pre-visit screening questionnaire is completed. Upon arrival to the office, the questionnaire was reviewed and an evaluation for the use of general anesthesia was conducted, resulting in the decision to proceed with the anesthetic and surgery upon obtaining the appropriate informed consents. After the initial administration of the anesthetic agent, the surgery was completed. The anesthesia start time was 10:05 A.M. and anesthesia services were completed at 11:07 A.M. The oral surgeon extracting the third molars is wondering how many units of anesthesia can be billed, or is it just a single flat rate procedure?

How would you code this care?

> **D9912** **pre-visit patient screening**
>
> **D9219** **evaluation for moderate sedation, deep sedation, or general anesthesia**
>
> **D9222** **deep sedation/general anesthesia – first 15 minutes**
>
> **D9223** **deep sedation/general anesthesia – each subsequent 15 minute increment**

A copy of the anesthesia record should be submitted with the dental claim to verify the anesthesia time. According to the D9220 descriptor (which is also applicable to D9223), anesthesia time begins when the anesthesia agent delivery and monitoring protocol start, and the procedure is completed when the patient may be safely left under the observation of trained personnel for recovery. In this scenario, 62 minutes elapsed between the procedure's start and completion, so the appropriate coding is:

> D9222 reported with a quantity of "1" for the initial 15 minutes
>
> D9223 with a quantity of "4" for the additional 47 minutes

Note: As anesthesia is reported in 15-minute (or portions thereof) increments, the D9223 claim documents delivery of <u>three</u> 15-minute increments and <u>one</u> two-minute increment (i.e., the additional 47 minutes and therefore a Quantity = "4" on the service line).

Clinical Coding Scenario #3:
Occlusal Equilibration

The patient says her spouse hears loud grinding sounds at night. However, the patient says that she has no pain in her jaws or joint area, but adds that she does have difficulty chewing food. There was not any time to do a pre-visit patient screening until the patient arrived at the office. The screening was completed via interview and the patient's temperature was taken. The dentist begins to consult with the patient who also says that her teeth seem to be sensitive when biting down and at times seem to make noise or "chatter" when chewing.

Based on this information and a limited problem-focused evaluation, the dentist determined that the patient needed her bite (occlusion) adjusted.

How would you code the "bite adjustment" procedure appointment?

> **D9912   pre-visit patient screening**
>
> **D0140   limited oral evaluation – problem focused**

Occlusal adjustment, also known as occlusal equilibration, refers to the reshaping of the occlusal surfaces of teeth to create a harmonious contact relationship between the upper and lower teeth. One of the following codes should be used, with selection based on the procedure's extent:

> **D9951   occlusal adjustment – limited**

or

> **D9952   occlusal adjustment – complete**

There is no formal definition of limited or complete occlusal adjustment. ADA claim completion instructions (i.e., "ADA Guide to Dental Procedures Reported with Area of the Oral Cavity or Tooth Anatomy (or Both)") indicate the applicable arch(s) should be reported along with either of these codes. A dentist selects the appropriate occlusal adjustment code after considering this guidance, time required, and clinical experience. The patient's record should include the reasons for selecting either code.

If the occlusal equilibration is associated with or to accommodate the placement of a restoration or prosthesis, the billing of the equilibration may be considered incidental to the restoration or prosthesis. Likewise, if the occlusal adjustment is associated with the final step of a comprehensive orthodontic treatment, it may be considered incidental to the orthodontic treatment.

Clinical Coding Scenario #4:
Occlusal Guard with Both Hard and Soft Attributes

In addition to the occlusal adjustment performed in clinical coding scenario #3, the dentist feels that a full arch occlusal guard should be fabricated and placed in the patient's mouth to prevent future damage to the teeth and jaws. The documentation dilemma is that the desired occlusal guard has a hard occlusal surface as well as other component parts that would also be found on a soft appliance.

There are three available occlusal guard procedure codes to use for this scenario, differentiated by extent of protection and the appliance material. But, none of the three clearly describe an appliance with both hard and soft attributes.

D9944 occlusal guard – hard appliance, full arch

D9945 occlusal guard – soft appliance, full arch

D9946 occlusal guard – hard appliance, partial arch

How would you code this care?

D9944 occlusal guard – hard appliance, full arch

A full arch code is appropriate as the dentist stated that a full arch guard should be fabricated to provide the necessary protection. The differentiation between hard and soft appliance is based on the knowledge that the operative part of an occlusal guard is the occlusal surface, and the key determinant of reporting the type of occlusal guard is what the material is on the occlusal surface. In this scenario the occlusal surface is hard.

To clarify further, occlusal guards that have any hard occlusal component, regardless of the presence of a soft component, should be coded as a hard occlusal guard.

Clinical Coding Scenario #5:
Pain following Oral Surgery Procedure

A student came home from college to have his third molars removed. He returned to college one week later, with complaints of worsening pain in the mandibular extraction sites, both right and left sides. He did not expect this, as at the time of surgery he had a new material, called Exparel®, injected in the extraction sites and had been experiencing minimal if any pain until now (eight to ten days post-surgery). He sought the care of a local dentist in the college town.

The receptionist asked the patient questions about COVID-19 and exposure prior to scheduling the appointment, as well as a brief history of the surgical procedure. Upon arrival, the COVID-19 question responses were verified with the patient and the patient's temperature, pulse, and oxygen levels were recorded.

The dentist examined the patient and diagnosed condensing osteitis, or dry socket, in both of the mandibular extraction sites. The dentist irrigated the sockets and placed a dry socket paste packing in both.

How would you code this care?

Condensing osteitis, or a dry socket, is the localized inflammation of the tooth socket following extraction due to failure of the development of a blood clot or the loss of the blood clot with resultant osteitis. The condition is very painful and characterized by bad breath and an unpleasant smell and taste in the mouth, as well as worsening pain each day. The dry socket treatment procedure is coded as:

D9930 treatment of complications (post-surgical) – unusual circumstances, by report

In addition to the treatment procedure code, there are two additional procedures to report:

D9912 pre-visit patient screening

D9912 documents the fact that the screening procedure occurred.

D0140 limited oral evaluation – problem focused

D0140 is appropriate as the dentist did perform a limited oral evaluation in determining the source of the chief complaint, before providing treatment (reported with D9930).

Clinical Coding Scenario #6:
Gingival Irritation around a Partially Erupted Third Molar

A patient reported to the dentist with a complaint of inflammation and pain from the gums around an unerupted third molar. The patient complained that food was getting stuck in the flap of tissue. The office asked the patient to complete a pre-visit screening form, and this was evaluated by the staff, then the pulse, oxygen levels, and temperature were recorded.

Once the patient passed the screening, the dentist evaluated the area and diagnosed pericoronitis. The dentist irrigated the area to remove and flush out the trapped food and to gain relief for the patient.

How would you code this treatment encounter?

D9912   pre-visit patient screening

D0140   limited oral evaluation – problem focused
and
D9110   palliative treatment of dental pain – per visit
> Treatment that relieves pain but is not curative; services provided do not have distinct procedure codes.

Using D9110 is appropriate as the procedure was the irrigation of the food entrapment solely to relieve pain and there are no distinct procedure codes for this service. D9110 does not define what procedure needs to be performed to qualify nor that the procedure be completed.

Curative treatment of the patient's diagnosed pericoronitis involves different procedures that are reported with their own discrete codes.

Note: There are some who erroneously think that the irrigation could be coded using **D4921 gingival irrigation – per quadrant**. This view is not correct as D4921's descriptor notes that the procedure is for irrigation of gingival pockets, which is not the case in this scenario and the reason why D4921 is not applicable.

Clinical Coding Scenario #7:
Sleep Apnea Appliance

A patient reports difficulty sleeping and that his significant other complains of his extreme snoring, then silence, where he seemingly stops breathing. The dental hygienist is scheduled to perform preventive services on this patient, but before doing so decides to involve the dentist due to the patient's comments on sleeping difficulties.

The dentist tells the patient that they have been trained in fabricating custom sleep apnea appliances and that the appliance will help eliminate the need for the CPAP machine. But, before doing so, the dentist adds that a sleep study needs to be ordered, performed, and reviewed before any potential benefits can be extended. The dentist refers the patient to their physician for the sleep studies and evaluation.

The study reveals severe sleep apnea based on findings of sleep fragmentation and repeated arousal during sleep, as well as periods of hypoxemia, acidosis, and alveolar hypoventilation. The physician recommended a custom sleep apnea appliance to address these issues.

During the next visit, the dentist updates and records patient information that includes a clinical examination, a perio evaluation, a visual oral cancer examination, and the capture of high-quality intraoral diagnostic images (photographic and periapical radiographs). Images and impressions are gathered for the fabrication of the appliance. The appliance is fitted, and the patient is checked to assure of proper fit, form, and function.

What CDT codes would be used to document the services provided related to fabricating the custom sleep apnea appliance?

The following procedure codes would be reported:

First visit:

    D0191 **assessment of a patient**

Next visit:

    D0140 **limited oral evaluation – problem focused**

    D9311 **consultation with a medical health care professional**

    D9947 **custom sleep apnea appliance fabrication and placement**

Clinical Coding Scenario #8:

Custom Sleep Appliance Adjustment and Reline

A patient with obstructive sleep apnea was given an appliance to wear that fits to the teeth and alters the position of the mandible. After some time passes the patient presents to the office stating that they feel some looseness or "play" in the appliance's fit.

The dentist determines that that there are some interferences and the appliance no longer properly fits the mandibular teeth. The dentist adjusts the appliance to eliminate the interferences, then takes new scans to send to accompany the appliance when it is sent back to the lab for repair and reline.

Three days later, the appliance is received back from the laboratory and checked to assure proper fit, form, and function.

What CDT codes would be used to document the procedures performed in this scenario (e.g., adjust, repair, and reline the custom sleep apnea appliance)?

The following procedure codes are applicable:

D9912 pre-visit patient screening

D0140 limited oral evaluation – problem focused

D9948 adjustment of custom sleep apnea appliance

D9949 repair of custom sleep apnea appliance

D9953 reline custom sleep apnea appliance (indirect)

Note: Some dental benefit plans may consider the repair and the adjustment as incidental to the more comprehensive procedure (namely the reline) and not be considered for individual reimbursement. A claim that lists the individual codes for all services performed is appropriate, regardless of reimbursement expectations or anticipation of benefit processing rules, exclusions, or limitations.

Coding Q&A

1. *Who could document and report a D9995 or D9996 CDT code?*

   A dental professional who oversees or performs the teledentistry event, and who, via diagnosis and treatment planning, completes the oral evaluation, may report the appropriate teledentistry procedure code. Applicable state regulations may also determine the oral health or general health practitioner who is permitted to document and report these CDT codes.

2. *What documentation should I maintain in my patient records, and what will be needed on a claim submission when reporting teledentistry codes D9995 and D9996?*

   The patient record should include the CDT code (or documentation to support the encounter) that reflects the type of teledentistry encounter, and there may be additional state documentation requirements to satisfy reporting. Treatment records should be very specific and document the scenario in which the encounter occurred. A claim submission must include all required information as described in the completion instructions for the ADA paper claim form and the HIPAA standard electronic dental claim format. Some government programs (e.g., Medicaid) may have additional claim reporting, security, and coding requirements.

3. *Are there any special teledentistry reporting rules when I am delivering care during a virtual encounter that occurs during a national health emergency or at other times under various environmental (e.g., health and safety) circumstances?*

   Some commercial health plans have benefit plan provisions or have established claim adjudication rules that pertain to reporting a teledentistry code and CDT codes for other services delivered during a virtual encounter. Plans may consider D9995 or D9996 to be for reporting the modality of how services are delivered and not a separately reimbursable service. All applicable CDT codes should be reported for services delivered during a virtual encounter—the appropriate teledentistry code and those for services delivered to the patient (e.g., evaluation procedures such as D0140, D0170, or D0171).

   Note: Most encounters during the COVID-19 pandemic have been real-time and documented with CDT code D9995.

4. *How may I report local anesthesia as a separate procedure?*

   D9215 local anesthesia in conjunction with operative or surgical procedures and **D9210 local anesthesia not in conjunction with operative or surgical procedures** are available CDT codes to report these local anesthesia services. Benefit plan limitations may exclude separate reimbursement benefits for local anesthesia when performed in conjunction with other covered procedures.

5. *I have administered Pacira's Exparel®, a sustained release pharmacologic agent, for pain control after third molar extractions, as well as in some periodontal and implant surgical procedures. How do I code for delivery of this non-opioid medicament for pain control?*

   D9613   infiltration of sustained release therapeutic drug, per quadrant

   As indicated in the nomenclature, procedure delivery is documented and reported by quadrant. If, for example, there were four third molar extractions on the same date of service and the therapeutic agent was placed in each, this procedure is reported four times. The same type of reporting also applies to other "per quadrant" (e.g., periodontal) procedures delivered and then followed by placement of the therapeutic drug.

6. *Should a dentist who sees a patient referred by another dentist for an evaluation of a specific problem report the consultation code (D9310) or a problem focused evaluation code (D0140 or D0160)? Also, does it matter if the consulting dentist initiates treatment for the patient on the same visit?*

   Typically, a consultation (D9310) is reported when one dentist refers a patient to another dentist for an opinion or advice on a problem encountered by the patient. According to this CDT code's descriptor, the dentist who is consulted may initiate additional diagnostic or therapeutic services for the patient. These services are to be reported separately using their own unique CDT codes, in addition to reporting D9310.

   Both D0140 and D0160 are problem-focused evaluations and may be reported if the consulting specialist believes either of these codes better describe the services that were provided. Please note that neither of these evaluation procedures' nomenclatures or descriptors contains language that prohibits the consulting dentist from initiating and reporting additional services.

   Note: D9310 may be reported by any dentist who is providing the consulting service within the scope of her or his state licensure. From the procedural and coding perspective, the presence of a specialty license or training is irrelevant for both the referring dentist and the consulting dentist.

© 2023 American Dental Association

7. *If a practitioner treats more than one patient in one nursing home on one day, is* **D9410 house/extended care facility call** *reported per patient or per facility?*

The descriptor for code D9410 states that it may be reported in addition to separate reporting of services provided to a patient seen at the facility. D9410 may be reported for every patient receiving service at the facility on a given day. However, benefit plan limitations and exclusions may place restrictions on reimbursement, such as once per facility visit, not per patient. It is important to remember to report what you do, not for what you intend to be paid or understand your dental benefit provider contract to be.

8. *A patient who is a college student was complaining of grinding their teeth. The symptoms are worsening as final examination week approaches. The dentist makes an anterior deprogrammer to provide relief and get this patient through finals. What CDT code should be used to report this?*

D9946 is appropriate for reporting the services performed.

D9946   occlusal guard – hard appliance, partial arch

This code properly represents the service delivered as the code's descriptor states that the procedure is for placement of a "...Removable dental appliance designed to minimize the effects of bruxism or other occlusal factors. Provides only partial occlusal coverage as an anterior deprogrammer..." would fit on a partial arch.

9. *How do I report external bleaching?*

You may use one of the following codes as applicable based on the extent of the service provided to the patient:

D9972   external bleaching – per arch – performed in office
or
D9973   external bleaching – per tooth

10. *How do I report the fabrication of trays and the provision of bleaching agent to my patients for their use at home?*

When trays and material are provided to a patient for application of bleach at home the following code is applicable:

D9975   external bleaching for home application, per arch; includes materials and fabrication of custom trays

11. *A patient with a diagnosis of obstructive sleep apnea (OSA) from his physician visits a dentist who has been trained in the treatment of OSA. The dentist fabricates a custom sleep apnea appliance and files a claim with the patient's dental benefit plan reporting* **D9947 custom sleep apnea appliance fabrication and placement**. *The claim is denied by a dental benefit plan even though the dental office used the proper CDT code to report the appliance. What happened?*

CDT code **D9947 custom sleep apnea appliance fabrication and placement** is the appropriate CDT code to report, but the plan may require additional documentation before adjudicating the claim. The additional documentation is likely proof of and results of the sleep study performed and interpreted by a certified sleep specialist (physician). An appeal of the denial that includes necessary documentation (after confirming the payer's requirements) would be the appropriate next action.

It is also possible that there are no dental benefits for this procedure. If so, the dentist may submit to the patient's medical benefit carrier for consideration using the medical claim format (e.g., 1500 paper/837P electronic claim) and coding system (e.g., CPT; HCPCS).

12. *After placing a custom sleep apnea appliance, the dentist asks patients to return for approximately three to four office visits, as needed, to adjust the appliance. What procedure code would be used to report visits to adjust the appliance after delivery?*

D9948 adjustment of custom sleep apnea appliance

This procedure code can be reported for each adjustment visit.

After four adjustments the dentist determines that the appliance would function better if it were relined. What procedure code should be used to report the reline?

D9953 reline custom sleep apnea appliance (indirect)

This procedure is indirect as the appliance was sent to the laboratory for completion.

Upon the appliance's return it was disinfected and the fit and function were verified before dismissing the patient. What procedure code may be reported for this procedure?

There is no specific code as placement of the relined appliance and all associated services are considered facets of the reline procedure.

13. *Is there a CDT code for air abrasion?*

    There is no procedure code specifically for air abrasion.

    If the procedure delivered is consistent with the nomenclature and descriptor of D9970, that code may be reported:

    D9970 enamel microabrasion
    > The removal of discolored surface enamel defects resulting from altered mineralization or decalcification of the superficial enamel layer. Submit per treatment visit.

    Many experts in the dental field view air abrasion as a technique utilized to perform or enable a restorative procedure. If there is a restorative procedure delivered on the same tooth on the same date of service, it is possible that D9970 may not be reimbursed separately as the dental benefit plan could consider it inclusive in the restorative procedure reimbursement.

14. *During a single or multi-surface restoration procedure I may place a desensitizer medicament as the base or liner. What code should I use to report placing the desensitizer—D9910?*

    Reporting **D9910 application of desensitizing medicament** is not appropriate in any restorative procedure, as noted in the third sentence of this code's descriptor:

    D9910 application of desensitizing medicament
    > Includes in-office treatment for root sensitivity. Typically reported on a "per visit" basis for application of topical fluoride. This code is not to be used for bases, liners or adhesives used under restorations.

    There is no discrete CDT code for reporting placement of a base or liner under a restoration as that action considered an integral part of the restoration procedure. Also, many dental benefit plans will not permit charges for desensitizer when it is performed on the same tooth receiving a restoration.

15. *How should I document in-office delivery, using custom trays, of the desensitizer referred to as "MI Paste?"*

    Fabrication of the tray "carrier" for medicament could be reported with the following code:

    D5999 unspecified maxillofacial prosthesis, by report
    > Used for a procedure that is not adequately described by a code. Describe the procedure.

Note: There are several products generally referred to as "MI Paste" and some contain fluoride. If the medicament being applied does include fluoride, then the following code should be considered.

D5986   fluoride gel carrier

Synonymous terminology: fluoride applicator.

A prosthesis, which covers the teeth in either dental arch and is used to apply topical fluoride in close proximity to tooth enamel and dentin for several minutes daily.

The medicament application procedure is reported with the following code:

D9910   application of desensitizing medicament

Includes in-office treatment for root sensitivity. Typically reported on a "per visit" basis for application of topical fluoride. This code is not to be used for bases, liners or adhesives used under restorations.

16. *There are times when I provide a tube of "MI Paste" for their home use. What CDT codes are appropriate to document this in the patient's dental record?*

Providing a tube of "MI Paste" that would be applied topically by the patient at home (e.g., via tooth brush; cotton swab; gloved finger) could be reported with the following code as the procedure reported involves only dispensing:

D9630   drugs or medicaments dispensed in the office for home use

Includes, but is not limited to oral antibiotics, oral analgesics, and topical fluoride; does not include writing prescriptions.

If you determine that this code does not adequately described the service you provide, that coding alternative is:

D9999   unspecified adjunctive procedure, by report

Used for a procedure that is not adequately described by a code. Describe the procedure.

Summary

The CDT Code's Adjunctive General Services category has proven to be an important part of a dental care treatment planning as these procedures support and enhance, when indicated, delivery of services documented with codes in other categories of service. In addition, procedures listed in the adjunctive category of service enable enhanced and more granular reporting of our treatments and procedures performed.

The value of this category of CDT codes was demonstrated during the COVID-19 pandemic. The teledentistry CDT codes were widely used and, based on program design, unlocked additional benefits as they helped identify the encounter as a telehealth event. This documentation can provide a valuable defense for a dental provider, if they ever were accused of violating a stay-at-home or safer-at-home order by performing dental services remotely.

Teledentistry is possible in many areas of dentistry, including diagnostic, preventive, restorative, prosthetics, and orthodontics. During the COVID-19 pandemic, the majority of the teledentistry claims were diagnostic in nature, with palliative procedures being the next most frequently used codes filed in conjunction with either a D9995 or D9996.

Equally exciting to the high utilization of the teledentistry codes is the consistent utilization of code D9613 infiltration of sustained release therapeutic drug – per quadrant. Reporting this code represents the delivery of medication that can impact and potentially eliminate the need for an opioid prescription historically associated with oral surgery periodontal or pediatric procedures. With education of both patients and dental providers, the use of medication represented by this procedure code can influence or eliminate one of the first potential exposures to an opioid by an adolescent or child, eliminating that first opioid prescription. The trend shows we are starting to achieve the goal of helping to address the current opioid epidemic, ultimately leading to the prevention of future generations of abuse.

The Adjunctive codes continue to be referenced regularly when other CDT codes do not seem to fit the procedure being performed. Many times, the use of an Adjunctive code can provide the clarity and granularity that makes the difference between a claim being paid or rejected, and between being able to defend the circumstances of treatment or not. The beauty of the CDT is that this code set is a living document which reflects the current state of and situations that impact the practice of dentistry.

Contributor Biography

Charles D. Stewart, D.M.D., is currently President, CEO, and Chairman of the Board of Directors for Aetna Dental of California, Inc. a CVS Health Company. He is also Senior Dental Director, for Aetna Inc. a CVS Health Company. Dr. Stewart is Chairman of the National Association of Dental Plans (NADP) Codes Workgroup, a part of the NADP Standards and Transactions Initiative, a role he has held since 2013. In this role, he represents NADP on the American Dental Association's Code Maintenance Committee. Dr. Stewart was recognized by NADP with the 2018 Don Mayes Leadership award for excellence in leadership and in 2021 with the Gabryl Award for excellence in advancing the NADP mission through volunteer leadership ("lifetime achievement award"). He is currently Chairman of California Association of Dental Plans (CADP) Quality Management Committee, member of the CADP Board of Directors, and the lead instructor for CADP's quality assurance consultant certification courses. Dr. Stewart also maintains a private practice on evenings and weekends. Dr. Stewart is a graduate of Oral Roberts University School of Dentistry.

By ADA Staff
Center for Dental Benefits, Coding and Quality, Practice Institute

This chapter addresses facets of a dental practice's business side, things a dentist should be aware of that will help anticipate or resolve problems. Topics covered include ascertaining a patient's benefits, becoming a participating dentist, claim processing problems, and audits. The chapter concludes with links to additional related resources available from the American Dental Association.

Dental Benefit Coverage

The majority of patients with private dental benefits coverage have their plans provided by employers or unions. Employers offer dental plans to help attract and retain employees and to help employees maintain good oral health. However, most dental plans are not designed to cover all dental procedures, and many procedures require the patient to meet a deductible or incur a high co-insurance payment. It is very important for dental offices to explain to their patients that a dental benefit plan is actually not insurance but simply a benefit. Thus, it is essential to educate your patients about costs and recommend they take their dental benefit grievances to their employer's human resources department when necessary.

Making the Decision to Participate with a Managed Care Plan

Making the decision to sign a managed care contract is one of the most important business decisions a dentist may make. When you sign a contract, you make promises that will be legally binding on you. Thus, it is extremely important that you carefully review any contract before you sign it.

It is highly recommended you consult your personal attorney before signing any contract. The ADA also offers an important resource for ADA members – the ADA Contract Analysis Service. Prior to signing a proposed contract, member dentists may submit a dental provider contract with a third-party payer or a dental management service organization to their state or local dental society who will forward it to the Service for a free analysis. This service provides a plain language explanation of proposed contract terms for each agreement analyzed; however, the service does not provide legal advice or recommend whether a contract should or should not be signed.

You have the right to negotiate the terms of a participating dentist agreement; however, the plan also has contractual rights that may affect your rights. It certainly doesn't hurt to ask if you have concerns with specific clauses in the participating dentist agreement.

Many times, if a dentist has contracted with a third-party payer, he or she may have agreed to abide by the carrier's processing policies, which may or may not appear in the contract itself. The processing policies of many carriers are published on their websites. Dentists should make it a point to understand the policies typically applied by payers.

And don't forget to ask for the plan's current dentist billing manual and be sure you understand how the plan processes the procedures that you most frequently perform.

Remember not to focus only on the contract itself – after all, you are making a business decision and data is very important. Your practice management software typically has reporting tools that many dentists may not be aware of and do not utilize to their own advantage. You may benefit from calling your software vendor to learn how to generate reports that will help you better understand your own practice metrics.

It is also important for dental offices to understand payer processing policies before treatment is started so that these policies can be adequately explained to patients. Patients often rely on their dentists and office staff to decode their dental benefits for them and the dentist-patient relationship can be affected by payer policies.

Treatment plans should cater to the needs of the patient rather than what is covered by the benefit plan. Always remember to "code for what you do." Although the payer may bundle codes for the purpose of benefit determination, the patient record should always accurately describe the services that the patient received. You always have the right to appeal the claim decision, especially in instances where the payer has made a judgment regarding the medical necessity of a treatment you provided your patient.

Helping You after You Sign the Contract

Sometimes legislation may be the best approach to dealing with issues related to dental benefit plans. The ADA's Washington, DC office has many efforts underway to address dental benefit issues through legislative remedies.

Examples of current efforts include:

1. Non-Covered Services
2. Assignment of Benefits
3. Coordination of Benefits
4. Flexible Spending Accounts

Non-Covered Services

A key concern reported to ADA by dental offices has been carriers' use of requiring dentists to charge patients the plan's maximum allowable fee for services not covered by the dental plan. The ADA is working closely with its state partners and has helped implement legislation in 42 states that prohibits dental plans from requiring dentists to accept the plan's maximum allowable fee for a non-covered procedure.

Bundling and Downcoding

Examples of provisions in the signed contract that limit reimbursement include bundling and downcoding, which has resulted in many dental offices calling the ADA asking for guidance. If the payer has applied some of these limitations and they are in accordance with the contract with which the dentist agreed, the dentist may be bound to the policies set forth by the payer.

The ADA defines bundling of procedures as the systematic combining of distinct dental procedure codes by third-party payers that results in a reduced benefit for the patient/beneficiary.

Downcoding is a practice of third-party payers in which the benefit code has been changed to a less complex or lower cost procedure than was reported, except where delineated in contract agreements.

Let's look at an example of downcoding. A 13-year-old patient with adult dentition is treated and the dentist has rendered a **D0120 periodic oral evaluation – established patient** and **D1110 prophylaxis – adult**.

The payer rejected the claim for D1110 and returned an explanation of benefits (EOB) statement indicating the correct code is **D1120 prophylaxis – child**, as this is the correct code because the dental benefit plan defines a patient under age 15 as a child, no matter what dentition is present. This is worth an appeal because the message implies that that the dentist miscoded the claim, which is not true.

An appeal could be avoided if the EOB acknowledged that the reimbursement was based on benefit plan design. It is important to note that appealing a claim may not always result in greater reimbursement but could simply help prevent misperceptions by the patient.

In this scenario, the claim was not adjudicated correctly as the payer ignored the D1110 descriptor and asked the dentist to report the wrong procedure code. The only proper action for the dentist is to code for what you do.

Now let's look at an example of bundling by a payer during claim adjudication. The dentist provided a **D0120 periodic oral evaluation – established patient, D1120 prophylaxis – child**, and **D1208 topical application of fluoride – excluding varnish** to a 6-year-old patient. The payer rejected the claim and the EOB implied that all three procedures were part of the same CDT code. Once again, this is a situation that should be appealed to correct the language within the EOB statement.

In this case, the payer ignored the nomenclatures and descriptors of these discrete codes and redefined procedure code D0120. A third-party payer is supposed to use the code number, its nomenclature, and its descriptor as written.

It is not acceptable when a payer says the procedure reported with D0120 includes other procedures, in this instance – D1120 and D1208 – that are appropriately reported separately on the claim form. In this particular example, the payer may even be in violation of its CDT Code license.

It is okay when a payer benefits procedures in combination with others as part of its payment policies, but the payer cannot claim that discrete procedures are actually part of other procedures.

Refund Requests and Overpayments

Some contracts may have clauses that contractually bind you to refund any overpayments. Many times when a third-party payer mistakenly pays a dentist, the payer will request a refund of the overpaid amount. In some cases, refund requests have been sent to dentists more than two years after the payment was made and the patient may no longer be a patient of record. In most instances, the overpaid amount is deducted from future benefits paid to the dentist. In other cases, overpayments made to other dentists for the same patient may be deducted from future benefit payments to the current treating dentist. Many members and the ADA question the fairness of this practice.

Several states have enacted legislation that restricts how far back a carrier can ask for a refund and a period of one year seems to be the most common. Ensuring you understand these clauses is of the utmost importance before signing a participating dentist agreement with a third-party payer.

Removal from Network Lists

If a dentist wants to terminate an agreement, there is usually a range of 30 to 90 days before a termination will take effect. Dental offices have reported that although a contract with a third-party payer was terminated previously, the carrier did not update its website with correct information. Patients were under the false impression that the dentist was still contracted with the plan and were expecting the carrier's discounted fees, not the dentist's full fees.

This can cause major problems for the patient and the dental office and may even interfere with the dentist-patient relationship. As a best practice, at the time of termination, dentists should submit in writing, to the carrier (sent via certified mail) a request specifically to remove their names from any participating dentist list.

Dentists should follow up with carriers who fail to remove their name in a timely manner.

What Fee Should I Submit?

A question frequently asked by dental offices is what fee to report on the claim form: the discounted fee or the dentist's full fee? Irrespective of whether you are contracted or not contracted, the ADA recommends that dentists always submit their full fee to carriers. Even when full fees are reported, carriers will reimburse based upon their fee schedules.

Tips to Negotiate a Contract

If you are a participating provider with one or more dental benefit plans, you may need to negotiate your fee increases. This negotiation should be done individually, between only you and your plan, and not with or on behalf of other dentists. Before you enter negotiations with a payer, prepare your talking points and do your homework.

- Your strengths: Do you have advantages in terms of access?
  - Number of dentists in your locality
  - Wait times for available appointments, impacting the patients covered under the plan
  - Influx of new patients covered under the plan
- Your numbers: What data do you need to effectively negotiate?
  - Know which procedure codes generate the highest total revenue for your practice, including:
    - Frequency with which each procedure is reported
    - Current allowed amount (i.e., your current discounted fee)
    - Extent of these procedure codes' contribution to your overall practice revenue
    - Your desired fee for each procedure code

- - Extent of preventive services that your office provides
  - Costs associated with operating your business
  - Patient satisfaction rates (most recent available)
  - Date when your fees were last revised
- Efficiencies you offer: Which of your business practices are favorable to the payer?
  - Electronic claims submission
  - Use of online portals to verify eligibility and benefits
  - EFT enabled for receipt of claim payments
- Review the *ADA Survey on Dental Fees*
- Use all of the above information you have gathered to "tell your story."
- Identify the payer's provider representative assigned to your region who you can contact to begin to make your case. This may be someone known to your business staff, typically with the title of "provider relations manager."
- Begin with email introductions. If comfortable, request a phone call or continue making your case in writing.
- Always be respectful. Let the provider relations representative know that you value the patients garnered from being a network dentist.
- Be patient and don't give up! The first offer you receive may not be the best offer.
- Request information on whether the carrier leases their network and whether the revised fees will apply to any networks you have been leased into.
- After you succeed, make sure you have copies of all signed documents.
- Check the next Explanation of Benefits (EOB) documents to ensure the fee changes are appropriately reflected.
- Remember to renegotiate periodically.

It is good practice to always review your contracted fee schedules annually. Additionally, don't forget that it is very important to always report your full fee on the claim form. Several payers set fees based on market rates and the charges you submit may be used by payers to determine maximum allowable fees.

The fee schedules are typically part of the participating provider agreement – a legal contract between the dentist and the third-party payer. There are other clauses in the contract (along with documents referenced in the contract, i.e., the provider's office reference manual) that impact the final payment from the third-party payer. For example, a policy that bundles the fee for a core buildup with the fee for the crown is typically detailed in the provider's office reference manual, along with other processing policies. It is important to review these documents carefully before trying to project revenues and negotiating fees with the payer.

Helping the Non-Contracted Dentist

Many dental carriers will not honor assignment of benefits to non-contracted dentists. These plans claim that assignment of benefits is a contracted dentist benefit. The good news is that 23 states have passed legislation requiring that assignment of benefits be honored. These laws generally apply only to fully insured plans which are governed by state insurance statutes, and approximately 52% of patients with a dental benefit have a plan that is insured and subject to state laws. If your state has not passed assignment of benefits legislation, it is recommended you talk to your state dental society about doing so.

Helping All Dentists

Payment Delay and Lost Submissions

One of the biggest complaints concerning third-party claim payment is lost claim forms and radiographs. Many dentists report sending in claim forms or radiographs several times before the dental plan will acknowledge receipt. Often radiographs are submitted with the claim, but the dentist will receive an EOB requesting the radiographs.

In some instances, the method by which claims are submitted increases the possibility of loss. Attachments that are not firmly affixed to a claim form can get separated when the mail is opened; this is especially true when multiple claims are submitted in one envelope. If radiographs are not labeled and get detached from claim forms, they may not be able to be matched back to the appropriate claim form. Privacy and security standards require that personal medical information be protected so unmatched attachments would most likely be destroyed.

When a payer does not require a radiograph for a claim, the process established by that payer may require that the radiograph be removed and returned or destroyed. If a subsequent issue moves the claim from auto-adjudication to a manual review, a radiograph may be requested at that time.

Submitting electronic claims and the appropriate attachments is the best way to avoid the loss of claims, radiographs and other attachments.

There is no uniformity within the payer community regarding submission of radiographs, partly due to different business structures within the industry. Some companies would prefer that no radiographs be sent unless requested. Others want to see images at the time specific procedure codes are reported.

Top Procedure Denials

Periodontal scaling and root planing (D4341, D4342) and periodontal maintenance (D4910)

Scaling and root planing (SRP) denials are one of the most reported concerns to the ADA. Dentists believe that submitted radiographs show bone loss substantial enough to warrant coverage for SRP and have reported that dentist consultants working for payers deny these claims indicating there is no radiographic evidence of bone loss. Upon appeal some of these claims have been paid.

Dentists and their staff may not always understand what appears to be inconsistent SRP claim adjudication as payer adjudication policies vary substantially. One plan may require at least 4 mm pocket depth while another may have different depth criteria. Many plans will require radiographic evidence of bone loss before paying an SRP claim. Some payers may not benefit more than two quadrants of scaling and root planing performed on the same date of service.

It is very difficult for a small dental office to be familiar with the various payer requirements for payment of SRP claims as it is typical for a dental office to have patients present with well over 100 different dental plans.

A major concern of dental offices is that the denial language used on the EOB statement may lead the patient to think that the procedure was not necessary. Denial of benefits may not mean the SRP was unnecessary – it simply means the patient's clinical condition did not satisfy the benefit plan's threshold for reimbursement.

In addition to radiographic evidence of bone loss, it is not uncommon for payers to request periodontal charting and a narrative description for SRP coverage consideration.

Claim denials for **D4910 periodontal maintenance** occur because some carriers have limited benefits for D4910. Some plans reimburse only if periodontal maintenance was delivered within 2 to 12 months of scaling and root planing while others may require a 3-month wait after therapy. Some plans deny benefits unless two or more quadrants have received prior therapy; however, there are no such limitations in the CDT Code.

It is recommended that dental office staff determine how a patient's plan covers this procedure before delivery in order to better inform the patient of the coverage parameters so as to avoid any claim surprises. If known, tell patients in advance that plan provisions may not provide for reimbursement of D4910 for extended periods of time and that the patient may be responsible for the costs.

Crowns (D2710–D2799) and core buildups (D2950)

The ADA receives many calls on crown and core buildup denials and there are myriad reasons for these denials. Some carriers use a policy for crowns that is along the lines of requiring that at least 50% of the incisal angle must need replacement due to decay or fracture. In addition, many carriers will deny crowns for a tooth with a poor prognosis and due to abrasion and attrition. Core buildups are typically covered once every 5 years if there is less than 50% tooth structure due to disease or fracture. Many payers will require documentation, including radiographs and a narrative description, for coverage consideration. In addition, many dentists have found that submitting photographs can also help in getting the claim properly adjudicated.

The ADA has received calls from dental offices where carriers' EOBs have stated that only the crown should be reported as it includes the core buildup. In this example, the payer is incorrect, per the CDT Code's perspective, as the buildup procedure and crown procedure are separate and distinct from each other as not all crowns require a buildup.

It is understood that the payer can make single reimbursement based on benefit plan design, and this should be made clear on the EOB statement sent to the patient. The dentist should be able to balance bill the patient; however, the ability to balance bill is subject to the participating dentist agreement, if any.

To avoid post-treatment complaints, dental offices should help patients understand the clinical basis for treatment and should appeal the benefit decision if it is thought the claim has not been properly adjudicated.

Compliance Audits and Utilization Review

Many dental offices call the ADA when confronted with a compliance audit or with questions on utilization review. When a dentist is placed under utilization review, the office is often required to submit additional documentation for the procedures being questioned. These claims are then manually reviewed to determine the benefit.

Some carriers require that claims being reviewed be sent to a different address than where you would normally send claims. If you are being audited, please be sure to send audit documentation to the correct address provided by the dental plan. Otherwise it will slow down the processing of your claim submission.

When you are notified of being placed under review or are suddenly receiving requests for additional documentation, it is recommended you contact the dental plan's consultant or your provider relations manager to determine if a review is being undertaken and, if it is, why you were placed on utilization review and what it will take to get you off of the plan's utilization review.

The plan is obligated to disclose the results of your review. Please do not forget your right to appeal. You have the right to appeal the reasons why you have been placed on utilization review.

It is recommended you work with the plan to explain and justify potential differences in practice patterns, e.g., a dental office that caters to elderly patients may indeed have higher utilization patterns for bridges. This is something that could be explained and taken into consideration by the dental plan. Helping the dental plan understand the rationale for your recommended treatment plans can help significantly.

Remember to properly and accurately document your patient records to the very last detail, even if something appears obvious to you. It may be a good idea to submit pre-treatment estimates when you are under review, so as to minimize any surprises.

Over time, if the payer is assured that treatment patterns are justified, then the payer will remove the dentist from further review. However, in some instances, the payer may choose to follow up with an in-office audit.

In the event of an in-office audit, plan representatives will personally visit your office to review patient files and records. The plan will request that a separate work area be set up for them to conduct the review and you will be asked in advance to have specific patient records available for review by plan representatives.

Auditors and plan representatives may look at claims as far back as state laws allow. Please note that in-office reviews can last one or more days depending on the number of records to be reviewed.

If you are contracted with the plan and have agreed to such audits, it is recommended that you read and familiarize yourself with your contract and the plan's policies before the audit begins.

The ADA also encourages dentists to obtain a written description of the scope of the audit procedures. Consulting with your personal attorney so that you understand your rights and obligations in such a situation is also recommended.

It may be a good idea to talk with your plan representative about the following before the audit begins:

- Clinical review criteria
- Analytical methods
- Time periods for conducting reviews
- Qualifications of individuals conducting the review
- Confidentiality
- Disclosure of the process to insureds
- Access to review staff
- Appeals process for adverse determinations

A question we often receive is whether the dentist is allowed to disclose a patient's record to the plan in cases of an audit. The HIPAA Privacy Rule permits a dental practice to disclose such information in response to such a request if the dental plan has or had relationships with the individuals who are the subjects of the requested information. An important point to note is that for patients who have been beneficiaries of the plan in the past and are no longer deriving benefits from that plan, the payer's auditor can only look at the patient's records for the time the patient was part of the plan.

Individual patients have a right to request that disclosures not be made to a health or dental plan for services that the patient has paid for out of pocket and in full. A covered dental practice may not disclose information regarding patients who are not, and have never been, beneficiaries of that plan, even if a participating dentist agreement requires it. Disclosing the information may be in violation of HIPAA.

When a patient has paid for a service in full and asks the practice not to disclose the service to the plan, the dental practice must comply with that request. As a best practice, a notice of privacy practices (NPP) should be given to individuals at their first visit. The NPP should contain information about the patient's rights with regards to HIPAA and how the patient may request restrictions on disclosures of information. Your practice must also have procedures for your staff to flag such requests in the event of such a request coming from a patient, written or otherwise.

Resources

- The ADA offers valuable, educational ready-to-use resources on innovative dental insurance solutions for dentists at *www.ADA.org/dentalinsurance*.

- Information on the Code on Dental Procedures and Nomenclature (CDT Code), as well as the review and revision process, is available at *ADA.org/cdt*.

- *CDT 2023: Current Dental Terminology* (J023) is the most up-to-date coding resource on the market and will help you document codes for dental procedures quickly and accurately. This book not only helps fill documentation gaps but can help reduce rejected dental claims. Available at *ADAstore.org*.

- *Why Doesn't My Insurance Pay for This?* (W265) is a brochure designed to help patients understand dental insurance plans by explaining why some procedures are not covered. It describes annual maximums, least expensive alternative treatment clauses, pre-existing conditions, exclusions, and more. Available at *ADAstore.org*.

- *What Every Dentist Should Know Before Signing a Dental Provider Contract* is a publication that answers common questions dentists may wish to consider before signing a dental contract with third-party payers. Available at *ADA.org/dentalinsurance*.

- *Third-Party Concerns* is a series of articles published in *ADA News* on third-party problems reported by dental offices. Available at *ADA.org/DentalInsuranceResources*.

- *Responding to Claim Rejection* is a publication that educates dentists and dental offices on the proper way to handle and respond to claim rejections from third-party payers. Available at *https://catalog.ada.org/catalog/responding-to-claim-rejection-2187*.

- *Dental Benefit Video Series* are short video tutorials, created by the ADA Center for Dental Benefits, Coding and Quality, are designed to help dental professionals understand a key issue in dentistry: how third-party programs interface with dental offices. Available at *ADA.org/dentalbenefitvideos*.

- Dental Insurance Webinars are a series of recorded webinars on various dental benefit topics. Available at *ADA.org/dentalbenefitwebinars*.

- ADA Contract Analysis Service (ADA members only) is available at *https://www.ada.org/resources/practice/dental-insurance/dental-insurance-resources/dental-insurance-contract-issues*.

Section 3
Appendices

Appendix 1: CDT Code to ICD (Diagnosis) Code Crosswalk

CDT Code(s)	
D0120	periodic oral evaluation – established patient
D0140	limited oral evaluation – problem focused
D0150	comprehensive oral evaluation – new or established patient
D0210	intraoral – comprehensive series of radiographic images
D0220	intraoral – periapical first radiographic image
D0230	intraoral – periapical each additional radiographic image
D0251	extra-oral posterior dental radiographic image
D0270	bitewing – single radiographic image
D0272	bitewings – two radiographic images
D0274	bitewings – four radiographic images
D0330	panoramic radiographic image
D0372	intraoral tomosynthesis – comprehensive series of radiographic images
D0373	intraoral tomosynthesis – bitewing radiographic image
D0374	intraoral tomosynthesis – periapical radiographic image
D0387	intraoral tomosynthesis – comprehensive series of radiographic images – image capture only
D0388	intraoral tomosynthesis – bitewing radiographic image – image capture only
D0389	intraoral tomosynthesis – periapical radiographic image – image capture only
D0701	panoramic radiographic image – image capture only
D0707	intraoral – periapical radiographic image – image capture only
D0708	intraoral – bitewing radiographic image – image capture only
D0709	intraoral – comprehensive series of radiographic images – image capture only
D0999	unspecified diagnostic procedure, by report
Suggested ICD-10-CM Diagnosis Code(s)	
Z01.20	Encounter for dental examination and cleaning without abnormal findings
Z01.21	Encounter for dental examination and cleaning with abnormal findings
Z13.84	Encounter screening for dental disorders
Z86.16	Personal History of CoVid-19
U07.1	COVID-19

CDT Code(s)	
D1110	prophylaxis – adult
D1120	prophylaxis – child
Suggested ICD-10-CM Diagnosis Code(s)	
E11.9	Type 2 diabetes mellitus without complications
K03.6	Deposits [accretions] on teeth
K05.1	Chronic gingivitis
K05.10	Chronic gingivitis, plaque induced
K05.11	Chronic gingivitis, non-plaque induced
K05.30	Chronic periodontitis
K05.311	Chronic periodontitis, localized, slight
K05.312	Chronic periodontitis, localized, moderate
K05.313	Chronic periodontitis, localized, severe
K05.319	Chronic periodontitis, localized, unspecified severity
Z33.1	Pregnant state, incidental
Z72.0	Tobacco Use

CDT Code(s)	
D1206	topical application of fluoride varnish
D1208	topical application of fluoride, excluding varnish
Suggested ICD-10-CM Diagnosis Code(s)	
K02.3	Arrested dental caries
K02.61	Dental caries on smooth surface limited to enamel
K02.62	Dental caries on smooth surface penetrating into dentin
K02.63	Dental caries on smooth surface penetrating into pulp
K02.7	Dental root caries
K03.1	Abrasion of teeth
K03.2	Erosion of teeth
M35.00	Sjögren* syndrome, unspecified
M35.0C	Sjögren* syndrome with dental involvement

* also known as Sicca Syndrome

CDT Code(s)	
D1330	oral hygiene instructions
Suggested ICD-10-CM Diagnosis Code(s)	
E11.9	Type 2 diabetes mellitus without complications
K02.3	Arrested dental caries
K02.52	Dental caries on pit and fissure surface penetrating into dentin
K02.61	Dental caries limited to enamel
K02.62	Dental caries on smooth surface penetrating into dentin
K02.63	Dental caries on smooth surface penetrating into pulp
K02.7	Dental root caries
K02.9	Dental caries, unspecified
K03.2	Erosion of teeth
K03.6	Deposits [accretions] on teeth
K05.00	Acute gingivitis, plaque induced
K05.01	Acute gingivitis, non-plaque induced
K05.10	Chronic gingivitis, plaque induced
K05.30	Chronic periodontitis, unspecified
K05.311	Chronic periodontitis, localized, slight
K05.312	Chronic periodontitis, localized, moderate
K05.313	Chronic periodontitis, localized, severe
K05.319	Chronic periodontitis, localized, unspecified severity
K05.5	Other periodontal diseases
M35.00	Sjögren* syndrome, unspecified
M35.0C	Sjögren* syndrome with dental involvement
Z33.1	Pregnant state, incidental
Z72.0	Tobacco use

* also known as Sicca Syndrome

CDT Code(s)	
D1351	sealant – per tooth
D1354	interim caries arresting medicament application – per tooth
D2990	resin infiltration of incipient smooth surface lesions
Suggested ICD-10-CM Diagnosis Code(s)	
K02.51	Dental caries on pit and fissure surface limited to enamel
K02.53	Dental caries on pit and fissure surface penetrating into pulp
K02.61	Dental caries on smooth surface limited to enamel
K02.62	Dental caries on smooth surface penetrating into dentin
K02.63	Dental caries on smooth surface penetrating into pulp
M35.00	Sjögren* syndrome, unspecified

* also known as Sicca Syndrome

CDT Code(s)	
D1352	preventive resin restoration in a moderate to high caries risk patient – permanent tooth
Suggested ICD-10-CM Diagnosis Code(s)	
K02.51	Dental caries on pit and fissure surface limited to enamel
K02.53	Dental caries on pit and fissure surface penetrating into pulp
K02.62	Dental caries on smooth surface penetrating into dentin
K02.63	Dental caries on smooth surface penetrating into pulp

CDT Code(s)	
D1701	Pfizer-BioNTech Covid-19 vaccine administration – first dose
D1702	Pfizer-BioNTech Covid-19 vaccine administration – second dose
D1703	Moderna Covid-19 vaccine administration – first dose
D1704	Moderna Covid-19 vaccine administration – second dose
D1705	AstraZeneca Covid-19 vaccine administration – first dose
D1706	AstraZeneca Covid-19 vaccine administration – second dose
D1707	Janssen Covid-19 vaccine administration
D1708	Pfizer-BioNTech Covid-19 vaccine administration – third dose
D1709	Pfizer-BioNTech Covid-19 vaccine administration – booster dose
D1710	Moderna Covid-19 vaccine administration – third dose
D1711	Moderna Covid-19 vaccine administration – booster dose
D1712	Janssen Covid-19 vaccine administration - booster dose
D1713	Pfizer-BioNTech Covid-19 vaccine administration tris-sucrose pediatric – first dose
D1714	Pfizer-BioNTech Covid-19 vaccine administration tris-sucrose pediatric – second dose
D1781	vaccine administration – human papillomavirus – Dose 1
D1782	vaccine administration – human papillomavirus – Dose 2
D1783	vaccine administration – human papillomavirus – Dose 3
Suggested ICD-10-CM Diagnosis Code(s)	
Z23	Immunization

CDT Code(s)	
D2140	amalgam – one surface, primary or permanent
D2150	amalgam – two surfaces, primary or permanent
D2160	amalgam – three surfaces, primary or permanent
D2161	amalgam – four or more surfaces, primary or permanent
Suggested ICD-10-CM Diagnosis Code(s)	
K02.51	Dental caries on pit and fissure surface limited to enamel
K02.52	Dental caries on pit and fissure surface penetrating into dentin
K02.53	Dental caries on pit and fissure surface penetrating into pulp
K02.61	Dental caries on smooth surface limited to enamel
K02.62	Dental caries on smooth surface penetrating into dentin
K02.63	Dental caries on smooth surface penetrating into pulp
K03.81	Cracked tooth
S02.5XXA	Fracture of tooth (traumatic), initial encounter for closed fracture

CDT Code(s)	
D2330	resin-based composite – one surface, anterior
D2331	resin-based composite – two surfaces, anterior
D2332	resin-based composite – three surfaces, anterior
D2335	resin-based composite – four or more surfaces or involving incisal angle (anterior)
Suggested ICD-10-CM Diagnosis Code(s)	
K00.2	Abnormalities of size and form of teeth
K02.51	Dental caries on pit and fissure surface limited to enamel
K02.52	Dental caries on pit and fissure surface penetrating into dentin
K02.53	Dental caries on pit and fissure surface penetrating into pulp
K02.61	Dental caries on smooth surface limited to enamel
K02.62	Dental caries on smooth surface penetrating into dentin
K02.63	Dental caries on smooth surface penetrating into pulp
K03.1	Abrasion of teeth
K03.2	Erosion of teeth
K03.81	Cracked tooth
S02.5XXA	Fracture of tooth (traumatic), initial encounter for closed fracture

CDT Code(s)	
D2391	resin-based composite – one surface, posterior
D2392	resin-based composite – two surfaces, posterior
D2393	resin-based composite – three surfaces, posterior
D2394	resin-based composite – four or more surfaces, posterior

Suggested ICD-10-CM Diagnosis Code(s)	
K02.51	Dental caries on pit and fissure surface limited to enamel
K02.52	Dental caries on pit and fissure surface penetrating into dentin
K02.53	Dental caries on pit and fissure surface penetrating into pulp
K02.61	Dental caries on smooth surface limited to enamel
K02.62	Dental caries on smooth surface penetrating into dentin
K02.63	Dental caries on smooth surface penetrating into pulp
K02.7	Dental root caries
K03.1	Abrasion of teeth
K03.2	Erosion of teeth
K03.81	Cracked tooth
S02.5XXA	Fracture of tooth (traumatic), initial encounter for closed fracture

CDT Code(s)	
D2740	crown – porcelain/ceramic
D2750	crown – porcelain fused to high noble metal
D2751	crown – porcelain fused to predominantly base metal
D2752	crown – porcelain fused to noble metal
D2753	crown – porcelain fused to titanium and titanium alloys
D2790	crown – full cast high noble metal
D2792	crown – full cast noble metal
D2794	crown – titanium and titanium alloys
D2950	core buildup, including any pins when required
D2951	pin retention – per tooth; in addition to restoration
D2952	post and core in addition to crown; indirectly fabricated
D2954	prefabricated post and core in addition to crown

Suggested ICD-10-CM Diagnosis Code(s)	
K00.2	Abnormalities of size and form of teeth
K02.52	Dental caries on pit and fissure surface penetrating into dentin
K02.53	Dental caries on pit and fissure surface penetrating into pulp
K02.62	Dental caries on smooth surface penetrating into dentin
K02.63	Dental caries on smooth surface penetrating into pulp
S02.5XXA	Fracture of tooth (traumatic), initial encounter for closed fracture

CDT Code(s)	
D2928	prefabricated porcelain/ceramic crown – permanent tooth
D2930	prefabricated stainless steel crown – primary tooth
Suggested ICD-10-CM Diagnosis Code(s)	
K00.2	Abnormalities of size and form of teeth
K02.52	Dental caries on pit and fissure surface penetrating into dentine
K02.53	Dental caries on pit and fissure surface penetrating into pulp
K02.62	Dental caries on smooth surface penetrating into dentine
K02.63	Dental caries on smooth surface penetrating into pulp
S02.5XXA	Fracture of tooth (traumatic), initial encounter for closed fracture

CDT Code(s)	
D2940	protective restoration
Suggested ICD-10-CM Diagnosis Code(s)	
K02.9	Dental caries, unspecified
S02.5XXA	Fracture of tooth (traumatic), initial encounter for closed fracture

CDT Code(s)	
D3110	pulp cap – direct (excluding final restoration)
D3120	pulp cap – indirect (excluding final restoration)
Suggested ICD-10-CM Diagnosis Code(s)	
K02.52	Dental caries on pit and fissure surface penetrating into dentin
K02.53	Dental caries on pit and fissure surface penetrating into pulp
K02.62	Dental caries on smooth surface penetrating into dentin
K02.63	Dental caries on smooth surface penetrating into pulp
K04.0	Pulpitis
S02.5XXA	Fracture of tooth (traumatic), initial encounter for closed fracture

CDT Code(s)	
D3220	therapeutic pulpotomy (excluding final restoration) – removal of pulp coronal to the dentinocemental junction and application of medicament
D3310	endodontic therapy, anterior tooth (excluding final restoration)
D3320	endodontic therapy, premolar tooth (excluding final restoration)
D3330	endodontic therapy, molar tooth (excluding final restoration)
Suggested ICD-10-CM Diagnosis Code(s)	
K02.53	Dental caries on pit and fissure surface penetrating into pulp
K02.63	Dental caries on smooth surface penetrating into pulp
K03.81	Cracked tooth
K03.89	Other specified diseases of hard tissues of teeth
K04.0	Pulpitis
K04.1	Necrosis of pulp
K04.5	Chronic apical periodontitis
K04.6	Periapical abscess with sinus
K04.7	Periapical abscess without sinus
K04.8	Radicular cyst
K04.90	Unspecified diseases of pulp and periapical tissues
K04.99	Other diseases of pulp and periapical tissues
K05.5	Other periodontal diseases
K08.8	Other specified disorders of teeth and supporting structures
K08.81	Primary occlusal trauma
K08.82	Secondary occlusal trauma
K08.89	Other specified disorders of teeth and supporting structures
S02.5XXA	Fracture of tooth (traumatic), initial encounter for closed fracture

CDT Code(s)	
D3346	retreatment of previous root canal therapy – anterior
D3347	retreatment of previous root canal therapy – premolar
D3348	retreatment of previous root canal therapy – molar
Suggested ICD-10-CM Diagnosis Code(s)	
K08.59	Other unsatisfactory restoration of tooth
M27.5	Periradicular pathology associated with previous endodontic treatment
M27.51	Perforation of root canal space due to endodontic treatment
M27.52	Endodontic overfill
M27.53	Endodontic undersell
M27.59	Other periradicular pathology associated with previous endodontic treatment

CDT Code(s)	
D4210	gingivectomy or gingivoplasty – four or more contiguous teeth or tooth bounded spaces per quadrant
D4211	gingivectomy or gingivoplasty – one to three contiguous teeth or tooth bounded spaces per quadrant
Suggested ICD-10-CM Diagnosis Code(s)	
K05.30	Chronic periodontitis, unspecified
K05.31	Chronic periodontitis, localized
K05.311	Chronic periodontitis, localized, slight
K05.312	Chronic periodontitis, localized, moderate
K05.313	Chronic periodontitis, localized, severe
K05.319	Chronic periodontitis, localized, unspecified severity
K05.32	Chronic periodontitis, generalized
K05.321	Chronic periodontitis, generalized, slight
K05.322	Chronic periodontitis, generalized, moderate
K05.323	Chronic periodontitis, generalized, severe
K05.329	Chronic periodontitis, generalized, unspecified severity
K06.1	Gingival enlargement

CDT Code(s)	
D4249	clinical crown lengthening – hard tissue
Suggested ICD-10-CM Diagnosis Code(s)	
K02.9	Dental caries, unspecified
K03.81	Cracked tooth
K05.5	Other periodontal diseases
S02.5XXA	Fracture of tooth (traumatic), initial encounter for closed fracture

CDT Code(s)	
D4260	osseous surgery (including elevation of a full thickness flap and closure) – four or more contiguous teeth or tooth bounded spaces per quadrant
D4261	osseous surgery (including elevation of a full thickness flap and closure) – one to three contiguous teeth or tooth bounded spaces per quadrant
D4263	bone replacement graft – retained natural tooth – first site in quadrant
D4264	bone replacement graft – retained natural tooth – each additional site in quadrant
Suggested ICD-10-CM Diagnosis Code(s)	
K05.211	Aggressive periodontitis, localized, slight
K05.212	Aggressive periodontitis, localized, moderate
K05.213	Aggressive periodontitis, localized, severe
K05.219	Aggressive periodontitis, localized, unspecified severity
K05.221	Aggressive periodontitis, generalized, slight
K05.222	Aggressive periodontitis, generalized, moderate
K05.223	Aggressive periodontitis, generalized, severe
K05.229	Aggressive periodontitis, generalized, unspecified severity
K05.30	Chronic periodontitis
K05.311	Chronic periodontitis, localized, slight
K05.312	Chronic periodontitis, localized, moderate
K05.313	Chronic periodontitis, localized, severe
K05.319	Chronic periodontitis, localized, unspecified severity
K05.321	Chronic periodontitis, generalized, slight
K05.322	Chronic periodontitis, generalized, moderate
K05.323	Chronic periodontitis, generalized, severe
K05.329	Chronic periodontitis, generalized, unspecified severity
K05.6	Periodontal disease, unspecified
K08.20	Unspecified atrophy of edentulous alveolar ridge
K08.21	Minimal atrophy of the mandible
K08.22	Moderate atrophy of the mandible
K08.23	Severe atrophy of the mandible
K08.24	Minimal atrophy of the maxilla
K08.25	Moderate atrophy of the maxilla
K08.26	Severe atrophy of the maxilla

CDT Code(s)	
D4270	pedicle soft tissue graft procedure
D4273	autogenous connective tissue graft procedure (including donor and recipient surgical sites) first tooth, implant or edentulous tooth position in graft
D4275	non-autogenous connective tissue graft (including recipient site and donor material) first tooth, implant, or edentulous tooth position in graft
D4276	combined connective tissue and pedicle graft, per tooth
D4277	free soft tissue graft procedure (including recipient and donor surgical sites) first tooth, implant or edentulous tooth position in graft
D4278	free soft tissue graft procedure (including recipient and donor surgical sites) each additional contiguous tooth, implant or edentulous tooth position in same graft site
D4283	autogenous connective tissue graft procedure (including donor and recipient surgical sites) – each additional contiguous tooth, implant or edentulous tooth position in same graft site
D4285	non- autogenous connective tissue graft procedure (including recipient surgical site and donor material) – each additional contiguous tooth, implant or edentulous tooth position in same graft site
Suggested ICD-10-CM Diagnosis Code(s)	
K06.010	Localized gingival recession, unspecified
K06.011	Localized gingival recession, minimal
K06.012	Localized gingival recession, moderate
K06.013	Localized gingival recession, severe
K06.020	Generalized gingival recession, unspecified
K06.021	Generalized gingival recession, minimal
K06.022	Generalized gingival recession, moderate
K06.023	Generalized gingival recession, severe

CDT Code(s)	
D4341	periodontal scaling and root planing – four or more teeth per quadrant
D4342	periodontal scaling and root planing – one to three teeth per quadrant
D4346	scaling in the presence of generalized moderate or severe gingival inflammation – full mouth, after oral evaluation
D4910	periodontal maintenance
D6081	scaling and debridement in the presence of inflammation or mucositis of a single implant, including cleaning of the implant surfaces, without flap entry and closure
Suggested ICD-10-CM Diagnosis Code(s)	
A69.1	Other Vincent's infections
E11.9	Type 2 diabetes mellitus without complications
K03.6	Deposits [accretions] on teeth
K05.20	Aggressive periodontitis, unspecified
K05.211	Aggressive periodontitis, localized, slight
K05.212	Aggressive periodontitis, localized, moderate
K05.213	Aggressive Periodontitis, localized, severe
K05.219	Aggressive periodontitis, localized, unspecified severity
K05.221	Aggressive periodontitis, generalized, slight
K05.222	Aggressive periodontitis, generalized, moderate
K05.223	Aggressive periodontitis, generalized, severe
K05.229	Aggressive periodontitis, generalized, unspecified severity
K05.30	Chronic periodontitis
K05.311	Chronic periodontitis, localized, slight
K05.312	Chronic periodontitis, localized, moderate
K05.313	Chronic periodontitis, localized, severe
K05.319	Chronic periodontitis, localized, unspecified severity
K05.321	Chronic periodontitis, generalized, slight
K05.322	Chronic periodontitis, generalized, moderate
K05.323	Chronic periodontitis, generalized, severe
K05.329	Chronic periodontitis, generalized, unspecified severity
K05.5	Other periodontal diseases
K05.6	Periodontal disease, unspecified
K06.1	Gingival enlargement
Z33.1	Pregnant state, incidental
Z72.0	Tobacco Use
Z87.891	Personal history of nicotine dependence

CDT Code(s)	
D4355	full mouth debridement to enable a comprehensive periodontal evaluation and diagnosis on a subsequent visit

Suggested ICD-10-CM Diagnosis Code(s)	
K03.6	Deposits [accretions] on teeth
Z72.0	Tobacco Use
Z87.891	Personal history of nicotine dependence

CDT Code(s)	
D5110	complete denture – maxillary
D5120	complete denture – mandibular

Suggested ICD-10-CM Diagnosis Code(s)	
K08.1	Complete loss of teeth
K08.10	Complete loss of teeth, unspecified cause
K08.11	Complete loss of teeth due to trauma
K08.12	Complete loss of teeth due to periodontal diseases
K08.13	Complete loss of teeth due to caries
K08.19	Complete loss of teeth due to other specified cause

CDT Code(s)	
D5211	maxillary partial denture – resin base (including any retentive/clasping materials, rests, and teeth)
D5212	mandibular partial denture – resin base (including retentive/clasping materials, rests, and teeth)
D5213	maxillary partial denture – cast metal framework with resin denture bases (including any retentive/clasping materials, rests and teeth)
D5214	mandibular partial denture – cast metal framework with resin denture bases (including any retentive/clasping materials, rests and teeth)
D6010	surgical placement of implant body: endosteal implant
D6056	prefabricated abutment – includes modification and placement
D6057	custom fabricated abutment – includes placement
D6059	abutment supported porcelain fused to metal crown (high noble metal)
D6240	pontic – porcelain fused to high noble metal
D6750	retainer crown – porcelain fused to high noble metal
D6752	retainer crown – porcelain fused to noble metal
Suggested ICD-10-CM Diagnosis Code(s)	
K00.00	Anodontia
K08.409	Partial loss of teeth, unspecified cause, unspecified class
K08.419	Partial loss of teeth due to trauma, unspecified class
K08.429	Partial loss of teeth due to periodontal diseases, unspecified class
K08.439	Partial loss of teeth due to caries, unspecified class
K08.499	Partial loss of teeth due to other specified cause, unspecified class

CDT Code(s)	
D7111	extraction, coronal remnants – primary tooth
D7250	removal of residual tooth roots (cutting procedure)
Suggested ICD-10-CM Diagnosis Code(s) – ICD-10-CM	
K03.9	Disease of hard tissues of teeth, unspecified

Appendix 1. CDT Code to ICD (Diagnosis) Code Crosswalk

CDT Code(s)	
D7140	extraction, erupted tooth or exposed root (elevation and/or forceps removal)
D7210	extraction, erupted tooth requiring removal of bone and/or sectioning of tooth, and including elevation of mucoperiosteal flap if indicated

Suggested ICD-10-CM Diagnosis Code(s)	
K02.53	Dental caries on pit and fissure surface penetrating into pulp
K02.63	Dental caries on smooth surface penetrating into pulp
K04.01	Reversible pulpitis
K04.02	Irreversible pulpitis
K04.1	Necrosis of the pulp
K04.5	Chronic apical periodontitis
K04.6	Periapical abscess with sinus
K04.7	Periapical abscess without sinus
K04.8	Radicular cyst
K05.211	Aggressive periodontitis, localized, slight
K05.212	Aggressive periodontitis, localized, moderate
K05.213	Aggressive periodontitis, localized, severe
K05.219	Aggressive periodontitis, localized, unspecified severity
K05.3	Chronic periodontitis
K05.311	Chronic periodontitis, localized, slight
K05.312	Chronic periodontitis, localized, moderate
K05.313	Chronic periodontitis, localized, severe
K05.319	Chronic periodontitis, localized, unspecified severity
K08.439	Partial loss of teeth due to caries, unspecified class
K09.0	Developmental odontogenic cysts
L02.91	Cutaneous abscess, unspecified
L03.90	Cellulitis, unspecified
L03.91	Acute lymphangitis, unspecified
R44.8	Other symptoms and signs involving general sensations and perceptions
R44.9	Unspecified symptoms and signs involving general sensations and perceptions
R69	Illness, unspecified
S02.5XXA	Fracture of tooth (traumatic), initial encounter for closed fracture
S02.5XXB	Fracture of tooth (traumatic), initial encounter for open fracture
S03.2XXA	Dislocation of tooth, initial encounter

CDT Code(s)	
D7220	removal of impacted tooth – soft tissue
D7230	removal of impacted tooth – partially bony
D7240	removal of impacted tooth – completely bony
Suggested ICD-10-CM Diagnosis Code(s)	
K00.1	Supernumerary teeth
K00.6	Disturbances in tooth eruption
K01.0	Embedded teeth
K01.1	Impacted teeth
K09.0	Developmental odontogenic cysts

CDT Code(s)	
D7953	bone replacement graft for ridge preservation – per site
Suggested ICD-10-CM Diagnosis Code(s)	
K02.53	Dental caries on pit and fissure surface penetrating into pulp
K02.63	Dental caries on smooth surface penetrating into pulp
K04.01	Reversible pulpitis
K04.02	Irreversible pulpitis
K04.1	Necrosis of pulp
K04.5	Chronic apical periodontitis
K04.6	Periapical abscess with sinus
K04.7	Periapical abscess without sinus
K04.8	Radicular cyst
K05.211	Aggressive periodontitis, localized, slight
K05.212	Aggressive periodontitis, localized, moderate
K05.213	Aggressive periodontitis, localized, severe
K05.219	Aggressive periodontitis, localized, unspecified severity
K05.30	Chronic periodontitis, unspecified
K05.311	Chronic periodontitis, localized, slight
K05.312	Chronic periodontitis, localized, moderate
K05.313	Chronic periodontitis, localized, severe
K05.319	Chronic periodontitis, localized, unspecified severity
K05.321	Chronic periodontitis, generalized, slight
K05.322	Chronic periodontitis, generalized, moderate
K05.323	Chronic periodontitis, generalized, severe
K05.329	Chronic periodontitis, generalized, unspecified severity
K09.0	Developmental odontogenic cysts
S02.5XXA	Fracture of tooth (traumatic), initial encounter for closed fracture
S02.5XXB	Fracture of tooth (traumatic), initial encounter for open fracture
S03.2XXA	Dislocation of tooth, initial encounter

Appendix 1. CDT Code to ICD (Diagnosis) Code Crosswalk

CDT Code(s)	
D8080	comprehensive orthodontic treatment of the adolescent dentition
Suggested ICD-10-CM Diagnosis Code(s)	
K00.0	Anodontia
K00.6	Disturbances in tooth eruption
K08.8	Other specified disorders of teeth and supporting structures
M26.212	Malocclusion, Angle's class II
M26.213	Malocclusion, Angle's class III
M26.24	Reverse articulation
M26.29	Other anomalies of dental arch relationship
M26.30	Unspecified anomaly of tooth position of fully erupted tooth or teeth
M26.31	Crowding of fully erupted teeth
M26.35	Rotation of fully erupted tooth or teeth
M26.39	Other anomalies of tooth position of fully erupted tooth or teeth
M26.4	Malocclusion, unspecified
M26.81	Anterior soft tissue impingement
M26.82	Posterior soft tissue impingement
M26.89	Other dentofacial anomalies
Q67.4	Other congenital deformities of skull, face, and jaw

CDT Code(s)	
D9110	palliative treatment of dental pain – per visit
Suggested ICD-10-CM Diagnosis Code(s)	
K02.53	Dental caries on pit and fissure surface penetrating into pulp
K02.63	Dental caries on smooth surface penetrating into pulp
K04.01	Reversible pulpitis
K04.02	Irreversible pulpitis
K04.6	Periapical abscess with sinus
K04.7	Periapical abscess without sinus
M26.601	Right temporomandibular joint disorder, unspecified
M26.602	Left temporomandibular joint disorder, unspecified
M26.603	Bilateral temporomandibular joint disorder, unspecified
M26.609	Unspecified temporomandibular joint disorder, unspecified side
M26.69	Other specified disorders of temporomandibular joint

CDT Code(s)	
D9230	inhalation of nitrous oxide/anxiolysis, analgesia
Suggested ICD-10-CM Diagnosis Code(s)	
F41.9	Anxiety disorder, unspecified

CDT Code(s)	
D9910	application of desensitizing medicament
Suggested ICD-10-CM Diagnosis Code(s)	
K03.0	Excessive attrition of teeth
K03.1	Abrasion of teeth
K03.2	Erosion of teeth

CDT Code(s)	
D9944	occlusal guard – hard appliance, full arch
D9945	occlusal guard – soft appliance, full arch
D9946	occlusal guard – hard appliance, partial arch
Suggested ICD-10-CM Diagnosis Code(s)	
F59	Unspecified behavioral syndromes associated with physiological disturbances and physical factors
K03.0	Excessive attrition of teeth
M26.601	Right temporomandibular joint disorder, unspecified
M26.602	Left temporomandibular joint disorder, unspecified
M26.603	Bilateral temporomandibular joint disorder, unspecified
M26.609	Unspecified temporomandibular joint disorder, unspecified side
M26.69	Other specified disorders of temporomandibular joint
M26.89	Other dentofacial anomalies

CDT Code(s)	
D9951	occlusal adjustment – limited

Suggested ICD-10-CM Diagnosis Code(s)	
K03.0	Excessive attrition of teeth
K03.81	Cracked Tooth
K04.0	Pulpitis
K06.010	Localized gingival recession, unspecified
K06.011	Localized gingival recession, minimal
K06.012	Localized gingival recession, moderate
K06.013	Localized gingival recession, severe
K06.020	Generalized gingival recession, unspecified
K06.021	Generalized gingival recession, minimal
K06.022	Generalized gingival recession, moderate
K06.023	Generalized gingival recession, severe
M26.601	Right, temporomandibular joint disorder, unspecified
M26.602	Left temporomandibular joint disorder, unspecified
M26.603	Bilateral temporomandibular joint disorder, unspecified
M26.609	Unspecified temporomandibular joint disorder, unspecified side

Appendix 2: Introduction to Medical Claim Form Completion

By Jean L. Stevens, RHIT, CCS-P

Most dentists and dental team members are familiar with the components of a dental claim form used to report dental services to a patient's dental benefit plan. However, there are scenarios in which a dentist may need to submit a medical claim form to a patient's medical insurance provider.

Claims submitted to medical insurance plans require the use of HIPAA-standard diagnosis and procedure codes and have myriad other guidelines and instructions for completion. This appendix is an introduction to one type of medical claim form, the Health Insurance Claim Form that is often referred to as the "1500", which is the paper standard. This form and its comparable HIPAA-standard electronic format (837P) may be submitted to both commercial and government sponsored medical benefit plans.

- Comprehensive "1500" form completion instructions are available online (download at no cost) at the National Uniform Claim Committee (NUCC) website (*https://www.nucc.org/*). These instructions are applicable to claims filed with commercial (private) medical insurance plans, and include special instructions when the claim is for dental procedures.

  "1500 Claim Form Reference Instruction Manual" *https://nucc.org/index. php/1500-claim-form-mainmenu-35/1500-instructions-mainmenu-42.*

- Additional information on medical claim form submission to federal medical benefit programs are available from the Centers for Medicare and Medicaid Services. A paper Medicare (or Medicaid) claim form is often called the "CMS 1500", and its format and content is the same as the "1500" Health Insurance Claim Form seen on the NUCC website.

  "Medicare Claims Processing Manual, Chapter 26: Completing and Processing Form CMS-1500 Data Set" – *https://www.cms.gov/regulations-and-guidance/ guidance/manuals/downloads/clm104c26pdf.pdf*

  "Medicare Billing: Form CMS-1500 and the 837 Professional" – *https:// www.cms.gov/Outreach-and-Education/Medicare-Learning-Network-MLN/ MLNProducts/Downloads/837P-CMS-1500.pdf.*

- Individual private (e.g., commercial) and public (e.g., Medicare; state Medicaid agency) may also have their own supplemental completion instructions, and should be contacted to understand what the requirements (if any) are in effect.

Preparation instructions for the HIPAA-standard electronic medical benefit claim for professional services (837P) cited above are quite technical and outside the scope of this appendix. It is likely that your dental practice management software vendor has included (or makes available) a program that will enable you to submit an 837P; please contact your vendor's customer service representative for assistance.

The following figure is a sample Health Insurance Claim Form (the "1500"). Special instructions for populating dental procedure related information on a service line (for Section 24) follows this figure.

Special Instructions for Reporting Dental Procedure Related Information

These instructions address how to report Tooth Numbers and Areas of the Oral Cavity on the shaded portion of a service line ("1500" form/Section 24). The code sets used for this reporting follow.

- Codes for tooth numbers (ADA's Universal/National Tooth Numbering System; same as on a dental claim form) that are reported with the JP qualifier:

1 – 32	Permanent dentition
51 – 82	Permanent supernumerary dentition
A – T	Primary dentition
AS – TS	Primary supernumerary dentition

- Codes for areas of the oral cavity (HIPAA standard; same as on the dental claim form) that reported with the JO qualifier:

00	Entire oral cavity
01	Maxillary arch
02	Mandibular arch
10	Upper right quadrant
20	Upper left quadrant
30	Lower left quadrant
40	Lower right quadrant

"1500" form completion instructions follow:

1. When reporting tooth numbers, add in the following order: qualifier, tooth number (e.g., JP16).

2. When reporting an area of the oral cavity, enter in the following order: qualifier, area of oral cavity code (e.g., JO10).

3. When reporting multiple tooth numbers for one procedure, add in the following order: qualifier, tooth number, blank space, tooth number, blank space, tooth number, etc. (e.g., JP1 16 17 32).

4. When reporting multiple tooth numbers for one procedure, the number of units reported in 24G is the number of teeth involved in the procedure.

5. When reporting multiple areas of the oral cavity for one procedure, add in the following order: qualifier, oral cavity code, blank space, oral cavity code, etc., (e.g., JO10 20).

6. When reporting multiple areas of the oral cavity for one procedure, the number of units reported in 24G is the number of areas of the oral cavity involved in the procedure.

Illustrations of special instructions coding:

Tooth Number:

24. A. DATE(S) OF SERVICE						B. PLACE OF SERVICE	C. EMG	D. PROCEDURES, SERVICES, OR SUPPLIES (Explain Unusual Circumstances) CPT/HCPCS MODIFIER					E. DIAGNOSIS POINTER	F. $ CHARGES	G. DAYS OR UNITS	H. EPSDT Family Plan	I. ID. QUAL.	J. RENDERING PROVIDER ID. #
From MM	DD	YY	To MM	DD	YY													
JPI															N	G2	12345678901
10	01	05	10	01	05	11		D7240					A	500 ¦ 00	1	N	NPI	0123456789

Multiple Tooth Numbers:

24. A. DATE(S) OF SERVICE						B. PLACE OF SERVICE	C. EMG	D. PROCEDURES, SERVICES, OR SUPPLIES (Explain Unusual Circumstances) CPT/HCPCS MODIFIER					E. DIAGNOSIS POINTER	F. $ CHARGES	G. DAYS OR UNITS	H. Family Plan	I. ID. QUAL.	J. RENDERING PROVIDER ID. #
From MM	DD	YY	To MM	DD	YY													
JPI 16 17 32															N	G2	12345678901
10	01	05	10	01	05	11		D7240					A	500 ¦ 00	4	N	NPI	0123456789

Area of Oral Cavity:

24. A. DATE(S) OF SERVICE						B. PLACE OF SERVICE	C. EMG	D. PROCEDURES, SERVICES, OR SUPPLIES (Explain Unusual Circumstances) CPT/HCPCS MODIFIER					E. DIAGNOSIS POINTER	F. $ CHARGES	G. DAYS OR UNITS	H. EPSDT Family Plan	I. ID. QUAL.	J. RENDERING PROVIDER ID. #
From MM	DD	YY	To MM	DD	YY													
JO10															N	G2	12345678901
10	01	05	10	01	05	11		41820					A	500 ¦ 00	1	N	NPI	0123456789

Multiple Areas of Oral Cavity:

24. A. DATE(S) OF SERVICE						B. PLACE OF SERVICE	C. EMG	D. PROCEDURES, SERVICES, OR SUPPLIES (Explain Unusual Circumstances) CPT/HCPCS MODIFIER					E. DIAGNOSIS POINTER	F. $ CHARGES	G. DAYS OR UNITS	H. EPSDT Family Plan	I. ID. QUAL.	J. RENDERING PROVIDER ID. #
From MM	DD	YY	To MM	DD	YY													
JO10 20															N	G2	12345678901
10	01	05	10	01	05	11		D7310					A	500 ¦ 00	2	N	NPI	0123456789

Numeric Index by CDT Code

CDT Code	Page #(s)
D0709	17, 23, 31, 380
D0801	17, 19, 30, 57, 62, 191, 192, 204, 313, 330, 331, 332, 341, 343
D0802	17, 19, 30, 57, 62, 330
D0803	17, 19, 30, 62, 204, 219, 330
D0804	17, 19, 30, 62, 219, 330
D0999	41, 211, 380
D1110,	14, 36, 42, 46, 52, 70, 74, 82, 83, 86, 91, 93, 108, 157, 158, 160, 174, 176, 177, 182, 239, 255, 256, 261, 280, 369, 381
D1120	14, 37, 40, 70, 74, 83, 91, 255, 277, 369, 370, 381
D1206	37, 40, 70, 76, 78, 86, 93, 96, 381
D1208	37, 70, 82, 370, 381
D1310	85, 88, 97
D1320	39, 82, 88, 95, 166
D1321	87, 95, 317
D1330	85, 97, 149, 150, 154, 160, 162, 163, 166, 167, 171, 173, 277, 382
D1351	50, 70, 80, 81, 93, 382
D1352	50, 70, 80, 93, 97, 383
D1353	81, 94, 97
D1354	71, 75, 76, 77, 93, 94, 95, 382
D1355	71, 78, 84, 85, 95, 96
D1510	71
D1517	73, 97
D1551	79
D1556	94–95, 97
D1557	37, 79, 94–95
D1558	94–95
D1575	71, 73
D1701	36, 383
D1702	383
D1703	383
D1704	383
D1705	383
D1706	383
D1707	383
D1708	18, 72, 383
D1709	18, 72, 383
D1710	18, 72, 383
D1711	18, 72, 383
D1712	18, 72, 90, 383
D1713	18, 72, 383

CDT Code	Page #(s)
D1714	18, 72, 383
D1781	17, 20, 72, 89, 383
D1782	17, 20, 72, 89, 383
D1783	17, 20, 72, 90, 383
D1999	46
D2140	384
D2150	384
D2160	384
D2161	384
D2330	113, 125, 176, 384
D2331	384
D2332	384
D2335	115, 384
D2390	115
D2391	50, 80, 93, 97, 112, 113, 124, 126, 131, 134, 137, 249, 385
D2392	385
D2393	385
D2394	115, 385
D2740	109, 111, 253, 385
D2750	114, 385
D2751	385
D2752	104, 385
D2753	104, 111, 385
D2790	385
D2792	106, 385
D2794	108, 111, 385
D2799	103
D2910	112
D2921	114
D2928	111, 386
D2930	386
D2934	107
D2940	104, 112, 113, 386
D2941	114
D2949	104
D2950	103, 123, 124, 273, 385
D2951	99, 385
D2952	113, 283, 385
D2954	108, 113, 283, 385
D2955	109, 114, 117, 141
D2960	105
D2961	105
D2962	110
D2971	106, 111
D2980	108, 114
D2990	382
D2999	5, 112, 113, 114, 115
D3110	386

CDT Code	Page #(s)
D5820	195, 232, 247
D5850	201
D5851	192, 201
D5862	6, 198, 257
D5865	198
D5875	192, 196, 238, 257
D5876	194, 199
D5899	247
D5911	219
D5912	219
D5913	213, 218
D5914	218
D5915	218
D5916	211
D5926	217
D5931	207, 210, 214, 217, 218
D5932	206, 207, 210, 214, 217, 218
D5933	207, 214
D5934	205, 218, 219
D5935	218, 219
D5936	206, 214, 217, 218
D5937	209, 216
D5950	213
D5951	215
D5952	217, 218
D5953	218
D5954	218
D5955	218
D5982	206, 254
D5984	207, 210
D5986	208, 215, 364
D5987	216
D5988	212, 218, 254
D5991	209, 216
D5993	210, 217
D5995	215
D5996	215
D5999	208, 215, 363
D6010	222, 232, 233, 235, 237, 240, 241, 252, 258, 264, 265, 295, 296, 298, 323, 391
D6011	185, 196, 213, 234, 236, 237, 246, 258, 265
D6013	222, 242, 253, 257, 265
D6015	191
D6016	228
D6040	264
D6050	264

CDT Code	Page #(s)
D6051	232
D6055	224, 249, 259, 265
D6056	223, 224, 237, 241, 249, 253, 255, 259, 261, 262, 263, 265, 391
D6057	223, 232, 253, 255, 259, 265, 391
D6058	224, 232, 265
D6059	224, 253, 265, 391
D6060	224, 265
D6061	224, 265
D6062	224, 265
D6063	224, 265
D6064	224, 265
D6065	225, 253, 260, 265
D6066	225, 253, 265
D6067	225, 265
D6068	225, 265
D6069	225, 265
D6070	225, 265
D6071	225, 265
D6072	225, 265
D6073	225, 265
D6074	225, 265
D6075	225, 251, 253, 265
D6076	225, 240, 265
D6077	225, 265
D6080	164, 229, 239, 245, 250, 256
D6081	155, 164, 245, 257, 390
D6082	225, 265
D6083	225, 265
D6084	225, 265
D6085	225, 232, 256, 265, 316
D6086	225, 265
D6087	225, 265
D6088	225, 265
D6090	229, 248, 260
D6091	197, 200, 234, 238, 248, 262
D6092	257
D6093	257
D6094	224, 265
D6095	265
D6096	238, 265, 324
D6097	224, 265
D6098	225, 265
D6099	225, 265
D6100	181, 228, 264, 280
D6101	245

CDT Code	Page #(s)
D7953	168, 181, 231, 243, 280, 297, 301, 321, 393
D7955	130, 293, 322
D7956	17, 21, 168, 181, 187, 231, 232, 291, 297, 322
D7957	17, 21, 181, 187, 291, 297–298, 322
D7961	170
D7962	324
D7970	312
D7971	324
D7979	324
D7983	325
D7993	213, 324
D7994	296
D7999	304, 307, 317, 319
D8010	326
D8020	326, 340
D8030	326
D8040	326
D8070	329, 334
D8080	329, 332, 333, 334, 335, 394
D8090	329
D8210	335
D8220	335
D8660	333, 336, 342
D8670	333, 334, 339, 342, 343
D8680	333, 334
D8681	333, 334, 335, 344
D8695	336, 337
D8696	337
D8697	343
D8699	338
D8702	343
D8703	343
D8704	343
D8999	341, 343
D9110	17, 22, 45, 75, 112, 148, 175, 348, 356, 394
D9120	278
D9130	311
D9215	110, 360
D9219	352
D9222	300, 310, 352
D9223	300, 310, 352
D9230	167, 395
D9239	153, 154, 300

CDT Code	Page #(s)
D9243	153, 154, 300
D9248	167, 300, 307
D9310	63, 309, 360
D9311	150, 316, 357
D9410	84, 361
D9430	162
D9440	103
D9450	17, 26, 331, 332, 348
D9610	307
D9613	312, 360, 365
D9630	47, 129, 149, 154, 316, 364
D9910	93, 363, 364, 395
D9912	352, 353, 355, 356, 358
D9930	355
D9932	250
D9933	250
D9934	250
D9935	250
D9941	307
D9943	316
D9944	354, 395
D9945	354, 395
D9946	354, 361, 395
D9947	208, 215, 316, 349, 357, 362
D9948	316, 349, 358, 362
D9949	316, 349, 358
D9951	160, 216, 353, 395
D9952	353
D9953	17, 26, 316, 348, 349, 358, 362
D9970	363
D9971	342
D9972	361
D9973	361
D9975	42, 361
D9995	56, 68, 339, 350, 351, 359, 365
D9996	56, 68, 339, 342, 351, 359, 365
D9999	364

Alphabetic Index by Topic

consultations vs. evaluations, 63, 360
oral cancer screening, 39, 41, 61, 67, 88
periodic, 61, 63, 64
problem focused, 38, 63, 125, 313, 350
remote. *See* teledentistry
vs. screening, 59
dental implants. *See* **implants**
dental offices
compliance audits, 375–377
mandatory closure of, 347, 348
removal from network lists, 371
top procedure denials, 374–375
utilization reviews, 375–377
dental pain. *See* **pain**
dental plans. *See* **dental benefit plans**
dental procedure codes, 1, 4, 5, 11.
See also **CDT codes**
dental records, 87, 286, 377
dental sealants, 70, 80, 81, 93, 94, 97
dental surface scan, 30, 57, 62, 204
dentin, 70, 80, 93, 113, 119
dentist billing manual, 368
dentists
compliance audits, 375–377
dental benefits basics, 367–377
lost submissions, 373
non-contracted, 370
patient privacy and, 373, 377
procedure coding, 16
provider agreements, 13
referrals, 63, 88, 125, 127, 360
remote care. *See* teledentistry
resources for, 378
responsibilities, 10
utilization review, 375–377
dentition
adolescent, 328, 332–333
adult, 328
considerations, 74
mixed, 52, 328
permanent, 52, 99, 328
primary, 328
prophylaxis codes and, 91
protecting during cancer treatment, 208
transitional, 52, 259–260, 328, 340
types of, 328

denture acrylic material, 198
dentures. *See also* **bridges**
"All-on-4," 260–261, 263
base reinforcement, 194
bone loss and, 193
cantilever bridge, 268, 270
complete, 190, 192, 199, 200, 201
described, 190
fixed, 224–225, 226, 227
fixed partial. *See* fixed partial denture
hybrid, 226–227
hyperplastic tissue excision, 312
immediate, 190, 193, 199
implant. *See* implant dentures
implant supported, 233–234, 254, 263, 295
interim, 200
locator attachment repair, 197
loose, 197, 238, 283
mandibular, 192, 197, 233–234, 249
modification of, 192
overdenture, 190, 198, 242
partial. *See* partial dentures
placement on implants, 192
removable, 190, 193, 195, 226
repair of, 194
retrofitting, 256–257
soft liner, 197, 201
descriptors, 5, 61, 63, 65
diabetic patients, 58
diagnosis codes. *See* **ICD codes**
diagnostic casts, 42
Diagnostic category, 29–68
changes, 30–31
clinical coding scenarios, 32–56
coding Q&A, 57–68
definitions/concepts, 29
introduction, 29
summary, 68
diagnostic models, 42
diet, 97
direct, 99
direct restorations, 99–100
distal shoe appliance, 97
distal shoe space maintainers, 71, 73, 97
distal wedge, 180, 186

interim, 286
pain caused by, 286
partial fracture of, 114
pediatric, 283
pontics, 254
re-bonding, 283
re-cementing, 276, 283
removal of, 278, 286
repair of, 279
replacing implant with, 280–281
retainers, 268
treatment plan, 272–273, 283
fixtures, 222, 269
flap, elevation of, 295
flap surgery, 168–169, 185
flap, surgical, 264, 306
flipper procedure, 231, 247
fluorescence oral cancer exam, 39
fluoride, 70, 71, 208
fluoride gel carrier, 215
fluoride varnish, 37, 40, 70, 93, 96
FMX (full mouth series), 31
fracture, orbital, 211, 299
fractured gold inlay, 114
fractured implant, 242
fractured partial denture, 114
fractured teeth
considerations, 318
infection, 274
interim prosthesis, 194
painful, 113, 274, 318
removable partial denture, 191, 192, 195
scenarios, 103–107
temporary crown for, 113
frenectomy, 170–171, 185, 324
frenum pull, 170–171
full bone impacted tooth, 290
full mouth debridement, 147, 157
full mouth series (FMX), 31

G

gastrointestinal (GI) tract, 347
general services. *See* **Adjunctive General Services category**
GI (gastrointestinal) tract, 347
gingival flap, 168–169, 180, 184, 185

gingival flap procedure, 146
gingival inflammation, 92
gingival irrigation, 147
gingival irritation, 356
gingival reshaping, 174
gingivectomy, 184
gingivitis
orthodontic treatment and, 182
overdue patient with, 156–157
subgingival decay, 172–173
treating, 242
glass ionomers, 100
glucose level, 53–54, 58
gold inlay, 114
graft procedures, 161, 170–171, 292
grafts/grafting
autogenous graft, 144, 290, 292, 298–299
connective tissue, 182, 258, 292
considerations, 143
hard tissue, 293
non-autogenous, 145, 161, 292
soft tissue, 144, 161–162, 182, 185, 258
grinding teeth, 200, 353, 361
GTR (guided tissue regeneration), 147, 228, 291, 302, 322
guide flange, 219
guided tissue regeneration (GTR), 147, 228, 291, 302, 322
gums, bleeding, 149

H

Hader bar, 248, 249
hard palate, cancer of, 210, 217–218
HbA1c testing, 66
HCPCS (Healthcare Common Procedure Code Set), 11
healing cap, 258
Health Insurance Portability and Accountability Act (HIPAA), 12, 13, 377
Healthcare Common Procedure Code Set (HCPCS), 11
heart disease, 315–316
HIPAA (Health Insurance Portability and Accountability Act), 12, 13, 377

surgical access to, 258
surgical removal of, 228
tightening screw, 239, 324
transosteal, 264
treatment plan, 283
unspecified procedure, 242, 243–244, 247, 296
zygomatic, 296
indirect, 100–101
indirect restorations, 100–101, 103–104
infection, 274, 304
inflammation, 92, 155, 157, 163, 164
inlay
described, 100
fractured, 114
gold, 114
provisional, 114
inlay restorations, 100
insurance. *See* dental benefit plans
interim, defined, 268
intermediate restorative material (IRM), 112
International Classification of Diseases. *See* ICD
intra-coronal attachment, 282
intraoral images, 29, 30–33, 57
intraoral tomosynthesis, 29, 30, 35, 57
intraorifice barrier, 118, 138
Invisalign aligner, 339, 341, 342, 343
IRM (intermediate restorative material), 112
irrigation, 118, 139

L

lab analog, 263
labial, 101
labial veneers, 105, 110
laboratory charges, 262, 284, 285
laboratory procedure, 100
"laser codes," 110
least expensive alternative treatment (LEAT), 14
LEAT (least expensive alternative treatment), 14
lesions, 46–48
carious, 49, 51, 77
cervical, 113, 131

painful, 209, 216
resorptive, 1 31
locator abutment, 200
locator attachment repair, 197
long-term care facilities, 60, 361
lost submissions, 370

M

male descriptor, 269
malocclusion/crowding, 335
mandibular arch, 163, 198, 259, 334, 343
mandibular arches scan, 204
mandibular cancer, 205
mandibular dentures, 192, 197, 233–234, 249
mandibular resection prosthesis, 219
marsupialization, 137, 291, 303
Maryland bridge, 270, 271
maxillary arch, 199
maxillary arches scan, 204
maxillary dentures, 235–236
maxillary hypoplasia, 212
maxillofacial prostheses, 218
Maxillofacial Prosthetics category, 203–220
changes, 203
clinical coding scenarios, 204–213
coding Q&A, 214–219
definitions/concepts, 203
introduction, 203
summary, 220
maxillofacial surgery. *See* Oral and Maxillofacial Surgery category
Medicaid, 11, 397
medical procedure codes, 11
medical/dental claims
denied claims, 12–15, 374–375
dental codes vs. medical codes, 11
filling out, 397–404
overview, 397
medicament carrier, 209, 215, 216
medicaments
caries arresting, 71, 75, 77, 93–95
caries preventive, 71, 84, 95
described, 346
desensitizing, 93, 363–364
Medicare, 9, 11, 397

Alphabetic Index by Topic

Alphabetic Index by Topic

extracting. *See* extractions

fractured. *See* fractured teeth

full bone impacted, 290

grinding, 200, 353, 361

impacted, 290, 301–302, 319

isolating, 118

missing, 34, 259, 272, 275–276, 285

pain. *See* pain entries

partial bone impacted, 290

replacement of, 275–276

reshaping, 342

soft tissue impacted, 290

submergence of, 308

unerupted, 71, 302–303, 325, 356

teledentistry

ADA publications for, 68

asynchronous, 347

considerations, 345, 346, 347, 359, 365

COVID-19 and, 359, 365

diagnostic images, 55–56

documenting encounters, 68

emergency treatment, 350–351

orthodontics, 339

resources, 56

scenarios, 350–351

synchronous, 347

temporary anchorage device (TAD), 253

temporomandibular disorder (TMD), 44, 311

temporomandibular joint (TMJ) disorder, 44

therapeutic drugs, 365

tissue conditioning, 201

tissue regeneration, 322

titanium crown, 104, 108

titanium/titanium alloys, 104, 111, 275, 284

TMD (temporomandibular disorder), 44, 311

TMJ (temporomandibular joint) disorder, 44

tobacco cessation guidance, 82, 88

tobacco counseling, 82, 88, 95

tobacco, smokeless, 88

tobacco use, 39, 82

tomosynthesis, 29, 30, 35, 57

tongue thrust appliances, 335

tongue thrust habit, 335

tooth. *See* teeth

tooth bounded spaces, 180

tooth decay, 106, 172–173, 184. *See also* caries

tooth surfaces, *101*

toothache, 121, 124, 136

torus/exostosis, 321

transillumination, 67

transitional dentition, 52, 259–260, 328, 340

transosteal implants, 264

traumatic wounds, 76–77, 307

treatment plans, 368, 376

Trefoil bar, 259

Trefoil system, 259

trismus appliance, 209, 216

two-part fixture, 269

U

UCLA-type crown, 259

ultrasonic scaler, 46, 149

"umbrella code," 333

unbundling, 139

unerupted tooth, 71, 302–303, 325, 356

unspecified procedure, 5, 285, 319

utilization reviews, 375–377

V

vacations, 350–351

vaccinations

COVID-19. See COVID-19 vaccinations

HPV. *See* HPV vaccinations

vaping, 87, 317

veneers, 105, 110

vesiculobullous diseases, 216

virtual 3D images, 43

virtual dentistry. *See* teledentistry

virtual patient encounters

See teledentistry

vital pulp therapy, 119

W

Wartons duct, 324

X

xerostomia, 51, 66, 149, 325

Z

Alphabetic Index by Topic

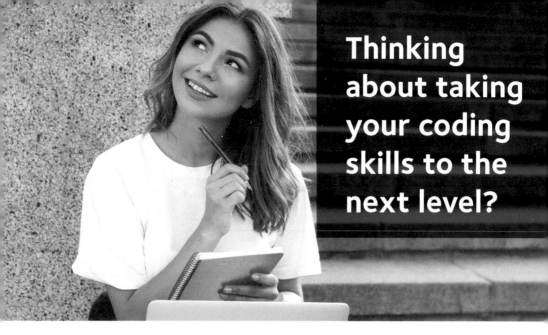

Thinking about taking your coding skills to the next level?

Take your learning to the next level by learning how to use codes in practice.

Mastery of ADA's CDT codes will make you a more valuable asset to the team and practice. Increase your coding skills and complete the **ADA Dental Coding Certificate: Assessment-Based CDT Program**. It helps new and experienced staff members achieve coding proficiency and helps the dental office run more smoothly.

Participants will:

- Gain thorough knowledge of coding terms and tools
- Understand dental procedure codes and how to apply them
- Accurately complete the ADA Dental Claim Form
- Use the *CDT 2023* and *CDT Companion* books correctly

As the official source for CDT® codes, the ADA has answered thousands of questions over the years. When dental teams have questions, we have the answers. Take advantage of our expertise and get up to code today!

Participants will earn 4 CE hours after successfully passing the online assessment. The course is available either with or without CDT books.

ADA American Dental Association®
America's leading advocate for oral health

This premier course is not included with CE Online Subscription and must be purchased separately.